Data Interpretation in Anesthesia

Tilak D. Raj
Editor

Data Interpretation in Anesthesia

A Clinical Guide

Springer

Editor
Tilak D. Raj, MD, MRCP, FRCA
Chairman of Anesthesia
Alliance Health Midwest
Midwest City, OK
USA

ISBN 978-3-319-55861-5 ISBN 978-3-319-55862-2 (eBook)
DOI 10.1007/978-3-319-55862-2

Library of Congress Control Number: 2017946757

Printed on acid-free paper

This Springer imprint is published by Springer Nature
The registered company is Springer International Publishing AG
The registered company address is: Gewerbestrasse 11, 6330 Cham, Switzerland

I would like to dedicate this book to my late parents, Arthur and Prema
and also to: Catherine, Vijay, Anushka, Kieran, and Roshan

Foreword

In their daily practice, anesthesiologists are faced with a tremendous amount of data during the clinical management of their patients. This textbook, *Data Interpretation in Anesthesia: A Clinical Guide*, focuses on the interpretation of data commonly available to an anesthesiologist.

The book is divided into five parts, including monitoring, laboratory testing, imaging, physiologic studies, and conceptual images. It consists of 83 chapters starting with a presentation of a data point, followed by relevant questions and answers with discussion. Pertinent references are provided in each chapter.

Another textbook in this format is not currently available for the discipline of anesthesiology. There are a variety of reviews that are vignette driven, or are discussions of general topics, but none that focus concisely on the individual data points that an anesthesiologist must quickly and astutely interpret for patient care. This format allows the consultant to efficiently reference areas of review.

The editor of this much needed book, Tilak D. Raj, MD, is a cardiothoracic and vascular anesthesia fellowship-trained, board-certified anesthesiologist (both in the UK and the USA), who has been involved in clinical practice and academic medicine for 20 years.

Contributors include an excellent selection of anesthesiologists, cardiologists, and an interventional neurologist.

Anesthesiology as a specialty is seeing amazing advancements in patient care. More and more advanced clinical algorithms emerge every day to help anesthesiologists understand data points, interpret results, and make decisions. This book will be very useful for all anesthesiologists, anesthesia residents, and practitioners involved in Maintenance of Certification in Anesthesiology (MOCA). It is not a book that just sits on a shelf collecting dust. It is a must read. I hope you enjoy it!

Carin A. Hagberg, MD
Division Head, Division of Anesthesiology,
Critical Care & Pain Medicine,
Helen Shaffer Fly Distinguished Professor
of Anesthesiology UT MD Anderson Cancer Center
1400 Holcombe Blvd, Faculty Center, Unit 409, Houston, TX 77030, USA

Preface

It is a pleasure to finally bring to fruition an idea I have had for a couple of years. As anesthesiologists, we come across a vast amount of clinical and investigative data during the perioperative care of our patients. This book should serve as a reference, providing information about the data we encounter in our daily practice. The current edition has 83 chapters and the list covers most of the data that we encounter. There is a basic layout for the chapters which start with a data point followed by discussion in a question and answer format. I chose this format to stimulate analytic thought and facilitate learning.

The chapters in the book are grouped into five parts. The "Conceptual Images" part has topics which are not strictly data but more topics of exam interest. They share the same format and provide additional knowledge in those areas.

This text should help residents and anesthesiologists striving to become board-certified and anesthesiologists in practice working toward Maintenance of Certification in Anesthesiology (MOCA).

The project could not have been completed without the expert and valuable contribution by authors from different specialties both from America and England, to whom I am extremely grateful. Editing and contributing to this book has provided a great learning experience for me, not just in medicine and anesthesiology but also in life and human nature.

Physicians should be passionate lifelong learners to provide good patient care, and physicians in academic settings should do the same not just for patient care but also to teach and act as good role models for students and residents. I shall close with the apt and inspiring quote by John Cotton Dana.

"Who dares to teach must never cease to learn."

Edmond, OK Tilak D. Raj

Acknowledgments

I would like to thank my colleagues in helping me with compiling the list of chapters and parts; Dwight Reynolds, MD, for the wonderful X-rays we used in Chap. 46 (CXR—CIED); Scott Tatum, R.N., B.S.I.T., for providing some ECGs used in the "ECG Quiz" chapter; and the "expert" Dan Mason from Haemonetics for his invaluable help in two chapters on TEG.

I am also greatly indebted to Carin Hagberg, MD, for kindly agreeing to provide a foreword for this book; my precious artist Gail Gwin, who provided the drawings for many chapters which she tirelessly worked on, outside of her busy work schedule; to Vijay Raj for his help with some images and graphs; to all the residents who provided valuable feedback; and last but not the least my wife Catherine who kept me focused and on track and to my children Vijay, Anushka, Kieran, and Roshan—"it can be done and you can do it!"

Contents

List of Contributors

Alberto J. de Armendi, MD, PhD, MBA Department of Anesthesiology, The Children's Hospital, University of Oklahoma Health Sciences Center, Oklahoma City, OK, USA

German Barbosa-Hernandez, MD Department of Anesthesia, Oklahoma University Health and Science Center, Oklahoma City, OK, USA

Daniel A. Biggs, MD, MSc Department of Anesthesiology, Oklahoma University Medical Center, Oklahoma City, OK, USA

John B. Carter, MD Department of Anesthesiology, Oklahoma University Medical Center, Oklahoma City, OK, USA

Pramod Chetty, MD Department of Anesthesiology, OU Health Sciences Center, Oklahoma City, OK, USA

Frederick van Damme, MB, ChB (Stell), FRCA Department of Anaesthesia, East Surrey Hospital, Redhill, UK

Gulshan Doulatram, MD Department of Anesthesiology, University of Texas Medical Branch, Galveston, TX, USA

Raghuvender Ganta, MD, FRCA Department of Anesthesiology, VA Hospital, OUMC, Oklahoma City, OK, USA

Ankur Garg, MD Orlando Neurosurgery, Orlando, FL, USA

Marcos E. Gomes, MD Department of Anesthesiology, University of Oklahoma Health Sciences Center, Oklahoma City, OK, USA

Ranganathan Govindaraj, MD, FRCA Associate Professor for Anesthesia and Pain, Department of Anesthesiology, UTMB, Galveston, TX, USA

Director for Ultrasound Guided Regional Anesthesia, Galveston, TX, USA

Mohammad A. Helwani, MD, MSPH Assistant Professor, Divisions of Critical Care and Cardiothoracic Anesthesiology, Washington University, St. Louis, School of Medicine, MO, USA

Edward Kosik, DO Department of Anesthesiology, University of Oklahoma Health Sciences Center, Oklahoma City, OK, USA

Abhinava S. Madamangalam, MBBS, MD Department of Anesthesiology and Perioperative Medicine, Augusta University Medical Center, Augusta, GA, USA

Deepinder Mann, DO Department of Anesthesiology, University of Texas Medical Branch, Galveston, TX, USA

Teodora Nicolescu, MD Department of Anesthesiology, Oklahoma University Health Sciences Center, Oklahoma City, OK, USA

Mehmet S. Ozcan, MD, FCCP Department of Anesthesiology, The University of Oklahoma Health Sciences Center, Oklahoma City, OK, USA

Aneesh Venkat Pakala, MD Section of Cardiovascular Disease, Department of Medicine, University of Oklahoma College of Medicine, Oklahoma City, OK, USA

Tilak D. Raj, MD, MRCP, FRCA Department of Anesthesiology, Alliance Health Midwest, Midwest City, OK, USA

Talla A. Rousan, MD, FACC Department of Medicine, The University of Oklahoma Health Sciences Center and the Veteran Affairs Medical Center, Oklahoma City, OK, USA

Madhumani Rupasinghe, MBBS, FRCA Department of Anesthesiology, University of Texas Health Science Center at Houston, Houston, TX, USA

Frederic J. Sage, MD, FRCA, FFICM John Hammond Department of Anaesthesia, East Surrey Hospital, Redhill, UK

Tanmay Shah, MD, MBBS Department of Anesthesiology, University of Oklahoma Health Sciences Center, Oklahoma City, OK, USA

Jacqueline J. Smith, MD Department of Anesthesiology, University of Oklahoma Health Sciences Center, Oklahoma City, OK, USA

John David Srinivasan, MD Assistant Professor, Department of Anesthesiology and Critical Care, Saint Louis University, School of Medicine, MO, USA

Robert C.M. Stephens, BA, MBBS, FRCA, MD, FFICM Department of Anaesthesia, University College London Hospitals, London, UK

Nicole T. Tran, MD Department of Cardiology, University of Oklahom Health Sciences Center, Oklahoma City, OK, USA

Kofi B. Vandyck, MD Department of Anesthesiology, University of Oklahoma Health Sciences Center, Oklahoma City, OK, USA

Abigail Whiteman, MA (Cantab), MB BChir., FRCA, PGCert Department of Anaesthesia and Perioperative Medicine, University College London Hospitals, London, UK

Casey Windrix, MD Department of Anesthesiology, OUHSC, Edmond, Oklahoma, USA

Part I
Monitoring

Chapter 1
CVP

Teodora Nicolescu

The below pressure waveform is obtained from an IV in the neck of a patient being monitored.

1. Identify the components labeled 1–5. Explain what they signify.
2. What information can be deduced from the central venous pressure measurements?
3. What determines the central venous pressure?
4. What factors influence the reading of central venous pressure?
5. What are the indications and contraindications of central venous catheter insertion?
6. Give some examples of CVP waveforms in pathological states.

T. Nicolescu, MD
Department of Anesthesiology, Oklahoma University Health Sciences Center,
750 NE 13th Street, Suite 200, Oklahoma City, OK, USA
e-mail: teodora-nicolescu@ouhsc.edu

T.D. Raj (ed.), *Data Interpretation in Anesthesia*,
DOI 10.1007/978-3-319-55862-2_1

Fig. 1.1 Central venous pressure waveform

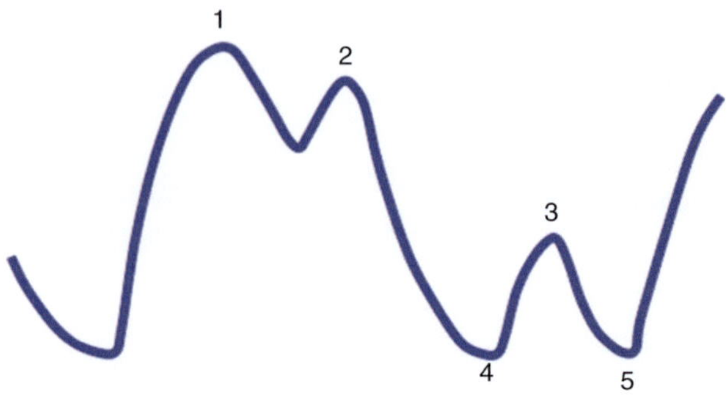

Fig. 1.2 Normal CVP

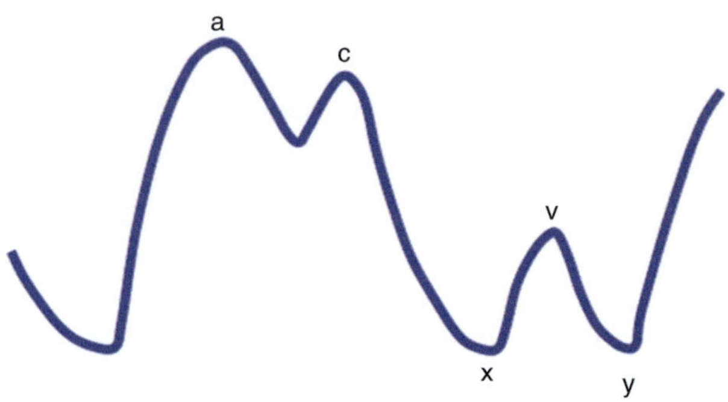

Answers

1. 1, a wave; 2, c wave; 3, v wave; 4, x descent; and 5, y descent.

   The **a wave** of the central venous pressure represents the **atrial contraction**. The right atrial pressure is at the highest value. It is mirrored by the PR interval on the ECG tracing. Notably, the a waves are absent in atrial fibrillation and are exaggerated in junctional rhythms and heart blocks (cannon waves). It is also enlarged in tricuspid and pulmonary stenosis as well as pulmonary hypertension.

   The **c wave** is due to the bulging of the tricuspid valve into the right atrium during early ventricular contraction (**ventricular systole**), while the **v wave** is due to the **rise in the atrial pressure** that occurs before the opening of the tricuspid valve. The v waves are prominent in tricuspid regurgitation.

   There are also two descents noted in the central venous pressure waveform.

   The **x descent** is due to the **atrial relaxation** or possibly by the tricuspid annular downward displacement during systole [1].

   The **y descent** represents the tricuspid valve displacement during diastole, as **atria start emptying** [2].

2. Central venous pressure measures right atrial pressure, which is a major determinant of right ventricular end-diastolic volume. It is used to assess (right) ventricular volume, filling, and therefore fluid status. It does however have limitations, mostly related to **ventricular compliance** which can be affected by a variety of

factors (**e.g., impaired relaxation**, **ischemia,** and **pharmacologic manipulation**). Of note, even in healthy patients, there is a wide variability in cardiac compliance. Although a very low CVP measurement may indicate volume depletion, a high value may be due to volume overload or poor ventricular compliance. Isolated central venous pressure measurements are not useful; instead, the trend of measurements over a given time and the response to a fluid challenge may provide useful information on the intravascular fluid status of a patient.

It is also important to keep in mind that filling pressure estimation is unreliable in predicting fluid responsiveness, particularly in septic patients. CVP measurement should be considered in the context of other parameters of a patient's volume status like heart rate, blood pressure, and urine output. In healthy hearts, right and left ventricular performances are parallel, therefore left ventricular filling can be approximated by the central venous pressure.

3. Determinants of the central venous pressure are as follows:
   (a) **Right ventricular function**
   (b) **Venous return** that in turn is determined by total blood volume, venous tone, cardiac output, right ventricular contractility, and intrathoracic pressure [3].

   It has to be understood that the central venous pressure can be overestimated, mainly due to fluctuations with respiration of the mean central venous pressure. Proper placement of the catheter just outside of the right atrium may insure more accurate readings. The pressure at the base of the c wave represents the right atrial pressure at the start of the right ventricular systole, making it the best estimate of right ventricular preload. Central venous measurements should be taken at end exhalation (lowest negative intrathoracic pressure) [5].

4. Several factors will influence the accuracy of the central venous pressure reading:
   (a) Changes in intrathoracic pressure (PEEP, ascites).
   (b) Cardiac rhythms disturbances.
   (c) Tricuspid valve disease.
   (d) Myocardial compliance changes (pericardial disease, tamponade). In tamponade there is equalization of diastolic pressures (in the absence of left ventricular dysfunction).

$$\mathrm{RAP} = \mathrm{RVEDP} = \mathrm{LAP} = \mathrm{LVEDP}$$

   Of note, the limited ventricular filling abolishes the y descent. In return the x descent (atrial relaxation) is accentuated or normal [4].

5. **Indications:**
   (a) Fluid management (particularly hypovolemia and shock)
   (b) Infusion of vasoactive drugs
   (c) Hyperalimentation
   (d) Insertion of pacemaker wires
   (e) In surgeries with air embolism potential
   (f) Difficult IV access

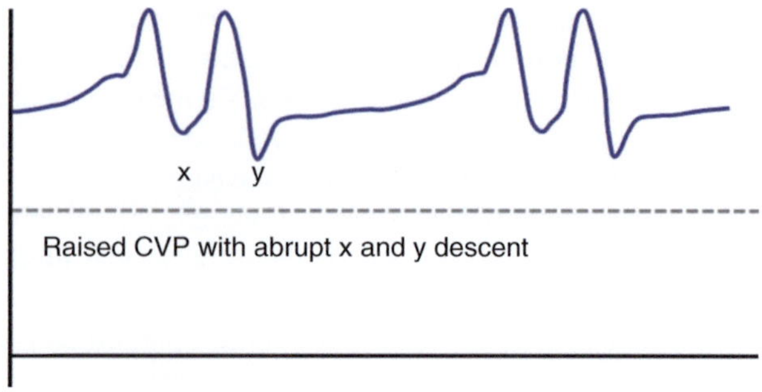

Fig. 1.3 Abnormal CVP—steep x and y descent (constrictive pericarditis)

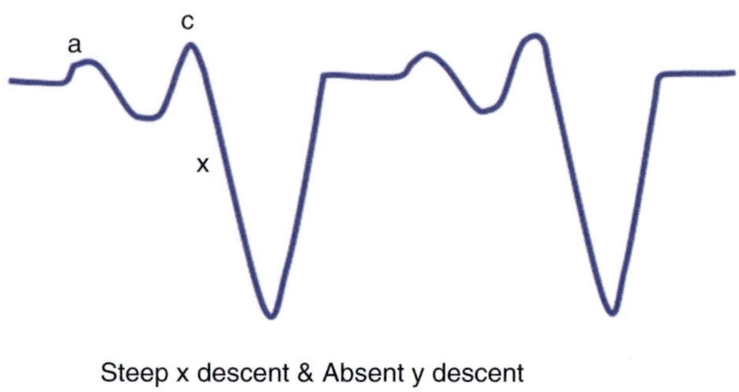

Fig. 1.4 Abnormal CVP—steep x descent (pericardial tamponade)

Contraindications:

(a) Right atrial tumor extension (renal cell carcinoma)
(b) Endocarditis (fungating valve vegetations)
(c) Relative presence of ipsilateral carotid endarterectomy

6. Waveform analysis

Large a waves	Pulmonary hypertension, tricuspid, and pulmonic stenosis
Cannon a waves	Irregular—complete heart block
	Regular—AV dissociation
Large v waves	Tricuspid regurgitation
Exaggerated x descent	Pericardial tamponade, constrictive pericarditis
Sharp y descent	Severe tricuspid regurgitation, constrictive pericarditis

References

1. Johnson B. Decrease in central venous pressure by lower body negative pressor or blood loss elicits similar responses. J Appl Physiol (1985). 2014;117(2):131–41.
2. Butterworth JF. Atlas of procedures in anesthesia and critical care D. Berlin-Starling curves and central venous pressure. Crit Care. 2015;19(1):55.
3. Avcil M. Comparison of estimating central venous pressure. Int J Clin Exp Med. 2015;8(7): 10586–94.
4. Carmona P, Mateo E, et al. Management of cardiac tamponade after cardiac surgery. J Cardiothorac Vasc Anesth. 2012;26(2):302–11.
5. Pittman JAL, Ping JS, et al. Arterial and central venous pressure monitoring. Int Anesthesiol Clin. 2004;42(1):13–30.

Chapter 2
Pulmonary Artery Catheters

Teodora Nicolescu

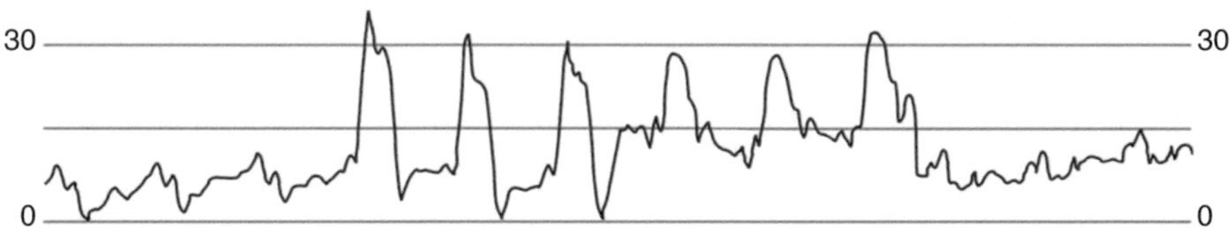

Fig. 2.1 Pulmonary artery catheter normal waveform

Questions

1. The above sequence of waveforms was encountered during a line placement in a patient. Describe what you see.
2. What information does the PA catheter provide?
3. How does ventilation management affect the accuracy of data from a PA catheter?
4. When is the pulmonary artery occlusion pressure (PAOP), also referred to as pulmonary capillary wedge pressure (PCWP), different from the left ventricular end-diastolic pressure (LVEDP)?
5. What do large v waves on the PA catheter tracing mean?
6. How can you accurately interpret mixed venous oxygen saturation?
7. What are the indications, complications, and evidence for PAC use?

T. Nicolescu, MD
Department of Anesthesiology, Oklahoma University Health Sciences Center,
750 NE 13th Street, Suite 200, Oklahoma City, OK, USA
e-mail: teodora-nicolescu@ouhsc.edu

T.D. Raj (ed.), *Data Interpretation in Anesthesia*,
DOI 10.1007/978-3-319-55862-2_2

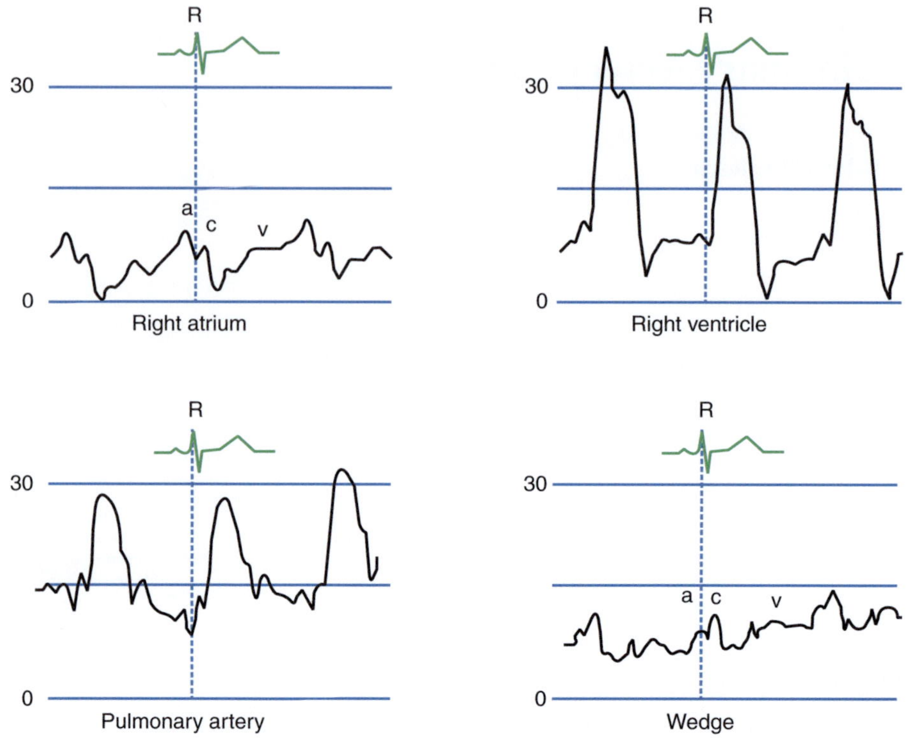

Fig. 2.2 Waveforms encountered during PAC advancement

Answers

1. When inserted, the PA catheter is first advanced through the sheath and at approximately 15–20 cm, the balloon is inflated. Along this path the catheter will pass through the (1) **right atrium**, (2) **the right ventricle**, and (3) **the pulmonary artery**, at which point, with slight advancement into a small arterial branch, it can obtain (4) the **pulmonary artery occlusion pressure**.

   The **right atrial pressures** (values 0–5 mmHg) will be similar to a **central venous tracing** that varies with respiration.

   A **sudden systolic pressure increase** (values 15–30 mmHg) confirms entrance into the **right ventricle**.

   Advancement into the **pulmonary artery** will result in a sudden **increase in diastolic pressures** (values 8–15 mmHg) confirming entrance into the pulmonary artery.

   The **pulmonary capillary wedge pressure** (values 8–12 mmHg) will rapidly fall once the balloon is inflated and reveal a left atrial pressure waveform with a, c, and v waves, just like a central venous tracing except the waves appear later.

2. The PA catheter provides a more precise left ventricular diastolic pressure estimation.

The right ventricular pressures do not correlate with pulmonary artery pressures distal to the occlusion point. However, this is not true for the relationship PAOP, LAP, and LVEDP which correlate.

Theoretically at least, at end diastole no pressure gradient should occur, making end diastole the best time for pressures correlation.

The values obtained from the PA catheter are as follows [2]:

(a) Cardiac output (CO)—the only value measured (all the rest are calculated values).

The cardiac output measurements are obtained by the **thermodilution method,** the basic principle being that the difference in temperature between the cold injectate and body temperature is inversely proportional to the pulmonary blood flow (cardiac output).

Accuracy of measurements is directly dependent on the speed of injection and precise quantification of injectate volume and temperature.

Once the average value of three measurements is obtained, calculations can provide the rest of the data derived from the PA catheter.

(b) Cardiac index(CO/BSA) where CO represents cardiac output and BSA is body surface area

(c) Systemic and pulmonary vascular resistance:

$$SVR(\text{systemic vascular resistance}) = \frac{(MAP - CVP) \times 80}{CO}$$

Normal: 900–1600 dynes.sec.cm^{-5}

where MAP represents mean arterial pressure, CVP central venous pressure, and CO cardiac output.

$$PVR(\text{pulmonary vascular resistance}) = \frac{(MPA - LAP\{\text{PAOP}\}) \times 80}{\text{Pulmonary flow}(CO)}$$

where MPA represents mean pulmonary artery pressures, LAP left atrial pressure (PAOP—pulmonary artery occlusion pressure), and CO cardiac output.

Normal: 20–130 dynes.sec.cm^{-5}

(d) Stroke volume and index:

$$\text{Stroke volume} = \frac{CO \times 1000}{HR}$$

$$\text{Stroke index} = \frac{\text{Stroke volume}}{BSA}$$

3. PA catheter data may be unreliable due **to intrathoracic pressure variations**. Balloon inflation will not occlude capillaries unless it is placed in West lung zone III (arterial pressure exceeds venous, which exceeds alveolar pressure), where

the capillaries can remain open. Placement in zone I or II can obstruct blood flow rendering the readings inaccurate, reflecting alveolar rather the pulmonary occlusion pressures.

Thus, it is important to remember that intravascular volume depletion or PEEP, for example, may convert a lung zone III to a zone II (alveolar pressure exceeds arterial pressure), thereby affecting the readings. This may also occur during any ventilation management in which there is insufficient expiratory time (air trapping or inverse ratio ventilation).

Pressures are evaluated at end expiration to minimize the effect of pleural pressures on intracardiac pressures.

4. There are conditions when PAOP **overestimates** or **underestimates** the LVEDP.

Overestimation:

(a) Tachycardia (shortened diastolic filling time). At rates greater than 115/min, the pulmonary artery end-diastolic pressure (PAEDP) is greater than the PAOP.
(b) Increase in pulmonary vascular resistance (sepsis, pulmonary disease, obstruction to venous drainage).
(c) Mitral stenosis, atrial myxoma.
(d) Increased intrathoracic pressures (mediastinal tumors).
(e) Conditions associated with large PA v waves (large v waves may obscure catheter wedging with pulmonary artery rupture being a real danger). The normal PA waveform has an arterial waveform with an upward slope, a downward slope, and a dicrotic notch associated with the pulmonic valve closure. While the peak systolic wave on the PA tracing corresponds to the electrographic T wave, by contrast, the large v waves occur after the electrocardiographic T wave. Large v waves on the PAC are seen in mitral regurgitation, VSD, and CHF.

Underestimation:

(a) Aortic regurgitation.
(b) Non-compliant left ventricle—transmyocardial filling pressure and LVEDP have a curvilinear relationship, therefore changes in left ventricular end-diastolic volume (LVEDV) will result in changes in the LVEDP based on the location on the curve. Of note, ventricular compliance is affected by vasoactive drugs, and beta-blockers.
(c) Pulmonary embolism.
(d) Right bundle branch block (delay in right ventricular systole).
(e) Pulmonary edema.

5. Large v waves are seen in (1) myocardial ischemia, (2) mitral regurgitation, (3) decreased atrial compliance, (4) or increased SVR. The diastolic PAOP offers the best approximation for the LVEDP when large v waves are present.

6. Fiber-optic PACs can be used to measure mixed venous oxygen saturation (SvO_2). Mixed venous oxygen saturation is the percentage of oxygen bound to the hemoglobin returning to the right side of the heart. It reflects the "leftover" oxygen after tissues have removed their needed oxygen (oxygen extraction). Normal SvO_2 values are 60–80% with a 10% change considered significant [3].

   Low **mixed venous oxygen saturation** (SvO_2) is caused by the following:

   - Decreased oxygen delivery
     - Low cardiac output
     - Decrease in arterial oxygenation (SaO_2)
     - Decrease in hemoglobin concentration
   - Increased oxygen consumption
     - Hyperthermia
     - Neuromuscular blocker re-dosing needed during anesthesia

   High SvO_2 is caused by the following:

- Increased O_2 delivery (high FiO_2, hyperoxia)
- Decreased O_2 demand (hypothermia, neuromuscular blockade)
- High flow states (sepsis, liver disease)

Changes in SvO_2 come early before changes in hemodynamics manifest. A surrogate of SvO_2 measurement the $SvcO_2$ (normally being over 70%) is obtained from the internal jugular vein or subclavian vein and used to identify changes in a patient's oxygen extraction. An increase in extraction is the way tissue oxygen needs are met when the amount of oxygen reaching tissues is decreased [4].

It is important to note, however, that a normal SvO_2 value does not always reflect adequate oxygenation. In situations such as carbon monoxide poisoning and sepsis, SvO_2 levels may be normal or high despite end-organ hypoxia.

The accuracy of the SvO_2 values is affected by the optical intensity of the reflected light at the end of the catheter. This may be affected by physical factors such as migration of the catheter, its kinking, occlusion, or clot at the end. Signal quality indicator is displayed continuously on the monitor which should be used to evaluate the accuracy of the measurement [5].

7. **Indications for PAC use include the following:**

Cardiac conditions—valvular disease, myocardial ischemia management, evidence of heart failure

Fluid management for shock, sepsis, acute burns

Pulmonary artery hypertension management

Obstetric conditions—placental abruption

Contraindications include left bundle branch block (insertion when this is present will trigger complete heart block) and certain arrhythmias such as WPW or Epstein's anomaly due to the possibility of inducing tachyarrhythmias.

Evidence, Outcome: UK National Health Service PAC-Man (PAC in patient management in ICU)—no difference in hospital mortality in groups managed with and without a PAC.

ESCAPE (Evaluation Study of Congestive Heart Failure and PAC Effectiveness) trial—no difference in hospital mortality and length of hospital stay in groups using clinical judgment and PAC compared with clinical judgment alone.

Complications: Incidence of complications was 10% in the PAC-Man and 5% in the ESCAPE studies. Any prolonged use, over 48 h, has been associated with complications that range from arrhythmias (particularly on insertion), clot development, or infections to serious ones rarely, such as pulmonary artery rupture [6].

Concluding comments:

Judicious data interpretation should be used when evaluating the PA catheter information. Aside from the potential errors mentioned above, there are a few **pitfalls** associated with hemodynamic indices' interpretation worth mentioning:

1. Adjusting SVR to body weight or using RAP in certain calculation (e.g., septic shock where large beds of capillaries are removed increase arteriolar resistance but not tone).
2. Careful evaluation of contractility indices (left and right ventricular stroke work indices) needs to be performed to avoid underestimation of contractility (when PAOP is different from LVEDP).

References

1. Jean Louis Vincent A. Clinical review: update on hemodynamic monitoring – a consensus of 16. Crit Care. 2011;15(4):229.
2. Marik PE. Obituary: pulmonary artery catheters from 1970 to 2013. Ann Intensive Care. 2013;3:38.
3. Journois D, Safran D. Continuous monitoring of mixed oxygen saturation. Ann Fr Anesth Reanim. 1993;12(4):393–408.
4. Raper R, Sibbald WJ. Misled by the wedge? The Swan Ganz catheter and left ventricular preload. Chest. 1986;89:427.
5. Tuman KJ, Caroll GC. Pitfalls in interpretation of pulmonary artery catheter data. J Cardiothorac Anesth. 1989;3(5):625–41.
6. Hadian M, Pinsky MR. Evidence based review of the use of pulmonary artery catheter: impact data and complications. Crit Care. 2006;10(Suppl 3):S8.

Chapter 3
ECG

Teodora Nicolescu

Questions

1. In the image above, mark the following—P, Q, R, S, T, and U and PR, QRS, and QT intervals.
2. Questions: Which cardiac electric activity are P-waves indicative of and why do we see biphasic P-waves in lead V1?
3. What cardiac electric cycle occurs during the PR interval? What can affect it?
4. What is the QT interval and what can prolong it?
5. How do we determine the heart axis from the EKG and what can it represent?
6. What is the Osborn wave and what does it represent?
7. What is right bundle branch block and the criteria for its diagnosis? What is its significance when present on EKG?
8. What is left bundle branch block? What are the diagnostic criteria and its significance?

T. Nicolescu, MD
Department of Anesthesiology, Oklahoma University Health Sciences Center, 750 NE 13th Street, Suite 200, Oklahoma City, OK, USA
e-mail: teodora-nicolescu@ouhsc.edu

T.D. Raj (ed.), *Data Interpretation in Anesthesia*,
DOI 10.1007/978-3-319-55862-2_3

Fig. 3.1 Normal EKG

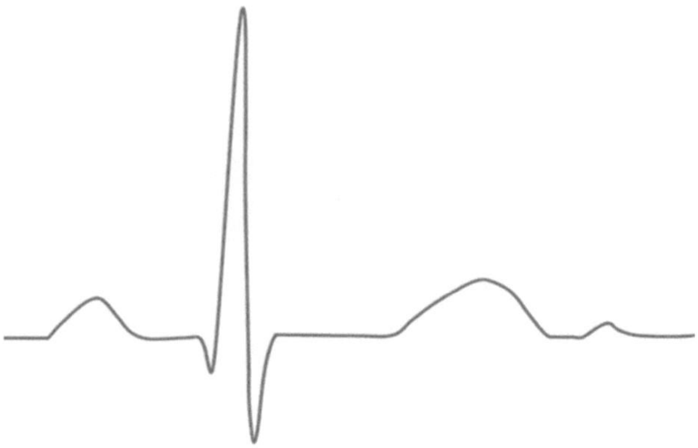

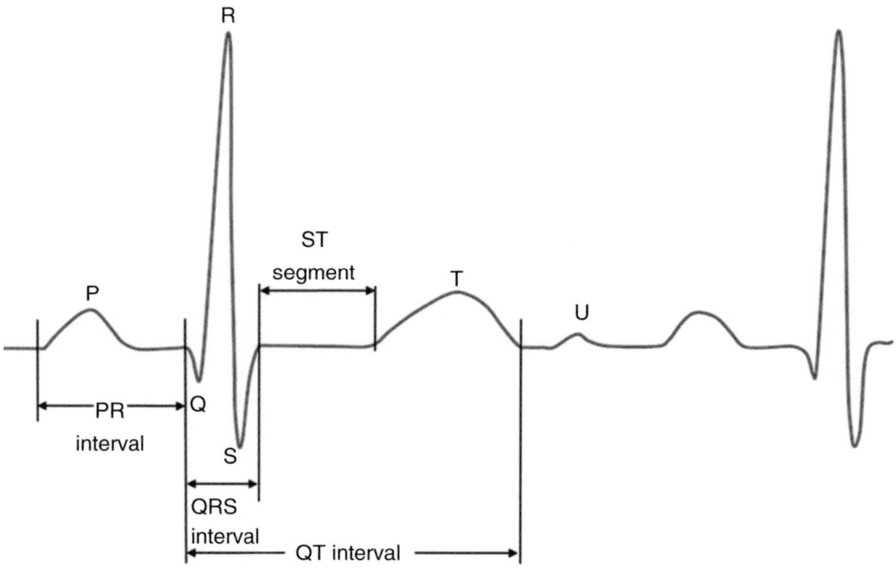

Fig. 3.2 Normal EKG (components labeled)

Answers

1. **P-waves** represent **atrial depolarizations**. The right atrial depolarization will precede the left one, due to the fact that the sinoatrial node is located in the right atrium. It is the minute difference between those depolarizations that is responsible for the biphasic P-wave in lead V1. P-waves are best visible in leads II and V1.

2. The **PR interval** encompasses **atrial depolarization** and **conduction** through the atrioventricular node and the Purkinje system. The normal duration is 0.12–0.2 s.

   Short PR interval less than 0.12 s occurs in preexcitation.

   A **long PR interval (over 200 ms)** is associated with first-degree blocks, electrolyte disturbances (hypokalemia), or Lyme disease myocarditis. PR segment depression on EKG represents a sign of atrial injury. A long PR interval has been considered a normal finding in older patients; however a study by McCabe and Newton Cheh that analyzed data of over 7500 patients at Massachusetts General Hospital suggested that when the PR interval is above 200 ms, patients had twice the overall risk of developing atrial fibrillation, three times the risk of needing a pacemaker, and one and a half times the risk of earlier death, when compared with patients of the same age with normal PR interval [1].

3. **QT interval** is composed of the QRS complex, ST segment, and T wave. In contrast to the **ST segment**, the **QT segment** is inversely proportional to the heart rate. QT interval shortens at faster heart rates and prolongs at slower heart rates. For this reason, QT corrected to heart rate (QTc) is calculated which allows comparisons at different heart rates. There are multiple ways to calculate QTc. Bazzett's formula, for example, is accurate at heart rates of 60–100 (QTc = QT measured/ $\sqrt{RR}$); however at heart rates above 100 or below 60, the Fredericia formula ($QT_C = QT/RR^{1/3}$) is the most accurate.
   Causes of prolonged QT:

   (a) Genetic: Romano Ward and Jervell Lange-Nielsen syndromes
   (b) Acquired: Antibiotics(macrolides), antidepressants/antipsychotics (phenothiazines), antihistamines, certain diuretics and diabetic medications, cholesterol-lowering medications, and antiarrhythmic medications will all cause QT prolongation. The same prolongation can be caused by electrolyte abnormalities such as hypokalemia, hypocalcemia, and hypomagnesemia [2].

   An abnormally prolonged QT interval increases the risk of ventricular arrhythmias especially torsades de pointes (treated with magnesium which shortens QT) and sudden cardiac death.

   There are two possible mechanisms that are responsible for the occurrence of the **torsades**:

   (a) Reentry due to the presence of different action potentials in adjacent myocardial cell units that have different durations—a phenomenon that is called "transmural dispersion of repolarization" [3].
   (b) Triggered activity initiated by early or delayed after depolarization [4].

4. Determining the **heart axis** will have to take into account leads I and II and AVF.

   If the QRS complex in leads I/II is positive—the heart axis is normal and between 30 and 90°.

   If the QRS complex is positive in lead I but negative in lead II, it is left axis (0–90°).

   If the QRS complex is negative in lead I but positive in lead II, it is right axis (+90 to 180°).

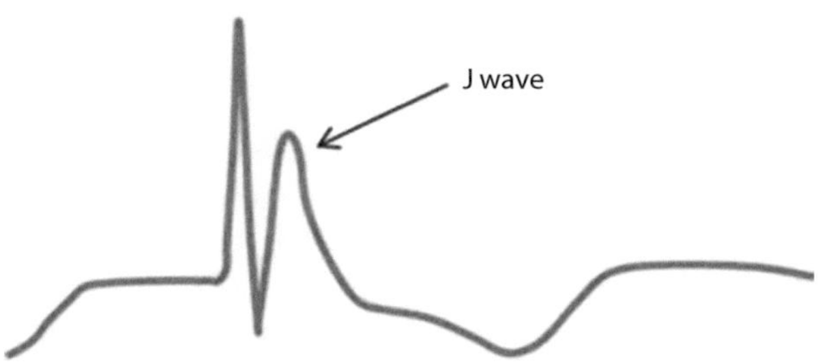

Fig. 3.3 J wave

If the QRS complex is negative in both leads I and II, there is an extreme axis shift (−90 to +180°)—northwest axis.

Causes that produce right-axis shift include but are not limited to physiologic inspiration, right bundle branch block, left posterior fascicular block, ASD secundum, or WPW syndrome.

Similarly, left-axis shift is produced by physiologic expiration, ascites, left ventricular hypertrophy, left bundle branch block, or left anterior fascicular block [5].

5. The **Osborn wave** or J wave is characterized by positive deflection at the J point (the point where the QRS complex finishes and the ST segment begins) [6].

Causes	Hypothermia (temp <30°C)
	Hypercalcemia
	Normal variant
	Neurological insults—head injury, subarachnoid hemorrhage
	Vasospastic angina
	Ventricular fibrillation

6. **Right bundle branch block (RBBB)** represents injury to the right branch of the His fascicle.

   EKG features include an RSR' QRS complex (M shaped) with a duration of over 120 ms (leads V1, V3) and the presence of a wide S wave in leads I, aVL, and V5, V6. ST depression and T wave inversions are visible in the right precordial leads (V1–V3).

   Causes of RBBB: pulmonary embolism, right ventricular hypertrophy, ischemic or rheumatic heart disease, cardiomyopathies, and the presence of a septal defect—ASD or VSD. Brugada syndrome (genetic sodium ion channel abnormality associated with sudden death) must be considered in the differential diagnosis.

7. **Left bundle branch block (LBBB)** is a conduction abnormality occurring in the left branch (the two divisions—left anterior and left posterior—may be individually affected) of the His fascicle. The electrocardiography of LBBB includes a QRS complex duration of over 120 ms, tall, monophasic, notched R waves (V6), and deep S waves (V1). Left axis deviation may be present. It is associated with organic cardiac disease [7].

   Causes of LBBB: aortic stenosis, hypertension, ischemic cardiac disease, and cardiomyopathies as well as certain drug toxicity, such as digoxin.

   Pacemakers have induced LBBB since the right ventricle is stimulated first. LBBB is an indication of diffuse myocardial disease and possibly of abnormal septal activity. There is evidence that LBBB is associated with worse outcomes than RBBB. The risk of heart failure is threefold higher in patients that have ECG evidence of LBBB vs RBBB. It is hypothesized that the relative conduction

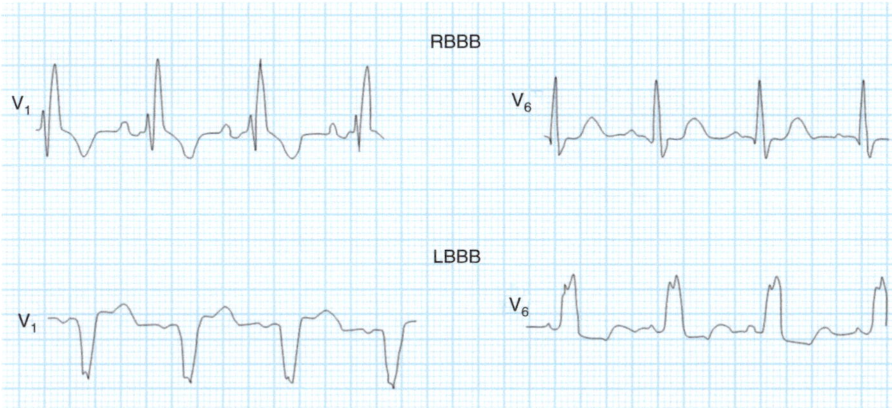

Fig. 3.4 Bundle branch block

delay is followed by mechanical asynchrony, regional workload differences, asymmetric hypertrophy, and early onset of heart failure as a result [8].

A newly diagnosed LBBB has been associated with a higher all-cause mortality and a higher risk of heart failure. At an ejection fraction of under 35%, the presence of LBBB induces a large drop in the cardiac output and cardiac efficiency.

The simultaneous presence of right and left bundle branch blocks leads to complete atrioventricular block and may require pacing.

BBB can be reproduced consistently at either high or very low heart rates. This is called rate dependent BBB and is due to damaged or inactivated sodium channels and lack of response during repolarization.

References

1. McCabe E, Newton CC. Long term outcomes in individuals with prolonged PR interval or first degree AVB. JAMA. 2009;24301(24):2571–7.
2. Estefanous FG, Barash PG, et al. Cardiac anesthesia, principles and clinical practice. 3rd ed. Lippincott Williams and Wilkin; 2001.
3. Wood M, Wood AJJ. Drugs and anesthesia-pharmacology for the anesthesiologist. 2nd ed. Lippincott Williams and Wilkins; 1999.
4. Napolitano C, Priori SG. Drugs. 1994;47(1):51–65.
5. Rodrigues JC, Erdei T, et al. Electrocardiographic detection of hypertensive left atrial enlargement in the presence of obesity: re-calibration against cardiac magnetic resonance. J Hum Hypertens. 2016; doi:10.1038/jhh.2016.63.
6. Omar HR, Mirsaeidi M. Cardiovascular complications and mortality determinants in near drowning victims a 5 year retrospective analysis. J Crit Care. 2016;37:237–9.
7. Eriksson P, Hansson PO. Bundle branch block in a general male population. Circulation. 1998;98:2494–500.
8. Van Dijk J, Mannaerts HFJ. Left bundle branch revised with novel imaging. Neth Heart J. 2006;14:372–80.
9. Cramer MMJ, De Boeck BW. 3-dimensional echocardiography: prime time in cardiology. Neth Heart J. 2007;15(3):87–8.

Chapter 4
A-Line

Teodora Nicolescu and Tilak D. Raj

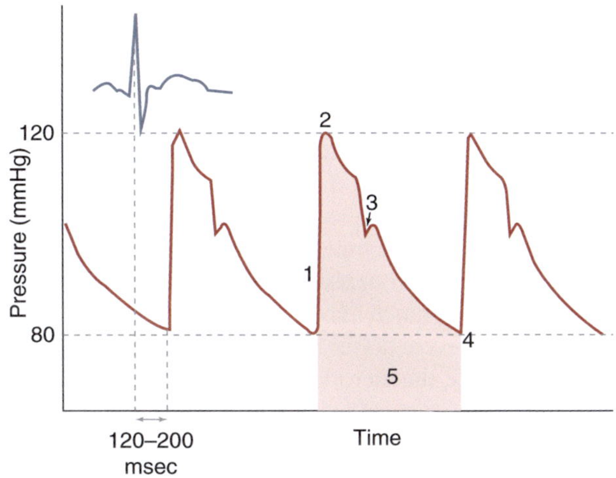

Fig. 4.1 Arterial waveform

Questions

1. In the Fig. 4.1, what are the components marked 1–5?
2. Describe the components of the arterial line waveform?
3. What are the indications and contraindications of arterial line placement?
4. What is damping and how does it affect an arterial line?
5. Does the site of monitoring affect the arterial waveform?
6. What other information can be derived from arterial line waveforms?

T. Nicolescu, MD (✉)
Department of Anesthesiology, Oklahoma University Health Sciences Center,
750 NE 13th Street, Suite 200, Oklahoma City, OK, USA
e-mail: teodora-nicolescu@ouhsc.edu

T.D. Raj, MD, MRCP, FRCA
Department of Anesthesiology, Alliance Health Midwest, Midwest City, OK, USA
e-mail: tilakdraj@gmail.com

T.D. Raj (ed.), *Data Interpretation in Anesthesia*,
DOI 10.1007/978-3-319-55862-2_4

Answers

1. 1, Systolic upstroke; 2, peak systolic pressure; 3, dicrotic notch; 4, end-diastolic pressure; 5, area under the curve—mean arterial pressure (MAP).

2. A correctly placed arterial line will have a sharp upstroke representing ventricular ejection, the **systolic phase,** whose peak denotes the **peak systolic pressure**. The systolic phase follows the R in the ECG after a 120–200 ms delay. This delay is due to the spread of depolarization, isovolumetric left ventricular contraction, aortic valve opening, ventricular ejection, transmission of the pressure wave to the monitored artery, and the pressure signal from the catheter to the transducer. In the hardened and atheromatous vascular tree, it's poor compliance increases the reflected wave causing a high systolic peak pressure. The steepness of the ascending limb is also related to heart rate increase, high peripheral resistance, or use of vasoconstrictors; conversely the use of vasodilators or impaired myocardial contractility will decrease the rate of upstroke. Aortic stenosis causes slurring and slowing of the upstroke.

   The peak systolic pressure is followed by the **systolic decline** as the ventricular contraction comes to an end.

   Systole ends with the closure of the aortic valves, and this is marked by the **dicrotic notch** when the tracing is obtained in the aorta. The appearance of the notch with its subsequent brief upstroke in pressure is due the elastic recoil of the aorta following the transient reversal of flow that precipitates closure of the aortic valve. A flat or nonexistent notch implies a dehydrated patient, or valve insufficiency. A low notch may be due to low systemic vascular resistance (SVR). In the setting of severe aortic insufficiency, a dual notch can appear (pulse bisferiens). Peripherally, the dicrotic notch and wave are due to a reflected pressure wave.

   Diastole starts at the dicrotic notch with a gradual downstroke slope corresponding to the **diastolic decline**. Its shape will be affected by changes in SVR. In patients with decreased arteriolar resistance, the dicrotic limb has a steep fall off due to reduced afterload. In contrast, patients with a high peripheral vascular resistance will have a prolonged fall off curve.

   The end of the downstroke marks the **end-diastolic pressure**. This is higher in hardened noncompliant vessels and lower in the presence of low SVR and aortic regurgitation.

   Mean arterial pressure (MAP) is the area under the pressure curve divided by its duration and averaged over several beats [1]. This determines perfusion to organs.

3. Indications:
   (a) Situations where beat-to-beat monitoring of blood pressure is required and where rapid hemodynamic changes is expected (surgeries with rapid blood loss potential, cardiovascular procedures)

(b) Use of intraoperative deliberate hypotension
(c) Surgeries or patient conditions requiring frequent arterial blood gases sampling or use of vasoactive drugs
(d) In patients where a noninvasive blood pressure monitoring could be difficult (burn patients, multiple limb injuries, morbidly obese patients)

Contraindications:

(a) Vascular concerns (Raynaud's syndrome, thromboangiitis obliterans, full thickness burns, and inadequate collateral circulation)
(b) Local infection
(c) Trauma distal to the site

Routine evaluation of collateral circulation is controversial as the incidence of ischemic injury is rare, and common testing such as the **Allen test** has both poor sensitivity and specificity [2].

4. The arterial waveform is the summation of numerous harmonic waves to form a single complex waveform by Fourier analysis. The monitoring system for the arterial pressure must have a frequency response that exceeds the natural frequency of the arterial pulse (1–3 Hz). Most commercially available systems have a frequency response in the several hundred Hertz. Factors that alter the energy in the oscillating monitoring system will alter the amplitude of oscillations. This is termed **damping**. Damping of the arterial line can be tested by its dynamic response which is a function of natural resonant frequency (how quickly the system vibrates to pressure change) and damping coefficient (how quickly those vibrations stop). This is done by the **square wave test**. When the flush valve is squeezed and released, it should produce a square wave with a sharp rise, plateau, and a sharp fall. A good arterial line trace would have a dicrotic notch and two oscillations after the flush test.

   An **overdamped** waveform would not demonstrate a dicrotic notch, and the square wave test would show only one oscillation. Factors such as debris, air bubbles, vasospasm, using a soft cannula or tubing, additional lengths of tubing, and three-way stopcocks decrease the resonant frequency of the monitoring system and cause overdamping.

   Overdamping (damping factor greater than 1.0) leads to under-reading of systolic blood pressure (SBP) and over-reading of diastolic blood pressure (DBP).

   An **underdamped** system would show many oscillations with the flush test.

   Underdamping (damping coefficient less than 0.7) occurs due to resonance and leads to overestimation of the SBP and underestimation of DBP. It is usually due to increased vascular resistance and stiff noncompliant tubing.

   In both scenarios, MAP is not affected [3].

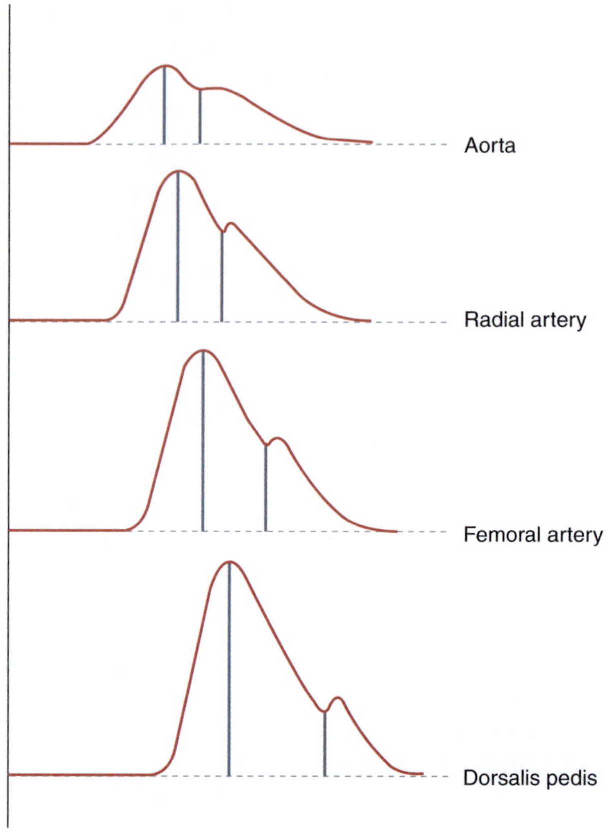

Fig. 4.2 Arterial waveforms at different locations

5. The arterial line waveform is different at different sites of measurement due to the physical characteristics (impedance and harmonics) of the vascular tree. As the pressure wave travels from the aorta to the periphery, one sees:
   - Delay in the waveform (60 ms later in the radial)
   - Steeped systolic upstroke
   - Higher peak systolic pressure
   - Dicrotic notch appearing later
   - Diastolic wave becoming more prominent
   - End-diastolic pressure lowering

   In summary, when compared to central aortic pressures, peripheral arterial waveforms have higher SBP, lower DBP, and a wider pulse pressure. MAP is only slightly higher in the aorta compared to the radial artery (Fig. 4.2).

6. Other than blood pressure, arterial line can provide the following information:
   - Pulse rate and rhythm.
   - Slope of the upstroke reflects myocardial contractility (dp/dt).
   - Pulse contour analysis allows calculation of certain derived parameters:
     - Stroke volume (SV)
     - Cardiac output (CO)
     - Vascular resistance
     - During positive pressure ventilation stroke volume variation (SVV) and pulse pressure variation (PPV) as a means of intravascular volume estimation
   - Specific waveform pattern might be diagnostic like pulsus alternans in tamponade and slow-rising upstroke with a delayed peak in aortic stenosis [4].

References

1. Magee P, Tooley M. The physics, clinical measurement and equipment of anaesthetic practice. Oxford University Press 2005.
2. MA J, Jarvis CL, Jones PR, Spyt TJ. Reliability of Allen's test in selection of patients for radial artery harvest. Ann Thorac Surg. 2000;70(4):1362–5.
3. Romagnoli S, Ricci Z. Accuracy of invasive arterial blood pressure monitoring in cardiovascular patients. Crit Care. 2014;18(6):644.
4. Esper SA, Pinsky MR. Arterial waveform analysis. Best Pract Res Clin Anaesthesiol. 2014;28:363–80.

Chapter 5
Intracranial Pressure

Jacqueline J. Smith

A 27-year-old male involved in a motorcycle accident. He presented to emergency room unresponsive and intubated. Vital signs: blood pressure 180/100, pulse 50, SaO_2 = 96%. Physical exam: unresponsive, intubated male. HEENT: facial abrasions, pupils were unequal, and sluggishly reactive; c-collar in place, and aside from a femur fracture, the remaining PE was unremarkable. He was sent for CT and found to have a large subdural hematoma requiring emergent evacuation in the operating room. Once taken to the operating room and the bone flap is removed, the surgeon notes the brain is "bulging and tense." Postoperatively, an intraventricular catheter was left in place to monitor ICP. In the ICU the ICP monitor showed the following (Fig. 5.1):

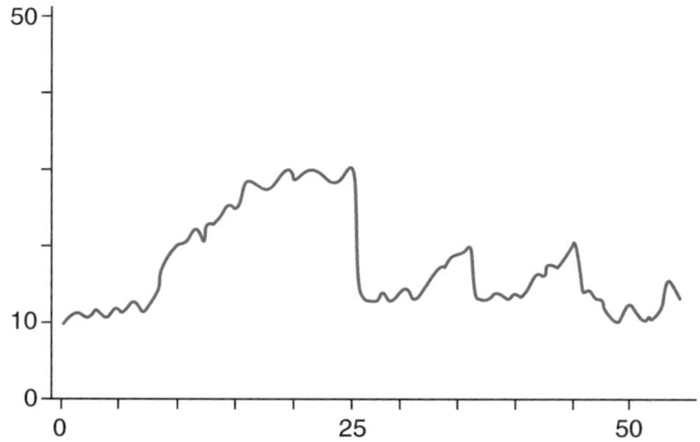

Fig. 5.1 ICP waveform

J.J. Smith, MD
Department of Anesthesiology, University of Oklahoma Health Sciences Center, 750 NE 13th Street, OAC 200, Oklahoma City, OK, USA
e-mail: Jacqueline-smith@ouhsc.edu

T.D. Raj (ed.), *Data Interpretation in Anesthesia*,
DOI 10.1007/978-3-319-55862-2_5

1. What are normal values for intracranial pressure?
2. How does a patient with intracranial hypertension present?
3. What is cerebral perfusion pressure?
4. What are the causes for intracranial hypertension?
5. What is the significance of increased intracranial pressure?
6. Describe the Monro-Kellie hypothesis and Cushing's Triad.
7. Name some indications and contraindications for invasive ICP monitoring.
8. Name some types of ICP monitors, and what kind of information can an invasive monitor display?
9. Name some therapeutic maneuvers that could be used to reduce intracranial hypertension?

Answers

1. Normal values for intracranial pressure (ICP) are 7–15 mmHg in supine adults. ICP is positional resulting in lower values with head elevation. ICP > 15 mmHg is considered abnormal, and >20 mmHg is considered pathological. ICPs over 20 mmHg, particularly if sustained can lead to worse outcomes.

2. Intracranial hypertension may present with headache, hypertension, bradycardia, and irregular respirations or apnea (Cushing's Triad). Rarely do these symptoms occur concurrently. A focused neurological exam may reveal papilledema, neurological deficits, and altered consciousness as assessed by the Glasgow Coma Scale.

   Uncontrolled intracranial hypertension may lead to brain herniation. Herniation can occur in the supratentorial or infratentorial region of the brain. Common sites for herniation include cingulum (subfalcine), medial temporal lobe (uncal), and inferior cerebellum (tonsillar) [1]. Signs of herniation include dilated and nonreactive pupils, asymmetric pupils, motor exam that demonstrates extensor posturing or no response, and progressive decline in neurologic condition (decrease in GCS > 2 points) that is not associated with non-TBI causes. Signs of uncal herniation specifically include acute loss of consciousness, ipsilateral pupillary dilation (CN III), and contralateral hemiparesis. Transtentorial herniation may cause ipsilateral cerebral infarction because of posterior cerebral artery occlusion.

3. Cerebral perfusion pressure (CPP) is the driving force of blood across the intracranial arterioles and a major determinant of cerebral blood flow (CBF). The relationship between CPP and CBF can be described by the expression CBF = CPP/CVR (cerebral vascular resistance). CPP can be estimated using the formula CPP = MAP–ICP since ICP is generally higher than CVP. Management of patients with intracranial hypertension focuses on optimizing cerebral perfusion by minimizing ICP and maximizing MAP and minimizing increases in CVR. CPP < 60–70 mmHg adversely affect brain tissue oxygenation and metabolism. Attempts to exceed a CPP of 70 mmHg are counterproductive (Level II), and a CPP of <50 mmHg should be avoided. [2]

4. Causes can be grouped into three processes: extra-axial, focal, and diffuse. Extra-axial process would include epidural hemorrhage, subdural hemorrhage, subdural empyema, extra-axial brain tumor, and pneumocephalus. Focal brain process would include brain tumor (primary, metastatic), ischemic stroke, primary intracerebral hemorrhage, brain abscess, traumatic brain injury, and hydrocephalus. Diffuse brain process would include traumatic brain injury, aneurysmal subarachnoid hemorrhage, infectious meningitides and encephalitides, noninfectious neuroinflammatory disorders, hepatic encephalopathy, and

toxic-metabolic encephalopathies. Additionally, an increase in venous pressure due to cerebral venous sinus thrombosis, heart failure, superior vena cava, or jugular vein thrombosis/obstruction can cause increased ICP. Metabolic disorders like hypo-osmolality, hyponatremia, or uremic encephalopathy may manifest with increased ICP. Pseudotumor cerebri, idiopathic intracranial hypertension, and choroid plexus tumors (increased CSF production) must also be considered in the differential [1].

5. The significance of increased ICP depends on its effect on cerebral perfusion pressure. A retrospective look at 427 patients in the NMDA antagonist Selfotel trial found that the most powerful predictor of neurological worsening was ICP > 20 mmHg either initially or during neurologic deterioration. There was no correlation with cerebral perfusion pressure (CPP) as long as it was greater than 60 mmHg. CBF is kept constant by autoregulation (Fig. 5.2). Autoregulation is a process of adjustment by the brain's arterioles to keep cerebral blood flow constant over a wide range of MAP or CPP. When MAP is high, those arterioles constrict increasing cerebral vascular resistance (CVR) and reducing the pressure. When MAP is low, CVR decreases and maintains CPP/CBF. When MAP is less than 65 mmHg or greater than 150 mmHg, the arterioles are unable to autoregulate, and CBF becomes dependent on the MAP, described as "pressure-passive flow" which also occurs in abnormal brain. MAP < 65 mmHg place the brain at risk for ischemia and MAP > 150 mmHg may cause excess CBF and may result in increased ICP and edema.

   Optimally the goal is to maintain CPP greater than 60 mmHg by either decreasing ICP or increasing MAP using vasopressors (only vasopressors that do not increase ICP). As long as CPP > 60 mmHg, ICP control is more important than further increases in CPP in terms of neurologic outcome [2].

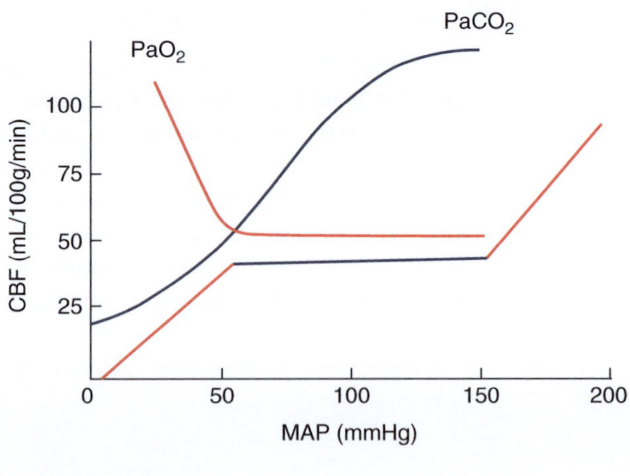

Fig. 5.2 Cerebral autoregulation

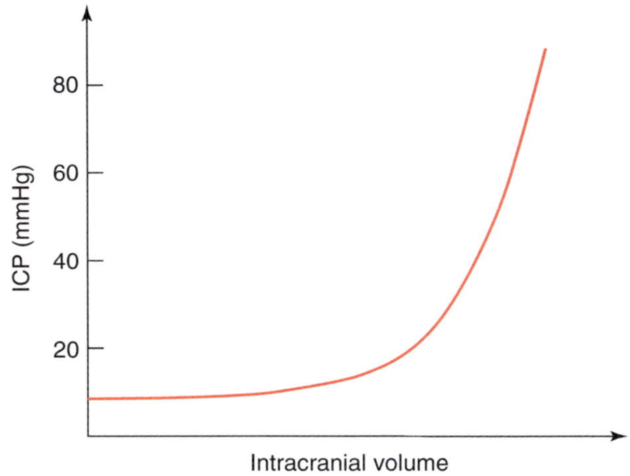

Fig. 5.3 Compliance curve

6. Normal or abnormal ICP is a function of the volume and compliance of each component of the intracranial compartment. Known as the Monro-Kellie hypothesis, this doctrine states that the cranial compartment is enclosed in a nonexpandable case of bone, and thus the volume inside the cranium is fixed. In an incompressible cranium, the blood, CSF, and brain exist in a state of volume equilibrium. A volume increase in one component is compensated by a reciprocal decrease in each of the other components. Once the compensation limits are exceeded, intracranial pressure rises, and CBF can fall (Fig. 5.3).

   In 1903, Cushing described as a clinical tool what is now widely known as the "Cushing's reflex." It consists of a widening pulse pressure (rising systolic, declining diastolic) and bradycardia [2]. When the arterial pressure is less than the intracranial pressure, a reflex called the "CNS ischemic response" or "Cushing's reflex" is initiated by the hypothalamus in the brain. The hypothalamus activates the sympathetic nervous system, causing peripheral vasoconstriction and an increase in cardiac output. These two effects serve to increase arterial blood pressure. When arterial blood pressure exceeds the intracranial pressure, blood flow to the brain is restored. The increased arterial blood pressure caused by the CNS ischemic response stimulates the baroreceptors in the carotid bodies, thus slowing the heart rate drastically often to the point of a bradycardia. The Cushing reflex helps save brain tissues during periods of poor perfusion. It's a late sign of increasing intracranial pressure and indicates that brainstem herniation is imminent. A related term is "Cushing's triad," which is the presence of hypertension, bradycardia, and irregular respirations in a patient with increased intracranial pressure. These findings are another manifestation of the Cushing reflex. The irregular respirations are due to reduced perfusion of the brainstem from swelling or possible brainstem herniation.

7. Indications: [6]
   - An ICP monitor should be placed in patients with a Glasgow Coma Score less than 8 T after resuscitation and after reversal of paralytics or sedatives that may have been used during intubation.

- GCS 3–8 and abnormal CT scan.
- GCS 3–8 with normal CT scan and 2 or more of the following:
  Age > 40 years
  Motor posturing
  SBP < 90 mmHg
- GCS 9–15 and CT scan:
  Mass lesion (extra-axial >1 cm thick, temporal contusion, ICH > 3 cm)
  Effaced cisterns
  Shift >5 mm
- Following craniotomy.
- A patient at risk for increased ICP undergoing a necessary non-neurosurgical procedure under general anesthesia rendering clinical observation impossible.
- Patients who have nonsurgical intracranial hemorrhage but are intubated for non-neurosurgical reasons preventing clinical examination.
- Patients with moderate head injury due to brain parenchymal contusions that are at risk of developing cerebral edema or continued hemorrhage. Extreme vigilance and clinical judgment must be used for lesions in the temporal fossa, since their proximity to the brainstem can lead to herniation and brainstem compression with little change in global ICP.
- Patients who have undergone tumor or arteriovenous malformation resection and are at risk for cerebral edema who cannot be assessed clinically.

Placement of an ICP monitor has no absolute contraindications because of its relatively low risk. The following conditions increase the risk for hemorrhage and merit careful clinical judgment.

(a) Patients with a known bleeding disorder
(b) Patients with thrombocytopenia (platelets count < 10,000/μL)
(c) Known platelets dysfunction (aspirin/clopidogrel or uremic encephalopathy)
(d) Prothrombin time > 13 s
(e) International normalized ratio greater than 1.3

Potential complications include intraparenchymal, interventricular, or subdural hemorrhage. Catheter-related hemorrhages occur in 1–33% of patients. Infection occurs in 1–12% of patients. Higher rates of ventriculitis/meningitis occur with longer duration of EVD placement [3]. Infection rates increase exponentially after 5 days [4].

8. Types of intracranial pressure monitors: invasive vs noninvasive
   - Epidural
   - Subarachnoid
   - Intraparenchymal fiber-optic
   - Intraventricular
   - Transcranial Doppler
   - Optic nerve sheath diameter

ICP monitoring allows measurement of ICP at a given point but also provides information about intracranial dynamics and brain compliance from waveform

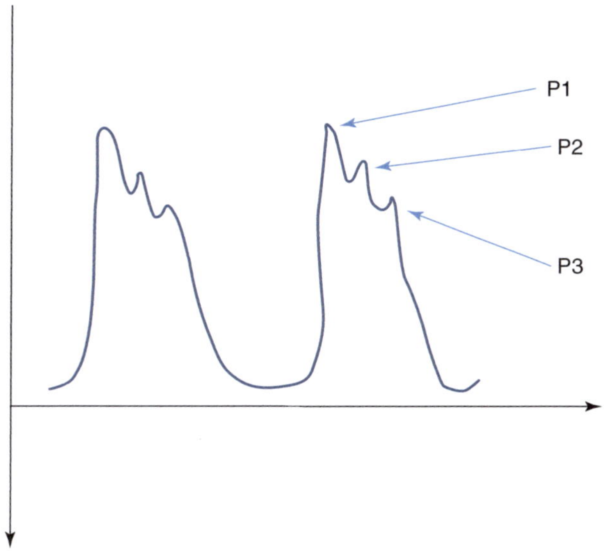

Fig. 5.4 Normal ICP waveform

analysis. Prognosis of survival following head injury and optimization of CPP-guided therapy can be based on parameter analysis.

A normal ICP trace is pulsatile and reflects cardiac and respiratory cycles. Amplitude reflects changes in intrathoracic pressure and varies between 2 and 10 mmHg (Fig. 5.4). Respiratory variation diminishes with rising ICP and eventually disappears entirely.

The pulse component of a normal ICP waveform consists of 3 peaks generally 1–4 mmHg in amplitude and correlate with the arterial waveform that occurs with each cardiac cycle.

The P1 wave or percussion wave reflects the arterial pulse transmitted through the choroid plexus into the CSF. The P2 or the tidal wave reflects cerebral compliance as the arterial pulse wave bounces off the springy brain parenchyma. The dicrotic wave or P3 correlates with aortic valve closure making the trough prior to P3 equivalent to the dicrotic notch.

Based on the morphology of the CSF pulsations, the state of brain compliance can be estimated. As ICP increases above resting level, the cardiac pulse component amplitude increases while the variability of the respiratory component decreases (Fig. 5.5). The waveform can provide information about altered intracranial dynamics and compliance such as increased waveform amplitude, elevated P2, waveform rounding, and plateau wave presence, all suggesting significant increase in ICP that would warrant intervention.

As intracranial compliance decreases, the greater the effect a 1 cc withdrawal of CSF has on ICP (>5 mmHg). Additionally, pathological waves or Lundberg A, B, and C waves appear (Fig. 5.6). Lundberg A waves or plateau waves are characteristic of conditions that lead to reduced intracranial compliance. With amplitude of 50–100 mmHg occurring for 5–10 min duration, they indicate a situation of low CPP and ischemia. If ICP is left untreated, they are an ominous sign for the development of brain herniation.

Fig. 5.5 ICP waveform reflecting decreased brain compliance

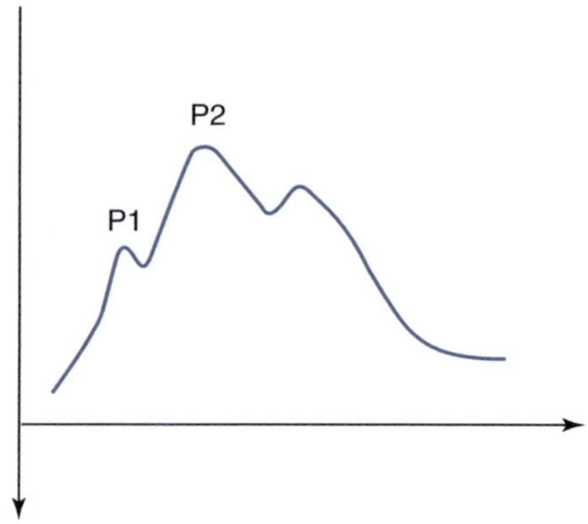

Fig. 5.6 ICP waveform with illustrated Lundberg waves

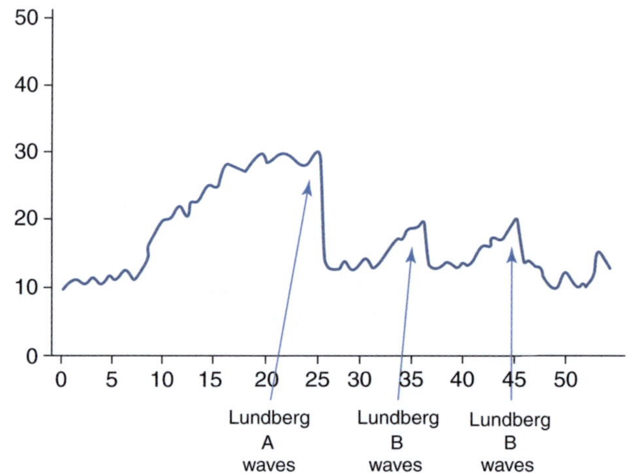

Lundberg B waves are rhythmic oscillations, sharply peaked occurring every 1–2 min. In a crescendo manner, ICP increases to 20–30 mmHg from a variable baseline and are not sustained.

Lundberg C waves have no clinical significance being documented in healthy patients. These waves correspond to fluctuations in arterial pressure brought about by oscillations in baroreceptor and chemoreceptor reflex control systems [5].

9. Management of increased intracranial pressure can fall along three tiers of therapy.

   (a) Tier 0: Standard measures which include assessment of adequate circulation, airway patency, and ventilation. The head of the bed should be elevated to 30° or higher to facilitate cerebral venous drainage. Any stimuli like tracheal suctioning should be minimized as it can raise ICP. Lower body and brain temperature if hyperthermia is present. Only iso or hyperosmotic fluids should be administered as intravenous solutions. Correct hyponatremia slowly. Vasogenic edema from brain tumors, abscesses, or noninfectious neuroinflammatory conditions should be treated with high-dose corticosteroid therapy. A non-contrast head CT should be obtained when patient can be safely transported.

(b) Tier 1: If acute obstructive hydrocephalus is present on CT, an external ventricular drainage (EVD) system should be placed emergently. If an EVD is in place, 5–10 mL of CSF should be drained. Mannitol should be administered as a 0.5–0.1 g/kg bolus and repeated every 4–6 h if monitoring serum osmolality. Stop osmotic therapy if serum osmolality is >320 mOsm/kg. A brief course of hyperventilation (<2 h) to a $PaCO_2$ of 30–35 mmHg may be considered. Hyperventilation is known to lower ICP but also decreases CBF 3–4% for every mmHg decrease in $PaCO_2$. This can lead to dangerous drops in CBF in TBI scenarios. Decompressive surgical options may be considered if Tier 1 interventions do not resolve clinical signs of herniation or increased ICP. If surgery is not appropriate, move to Tier 2 therapies.

(c) Tier 2: Hypertonic saline in concentrations ranging from 2–23.4% can effectively treat brain edema and ICP. Concentrations > 3% are preferably administered via a central venous catheter. However, with careful monitoring of the peripheral IV site, 3% and 7.5% saline solutions should not be withheld when treatment indicated. Bolus 23.4% saline has been associated with ICP reduction and transtentorial herniation reversal. A target serum sodium level should be identified and checked every 4–6 h when using hypertonic saline therapies.

Propofol reduces cerebral metabolic oxygen consumption ($CMRO_2$) and cerebral blood volume (CBV) consequently reducing ICP. Administer as a bolus of 1–3 mg/kg and continue as an infusion at 25–200 μg/kg/min titrated as vital signs allow. CPP may be supported with intravenous fluids and/or vasopressors/inotropes. If these fail reconsider decompressive surgery.

(d) Decompressive surgical interventions include:
   - Placement of a ventricular drain
   - Evacuation of extra-axial lesion (epidural hematoma)
   - Resection of intracerebral lesion (lobar hemorrhage)
   - Removal of brain parenchyma (cerebellar mass)
   - Uni- or bilateral craniectomies

(e) Tier 3: This is the most aggressive level of management. These guidelines are consensus driven.
   - Barbiturate coma induction can be administered while following EEG continuous monitoring. Using pentobarbital, induction is started with a 10 mg/kg bolus over 30 min, and then 5 mg/kg/h × 3 h, followed by a maintenance infusion of 1–4 mg/kg/h titrated to ICP goal. The infusion rate is adjusted according to either burst suppression of 5–20 s or ICP. This infusion can be continued for 24–96 h while the underlying processes causing the ICP issues are managed. This therapy is not without complications. Pentobarbital is associated with respiratory depression, circulatory instability, immune

suppression, and paralytic ileus. Pupillary reactivity is the only neurologic assessment finding, and drug clearance may take days after infusion has stopped.

- Moderate hypothermia to a target core temperature of 32–34°C can be induced with external cooling or cold intravenous fluids to decrease CMO_2 and theoretically achieve some brain protection. Treatment may be associated with shivering, cardiac dysrhythmias, sepsis, coagulopathy, and electrolyte disturbances.
- Moderate hypocapnia to a $PaCO_2$ of 25–35 mmHg thru hyperventilation can be used if patients have not responded to other therapeutic maneuvers to decrease ICP. Cerebral ischemia can be avoided if some cerebral oxygenation monitor like jugular venous oximetry or a brain tissue oxygen probe is used along with hyperventilation. Prolonged hyperventilation for >6 h is not beneficial and may cause ischemic brain injury [1].

References

1. Stevens RD, Huff JS, Duckworth J, Papangelou A, Weingart SD, Smith WS. Emergency neurological life support: intracranial hypertension and herniation. Neurocrit Care. 2012; doi:10.1007/s12028-012-9754-5.
2. Gupta G. Intracranial pressure monitoring: background, indications, and contraindications. Emedicine. Medscape.com/article/1829950-overview.
3. Brain Trauma Foundation, American Association of Neurological Surgeons, Congress of Neurological Surgeons, et al. Guidelines for the management of severe traumatic brain injury. VI. Indications for intracranial pressure monitoring. J Neurosurg. 2001;95:560–8.
4. Kirmani AR, Sarmast AH, Bhat AR. Role of external ventricular drainage in the management of intraventricular hemorrhage; its complications and management. Surg Neurol Int. 2015;6:188.
5. Abraham M, Singhal V. Intracranial pressure monitoring. J Neuroanaesthesiol Crit Care. 2015;2:193–203.
6. Brain Trauma Foundation, American Association of Neurological Surgeons, Congress of Neurological Surgeons, et al. Guidelines for the management of severe traumatic brain injury. VIII. Intracranial pressure thresholds. J Neurotrauma. 2007;24(Suppl 1):s55–8.

Chapter 6
Capnography I

Raghuvender Ganta and Tilak D. Raj

Fig. 6.1

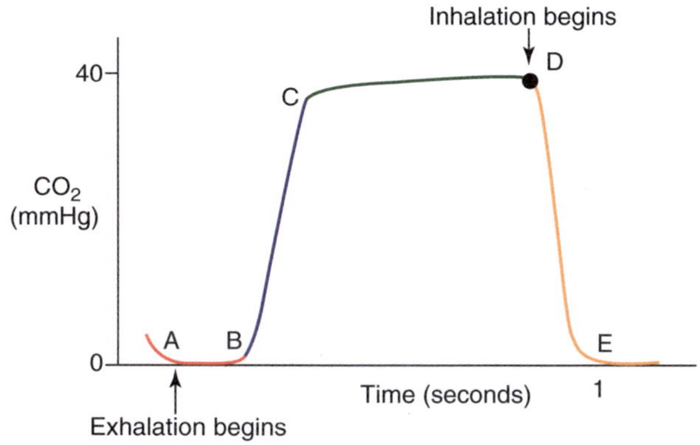

Questions

1. What does the picture (Fig. 6.1) above depict?
2. In the picture above, what do points A and D denote?
3. Differentiate between capnometry, capnogram, and capnography.
4. Explain the phases of capnography.
5. How do capnographs work?
6. What are the types of capnometers?
7. Name some uses of capnography?
8. What are the factors that affect $ETCO_2$?
9. What is the principle of calorimetric CO_2 detector?

R. Ganta, MD, FRCA (✉)
Department of Anesthesiology, VA Hospital, OUMC, 921 NE 13th Street, Oklahoma City, OK 73104, USA
e-mail: raghuvender-ganta@ouhsc.edu

T.D. Raj, MD, MRCP, FRCA
Department of Anesthesiology, Alliance Health Midwest, MIdwest City, OK, USA
e-mail: tilakdraj@gmail.com

T.D. Raj (ed.), *Data Interpretation in Anesthesia*,
DOI 10.1007/978-3-319-55862-2_6

Answers

1. The picture above shows a normal capnography.

2. Point A denotes the beginning of exhalation and D denotes the end-tidal CO_2 level and the start of inhalation of CO_2 free gas.

3. Capnometry is the measurement and numeric representation of the CO_2 concentration during inspiration and expiration. A capnogram is a continuous concentration-time display as a waveform, of the CO_2 sampled at a patient's airway during ventilation (Fig. 6.2). Capnography is the continuous monitoring of the patient's capnogram. Capnograph is the machine that generates a waveform and the capnogram is the actual waveform.

4. The capnogram is divided into four distinct phases (Fig. 6.3).
   Phase I: Exhalation of CO_2 free gas from dead space A–B
   Phase II: Combination of dead space and alveolar gas B–C
   Phase III: Exhalation of mostly alveolar gas C–D
   Phase IV: Inhalation of CO_2 free gas D–E

5. Capnographs usually work on the principle that CO_2 absorbs infrared radiation. A beam of infrared light is passed across the gas sample to fall on a sensor. The presence of CO_2 in the gas leads to reduction in the amount of light falling on the sensor changing the voltage in a circuit.

6. Types of capnometers:
   (a) Mainstream: A cuvette containing the CO_2 sensor which is heated to 40 °C is placed between the ET tube and the breathing circuit. Response time is fast.
   (b) Sidestream: The CO_2 sensor is in the main unit away from the patient and expiratory gas is sampled by means of a long capillary tube which is connected to a T-piece placed between the ET tube and the breathing circuit. The rate of gas sampling is usually between 50 and 500 mL/min. If the sampling rate is more than the expired gas flow, then contamination from fresh gas occurs. Due to the sampling, there is a certain delay in detection. Advantages include ability to monitor in non-intubated, spontaneously breathing patients and also in prone positions.

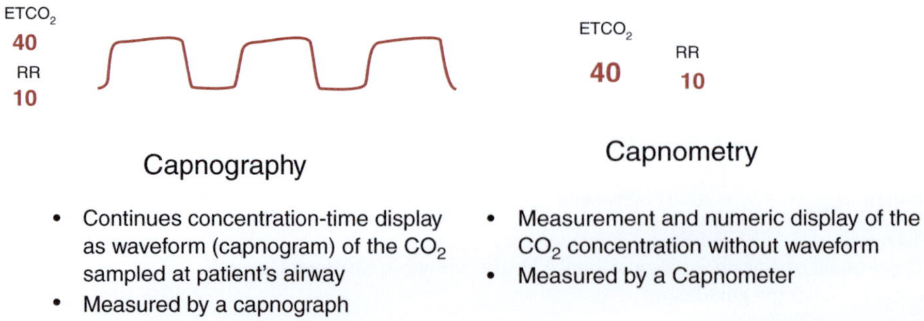

Fig. 6.2 Capnography and capnometry

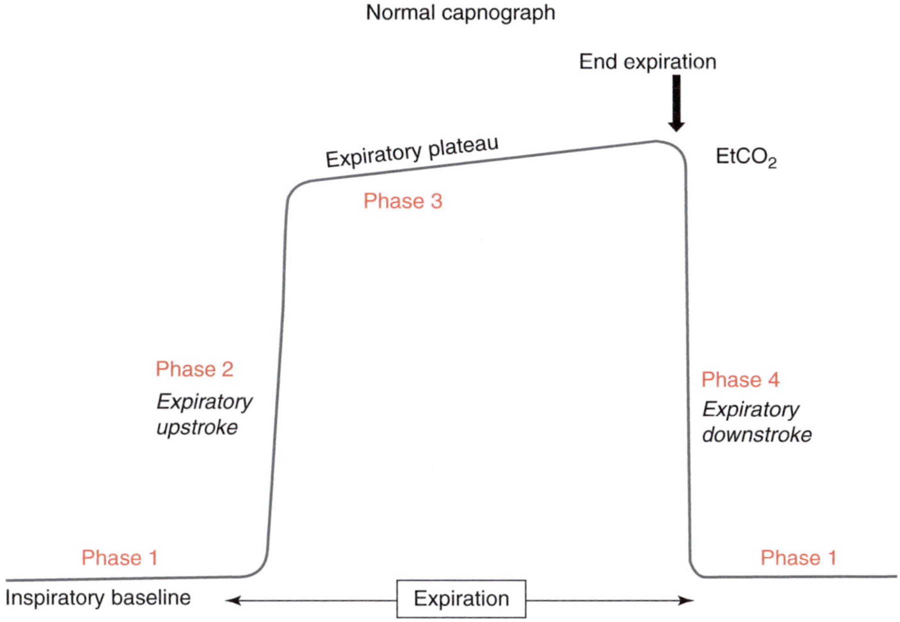

Fig. 6.3 Four phases of capnogram

7. Capnography is used in the following areas:

   It is essential in determining the appropriate placement of endotracheal tubes and is part of ASA standard in monitoring.

   As a clue to valve/ CO_2 absorber dysfunction/exhaustion.

   To monitor adequacy of ventilation and cardiac compression during resuscitation.

   Detection of adverse respiratory events such as hypoventilation, esophageal intubation, endotracheal dislodgement, and circuit disconnection [1, 2].

   During procedures done under sedation, capnography provides useful information, e.g., on the frequency and regularity of ventilation, than pulse oximetry.

   Monitoring during postoperative patient-controlled analgesia can improve patient safety and reduce adverse events by early detection of respiratory depression [3, 4].

8. The factors that affect $ETCO_2$ are:
   (a) The factors that increase ET CO_2 are:
   - Hyperthermia including malignant hyperthermia
   - Hyperthyroidism including “thyroid storm”
   - Rebreathing (baseline elevation)
   - Hypoventilation
   - Release of cross-clamp/tourniquet

   (b) The factors that decrease $ETCO_2$ are:
   - Hypothyroidism
   - Pulmonary/air Embolism
   - Hyperventilation
   - Low cardiac output

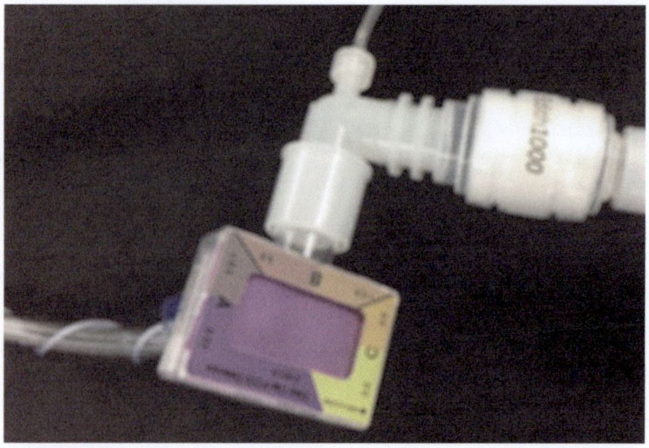

Fig. 6.4 Calorimetric CO_2 detector

9. Calorimetric CO_2 detector (Fig. 6.4) acts as a "detector" and not a monitor. The detector uses chemically treated paper that changes color when exposed to CO_2. A typical device has three color ranges based on the amount of CO_2 detected, and it requires six breaths for detection.
   Purple—$EtCO_2$ is less than 0.5%
   Tan—$EtCO_2$ is 0.5–2%
   Yellow—$EtCO_2$ is greater than 2%
   Normal $ETCO_2$ is greater than 4% hence the device has to turn yellow in people with intact circulation. It may change color due to acidic contaminants like stomach acid, lidocaine, or epinephrine.

References

1. Burton JH, Harrah JD, Germann CA, Dillon DC. Does end-tidal carbon dioxide monitoring detect respiratory events prior to current sedation monitoring practices? Acid Emerg Med. 2006;13(5):500–4.
2. Langhan ML, Ching K, Northrup V, Alletag M, et al. A randomized controlled trial of Capnography in the correction of simulated endotracheal tube dislodgement. Acad Emerg Med. 2011;18(6):590–6.
3. Gravenstein JS, Paulus DA, Hayes TJ. Capnography in clinical practice. Boston: Butterworths; 1989.
4. McCarter T, Shaik Z, Scarfo K, Thompson LJ. Capnography monitoring enhances safety of postoperative patient-controlled analgesia. Am Health Drug Benefits. 2008;1(5):28–35.

Suggested Readings

5. Jaffe MB. Infrared measurement of carbon dioxide in the human breath: "breathe-through" devices from Tyndall to the present day. Anesth Analg. 2008;107(3):890–904.
6. Raemer DB, Calalang I. Accuracy of end-tidal carbon dioxide tension analyzers. J Clin Monit. 1991;7(2):195–208.

Chapter 7
Capnography II

Raghuvender Ganta

Fig. 7.1

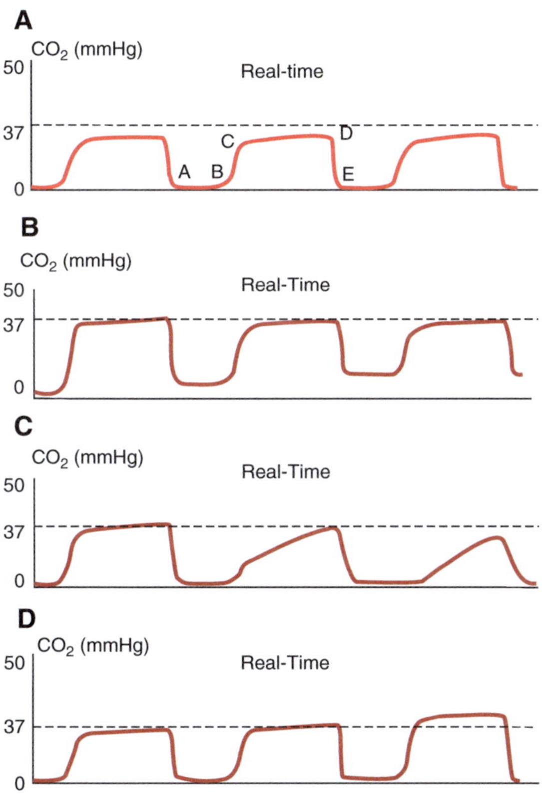

R. Ganta, MD, FRCA
Department of Anesthesiology, VA Hospital, OUMC,
921 NE 13th Street, Oklahoma City, OK 73104, USA
e-mail: raghuvender-ganta@ouhsc.edu

T.D. Raj (ed.), *Data Interpretation in Anesthesia*,
DOI 10.1007/978-3-319-55862-2_7

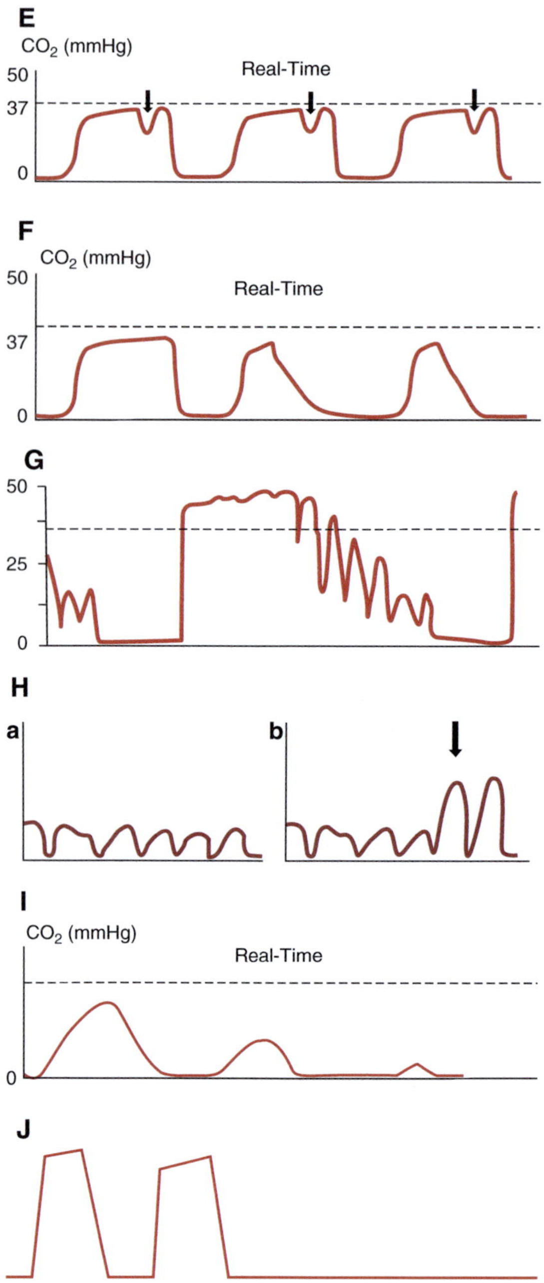

Question

What do the above waveforms A to J depict?

Answers

A. **Normal capnograph** (Fig. 7.1A)

A–B: baseline
B–C: expiratory upstroke
C–D: expiratory plateau
D: $ETCO_2$ value
D–E: inspiration begins

B. **The baseline of the capnogram does not return to zero, e.g., rebreathing** (Fig. 7.1B)

- An exhausted co_2 absorber [1]
- Channeling of the gas within the co_2 absorber
- An incompetent unidirectional inspiratory or expiratory valve [1]
- Accidental administration of co_2
- Inadequate fresh gas flow

C. **Obstruction in airway or breathing circuit** (Fig. 7.1C)

- Partially kinked or occluded artificial airway
- Obstruction in expiratory limb of breathing circuit [2]
- Bronchospasm
- Presence of foreign body in the airway.

D. **Increased end-tidal CO_2** (Fig. 7.1D)

- Hypoventilation [2]
- Increased metabolic rate
- Hyperthermia

E. **Curare cleft** (Fig. 7.1E)

- Inspiratory efforts of patient
- Hiccups
- Inadequate muscle relaxation [3]

F. **Endotracheal cuff leak** (Fig. 7.1F)

- Leak around the endotracheal tube
- Leakage of the sampling line [3, 4]

G. **Cardiac oscillations** (Fig. 7.1G)

- Movement of the heart produces small tidal volumes
- Capnograph can be affected by perfusion and cardiac function [4]

H. **ROSC (return of spontaneous circulation) during cardiac arrest** (Fig. 7.1H)

- HA: hypoperfusion, marked hypotension.
- HB: Correction of ET tube obstruction.

Increase in pulmonary circulation brings more CO_2 into the lungs for elimination.

I. **Esophageal intubation** (Fig. 7.1I)

- Endotracheal tube in the esophagus
- Little or no CO_2 present

J. **Flat ETCO$_2$ trace** (Fig. 7.1J)

- Ventilator disconnection
- Airway misplaced extubation, oesophageal intubation
- Cardiac arrest

References

1. Kodali BS. Capnography outside the operating rooms. Anesthesiology. 2013;118:192–201.
2. Gravenstein JS, Jaffe MB, Gravenstein N, Paulus DA. Capnography. 2nd ed. New York: Cambridge University Press; 2011.
3. Kodali BS. 2014. http://www.capnography.com
4. Kodali BS. Capnography during cardiopulmonary resuscitation: current evidence and future directions. J Emerg Trauma Shock. 2014;7(4):332–40.

Chapter 8
Pulse Oximetry

Alberto J. de Armendi and Ranganathan Govindaraj

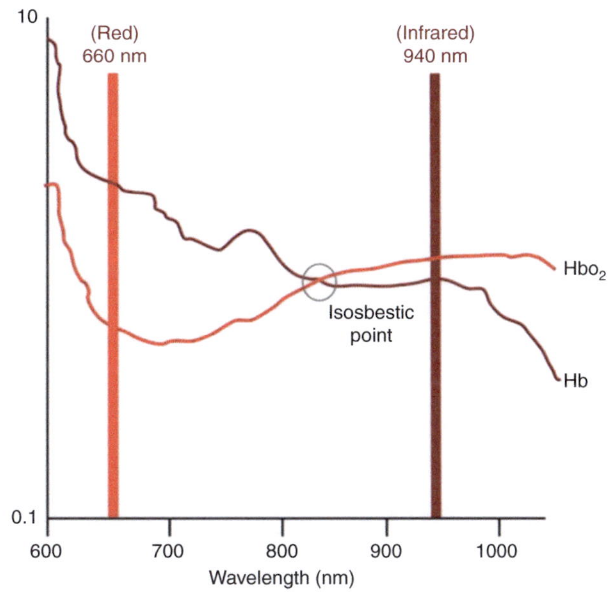

Fig. 8.1 Absorption spectra for oxyhemoglobin and reduced hemoglobin

A.J. de Armendi, MD, PhD, MBA (✉)
Department of Anesthesiology, The Children's Hospital, University of Oklahoma Health Sciences Center, 750 NE 13th Street, Suite 200, PO Box 5318, Oklahoma City, OK 73104, USA
e-mail: Alberto-dearmendi@ouhsc.edu

R. Govindaraj, MD, FRCA
Associate Professor for Anesthesia and Pain, Department of Anesthesiology, UTMB, Galveston, TX, USA

Director for Ultrasound Guided Regional Anesthesia, Galveston, TX 77555,USA
e-mail: gorangan@utmb.edu

T.D. Raj (ed.), *Data Interpretation in Anesthesia*,
DOI 10.1007/978-3-319-55862-2_8

Questions

1. How is the pulse oximeter value obtained?
2. What principle does it utilize?
3. What is isosbestic point?
4. What are the normal pulse oximeter values and how accurate is it?
5. What are the common sources of error?
6. What are the signs and symptoms of hypoxemia?
7. What other information can you obtain from a pulse oximeter?
8. What is perfusion index?

Answers/Discussion

1. A sensor in the form of a probe is generally placed on the finger, toe, or earlobe of the patient. The probe has diodes which emit light of two different wave lengths—660 nm in the visible red light range and 940 nm in the infrared range in a rapid on—off mechanism. The oxygenated hemoglobin allows red light through and absorbs infrared light, while the deoxygenated hemoglobin allows infrared light through and absorbs more red light. The ratio of oxygenated to deoxygenated hemoglobin determines the amount of red and infrared light absorbed which is read by a sensor attached to a photodetector. Comparison of their absorption at these wavelengths enables the oximeter to calculate the oxygen saturation which is read during the pulsatile component of the blood. The microprocessor displays SpO_2, heart rate, and a plethysmograph on the screen [1].

2. Pulse oximeters work on the principle of absorption spectrophotometry explained by Beer's and Lambert's laws. Beer's law states that the absorption of radiation by a given thickness of a solution of a given concentration is the same as that of twice the thickness of a solution of half the concentration [5]. Lambert's law states that each layer of equal thickness absorbs an equal fraction of radiation which passes through [3].

3. Isosbestic points are wavelengths at which both oxyhemoglobin and deoxyhemoglobin absorption is similar which is 808 nm, and the absorbance at this point depends only on the hemoglobin concentration. Earlier pulse oximeter models used a wavelength at an isosbestic point to compensate for hemoglobin concentration but newer models use various wavelengths.

4. Pulse oximeter data are accurate on average to ±2% of a simultaneously obtained arterial blood gas value. The SpO_2 values correlate with PO_2 values in the range from 70 to 100% given the variability between individuals, where the pulse oximeter probe is placed (finger versus earlobe, distal versus closer to the heart) and the manufacturer's variability range for healthy volunteers at sea level. Values greater than 95% are considered to be within the normal range. In healthy subjects, hypoxemia is defined as a pulse oximeter value less than 92% at sea level when breathing room air [2].

5. Common sources of error [4]:
   - Strength of Arterial Pulse: Any factor that reduces arterial pulsations will reduce the ability of the instrument to obtain and analyze the signal—hypothermia, hypotension, and vasopressor use.
   - Body Movement: Extraneous movements can cause interference—shivering and Parkinsonian tremors [6].
   - Carboxyhemoglobin (CoHb): CO binds to heme competitively with 250 times the affinity of oxygen, and COHb has the same absorption pattern of 660 nm light as O_2Hg causing artificial high SpO_2 readings.
   - Methemoglobin: Methemoglobin absorbs as much 660 nm red light as it does the 940 nm infrared. Saturation approaches 85% and is falsely low at high SpO_2 and falsely high at low SpO_2.

- Methylene blue, indigo carmine, and indocyanine green cause a drop in SpO_2.
- Color Interference: Pulse oximetry is not affected by skin color but is affected by artificial or opaque nail finishes that may interfere with transmission of light.
- Physical factors like electrocautery and restriction of blood flow during BP cuff inflation.
- Venous pulsations secondary to AV fistulas.
- Saturations below 80% are inferred and the saturation is overestimated.

6. Some of the common signs and symptoms of hypoxemia are:

   - Restlessness
   - Altered or deteriorating mental status
   - Increased or decreased pulse rate
   - Increased or decreased respiratory rate
   - Decreased oxygen oximetry readings
   - Cyanosis (late sign)

7. Additional information received from pulse oximeter include heart rate and perfusion index if the oximeter is designed with this special feature. Pleth variability index (PVI) is an automatic and continuous monitor of the respiratory variation of the pulse oximeter's plethysmographic waveform amplitude [7]. This has been shown to predict fluid responsiveness noninvasively in mechanically ventilated patients.

8. Ratio between the pulsatile and the nonpulsatile blood is used to measure the (3) perfusion index (PI) in the peripheral tissues. Optimum monitoring sites may be chosen based on relatively high PI. Another use would be a spike in PI indicating that epidural anesthesia has initiated peripheral vasodilatation which occurs before the onset of anesthesia.

References

1. Pulse Oximeter. American Thoracic Society. Patient Information *Series*. Am J Respir Crit Care Med. 2011;184:1. Online Version: www.thoracic.org. ATS Patient Education Series © 2011 American Thoracic Society. 2013;1–2.
2. Pulse Oximetry Training Manual. Lifebox. WHO surgical safety checklist. Safe surgery saves lives. World Health Organization. Patient safety. A World Alliance for Safer Health Care. ISBN 979 92 4 150113 2. NLM Classification: WO 178. 1–24. http://www.who.int/patientsafety/safesurgery/en/index.html. http://www.who.int/patientsafety/safesurgery/pulse_oximetry/en/index.html
3. Fearnley SJ. Pulse oximetry. Update in anaesthesia. http://www.nda.ox.ac.uk/wfsa/html/u05/u05_003.htm
4. Hill E, Stoneham MD. Practical applications of pulse oximetry. http://www.nda.ox.ac.uk/wfsa/html/u11/u1104_01.htm
5. Principles of pulse oximetry. http://www.oximeter.org/pulseox/principles.htm
6. Goldman JM, Petterson MT, Kopotic RJ, Barker SJ. Masimo signal extraction pulse oximetry. J Clin Monit Comput. 2000;16:475–83.
7. Cannesson M, Desebbe O, Rosamel P, et al. Pleth variability index to monitor the respiratory variations in the pulse oximeter plethysmographic waveform amplitude and predict fluid responsiveness in the operating theatre. Br J Anaesth. 2008;101(2):200–6.

Chapter 9
Cooximetry

John B. Carter

A patient is in pre-op holding with these vital signs.

HR 102 BP 135/88 RR 22 SaO_2 89%.

Supplemental O_2 6 L/min is administered by face mask with no improvement.

ABG: pH 7.42 PaO_2 206 $PaCO_2$ 35 SaO_2 100%.

The patient is asymptomatic with cyanosis, but an otherwise normal physical exam.

1. Why is the O_2 saturation different between the pulse oximeter and the blood gas?
2. How would cooximetry be helpful?
3. What variants of hemoglobin are detected by the cooximeter?
4. Describe the pathology and treatment of methemoglobinemia (MetHb).
5. Describe the pathology and treatment of carboxyhemoglobinemia (COHb).

J.B. Carter, MD
Department of Anesthesiology, Oklahoma University Medical Center,
750 NE 13th Street, OAC 200, Oklahoma City, OK 73104, USA
e-mail: John-b-carter@ouhsc.edu

T.D. Raj (ed.), *Data Interpretation in Anesthesia*,
DOI 10.1007/978-3-319-55862-2_9

Answers

1. There are three distinct methods of determining the oxygen saturation of blood. The results may be interchangeable in healthy people, but different in dyshemoglobinemias.

   (a) Pulse oximetry utilizes the Beer-Lambert law, which states that light absorbance is proportionate to the concentration (c) of the light attenuating substance. Oxyhemoglobin (O_2Hb) and deoxyhemoglobin (HHb) have differing absorption of light. Oxyhemoglobin (O_2Hb) absorbs more at 940 nm and deoxyhemoglobin (HHb) more at 660 nm, and it is the ratio of absorption of light at 660 nm to 940 nm that determines the saturation, using an algorithm derived from healthy controls. The SaO_2 assumes the presence of only O_2Hb and HHb, thus

   $$SaO_2 = \frac{cO_2Hb}{cO_2Hb + \mathrm{cHHb}}$$

   cO_2HB is content of oxy Hb and cHHb is deoxy Hb. It will be inaccurate if abnormal hemoglobin's such as methemoglobin (MetHb) and carboxyhemoglobin (COHb) are present. MetHb is absorbed at both 660 and 940 nm. COHb is absorbed at 940 nm, similar to O_2Hb.

   (b) In the arterial blood gas (ABG) analysis, the pH and partial pressure of oxygen in the blood are measured, and the saturation is calculated from the standard oxygen dissociation curve.

   (c) Cooximetry also utilizes the Beer-Lambert law. Using multiple wavelengths of light, the concentrations of O_2Hb and other Hb species are determined by their different absorption at various wavelengths (Fig. 9.1). This allows the calculation of a fractional SaO_2 or percentage of oxyhemoglobin as a percent of total Hb including abnormal species.

   $$\text{Fractional } SaO_2 = \frac{O_2Hb \times 100}{O_2Hb + HHb + \mathrm{COHb} + \mathrm{MetHb}}$$

   Cooximetry results for this patient measured 70% O_2Hb, 29% MetHb, and 1% COHb; thus, the fractional SaO_2 would only be 70%. Only 70% of the Hb is available for O_2 transport [1].

2. Cooximetry may be indicated if cyanosis or hypoxia measured by pulse oximetry fails to improve with O_2 administration or if there are discrepancies between O_2 sat and PaO_2 by ABG. It is also indicated for suspected carbon monoxide exposure. The cooximeter measures absorption at multiple wavelengths and can measure the concentration of many different Hb species. Pulse cooximetry applies multiple wave lengths of light to measure dyshemoglobins such as COHb and total hemoglobin concentration. They are not yet as accurate as a lab cooximeter and should be confirmed by the lab.

3. Cooximeters measure absorbance at more than two wavelengths from a minimum of six to as many as 128. Fractions of HHb, O_2Hb, COHb, and MetHb are

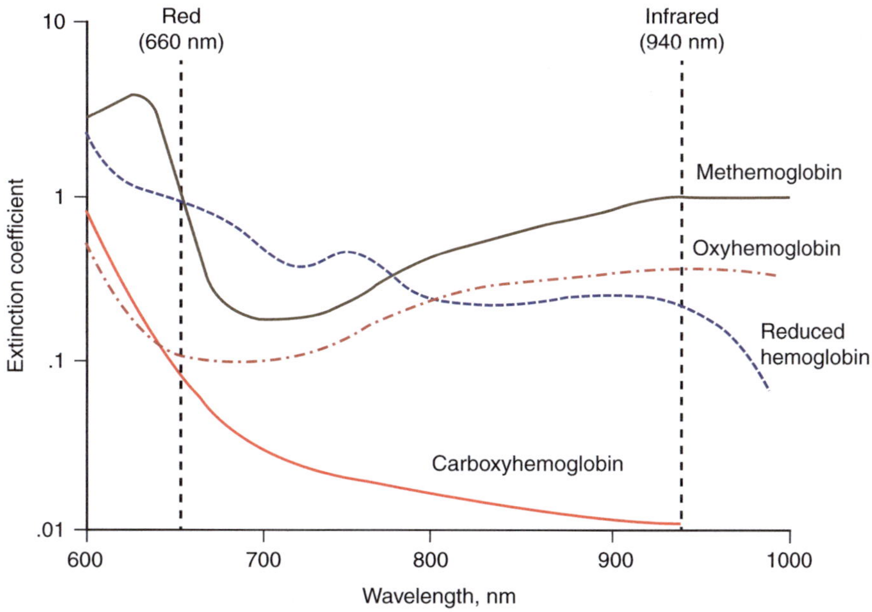

Fig. 9.1 Absorbance spectra of oxyhemoglobin, reduced hemoglobin, carboxyhemoglobin, and methemoglobin. Jubran. Critical Care.2015.19:272 (Open Access under terms of the Creative Commons Attribution License)

routinely measured. Arterial or venous blood may be used. It is important to note the difference of O_2 saturation versus fractional oxyhemoglobin in the presence of increased COHb or MetHb.

4. In methemoglobinemia the normal ferrous (Fe^{++}) in the hemoglobin (Hb) is oxidized to the ferric (Fe^{+++}) state which cannot bind oxygen and also shifts the oxygen dissociation curve to the left. Autoxidation of Hb to MetHb occurs spontaneously with a normal level of <2%. This is balanced by its reduction back to the ferrous state by cytochrome b5 reductase; an alternative is the NADPH generated by G6PD in the RBC, requiring an exogenous electron donor such as methylene blue. Methemoglobinemia may be hereditary, but it is more commonly acquired.

   Substances which may cause methemoglobinemia include:

   With high levels of MetHb, the pulse oximeter reading trends toward 85%; the O_2 dissociation curve shifts to the left. The fractional oxyhemoglobin will be lower than the SaO_2. When acutely acquired, MetHb levels <20% maybe asymptomatic. Symptoms include headache, fatigue, dyspnea, and lethargy. At levels >40%, altered consciousness, seizures, and death may occur. The diagnosis should be considered if the pulse oximetry is lower than the O_2 sat from an ABG. This can be confirmed with cooximetry.

Dapsone	Aniline dyes
Benzocaine	Primaquine
Lidocaine	Chloroquine
Prilocaine	Sulfonamides
Inhaled nitric oxide	Chlorates
Nitrites	Benzene derivatives
Nitroglycerin	Methylene blue

The treatment is to identify and stop the causative agent and administer methylene blue (MB) 1 to 2 mg/kg IV over 5 min. The response is usually rapid, and the MB may be repeated after 1 h if MetHb persists. MB will be ineffective and should be avoided in individuals with G6PD deficiency, more common in those of African or Mediterranean or Southeast Asian descent. If MB is contraindicated, ascorbic acid may be given 300–1000 mg/day orally. Supportive care as indicated may include ventilation, high inspired oxygen, and exchange transfusion [2].

5. Carbon monoxide poisoning is common and causes include faulty home heaters, inadequate home ventilation, auto exhaust, and house fires. Exposure may be chronic or acute. Iatrogenic carbon monoxide poisoning may result from the reaction of halogenated volatile agents, particularly desflurane and isoflurane with desiccated soda lime or baralyme. This has typically occurred on a Monday morning after O_2 was left flowing through the circuit drying out the absorbent canister [3]. Carbon monoxide has 200 times the affinity for Hb as O_2; thus low concentrations can produce significant COHb. COHb is normally 0–2% in non-smokers and up to 9% in smokers. High levels of COHb reduce oxygen carrying capacity of the blood and will give a falsely high pulse oximetry reading. CO causes inflammatory response and binds to cytochrome c oxidase at the mitochondrial level, impairing cellular respiration. There are high rates of early and late neurocognitive and cognitive deficits, as well as cardiovascular dysfunction and acidosis. Symptoms are nonspecific and range from mild such as headache to severe such as confusion, loss of consciousness, or death.

   Treatment is administration of 100% O_2 at high flow rates. This hastens the release of CO from the Hb. Hyperbaric oxygen has been demonstrated to decrease late neurologic sequelae and may be indicated if COHb > 25% [4].

References

1. Haymond SC, Cariappa R, Eby C. Laboratory assessment of oxygenation in Methemoglobinemia. Clin Chem. 2005;51(2):434–44.
2. Prchal J. Clinical features, diagnosis, and treatment of Methemoglobinemia. UpToDate 2015.
3. Weaver L. Carbon monoxide Poisoning. NEJM. 2009;360(12):1217–25.
4. Berry P. Severe carbon monoxide poisoning during Desflurane anesthesia. Anesth. 1999;90(2):613–6.

Chapter 10
Cerebral Oximetry

Jacqueline J. Smith

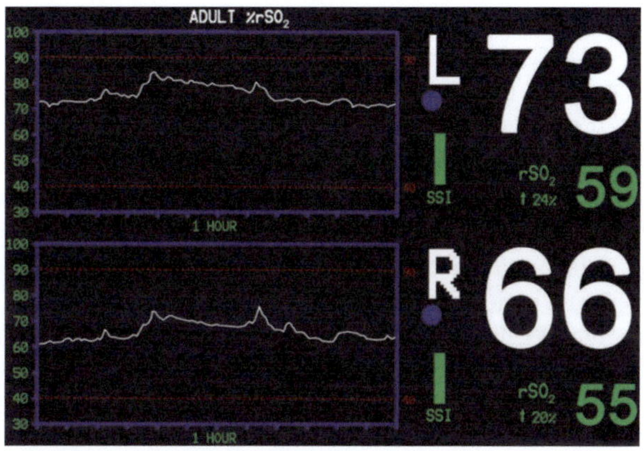

Fig. 10.1 An example of a cerebral oximeter monitor with normal values

Questions

1. What is cerebral oximetry?
2. How does it work? Is it similar to pulse oximetry?
3. In what clinical scenarios might the cerebral oximetry be used?
4. What are normal values? What are abnormal values?
5. What interventions can be performed to improve rSO_2 values?
6. What are some interference sources for NIRS?
7. What are the current FDA-approved cerebral oximetry devices in the United States?

J.J. Smith, MD
Department of Anesthesiology, University of Oklahoma Health Sciences Center, 750 NE 13th Street, OAC 200, Oklahoma City, OK, USA
e-mail: Jacqueline-smith@ouhsc.edu

T.D. Raj (ed.), *Data Interpretation in Anesthesia*,
DOI 10.1007/978-3-319-55862-2_10

Answers

1. Cerebral oximetry (CO) has been available to clinicians for more than two decades [1, 2]. Currently this monitor can be used as a "first alert" of impending organ dysfunction [3]. The cerebral cortex is an area of the brain that is particularly susceptible to changes in the demand and supply of oxygen and has a limited oxygen reserve. CO estimates the oxygenation of regional tissue by transcutaneous measurement thru the cerebral cortex.

2. Cerebral oximeters consist of adhesive sensors applied over the frontal lobes which both emit and capture reflected light based on near-infrared spectroscopy (NIRS). CO depends on the ability of light to penetrate the skull to determine hemoglobin oxygenation from the underlying brain tissue according to the amount of light absorbed by hemoglobin [4]. NIRS uses two photodetectors with each light source. Selective sampling of tissue beyond a specified depth beneath the skin is measured by the technology. Near-field photodetection can be subtracted from far-field photodetection to provide selective measurements of tissue oxygenation. Tissue sampling is mainly from venous (70–75%) rather than arterial (25%) blood (Fig. 10.1). It is independent of pulsatile blood flow. As opposed to pulse oximetry, which monitors arterial blood hemoglobin saturation (SpO_2), cerebral oximetry monitors hemoglobin saturation in mixed arterial, venous, and capillary blood in cerebral tissue ($SctO_2$). As a result $SctO_2$ is determined by two physiologic considerations. The first is the proportional volumes of arterial, venous, and capillary blood in the brain region illuminated by cerebral oximetry. $SctO_2$ is higher if the sample has an increased ratio of saturated arterial blood to desaturated venous blood and conversely lower if the ratio is decreased. The volume percentage of each blood compartment is not fixed. It varies interindividually and possibly between different brain regions of the same individual. It may also change with hypoxia, hyper-/hypocapnia, neural excitation, and vasoconstrictor administration [5].

   The second consideration is the balance between cerebral oxygen supply and demand. Cerebral oxygen supply is determined by cerebral blood flow and arterial blood oxygen content. If arterial blood content is stable, an increase in CBF will expand arterial blood volume and shift the volume ratio toward more arterial blood. Cerebral oxygen demand is determined by cerebral metabolic rate of oxygen. If cerebral oxygen supply is stable, an increase in cerebral metabolic rate of oxygen will expand venous blood volume ratio toward more venous blood. These physiologic processes alter $SctO_2$ readings. When $CMRO_2$, arterial blood content, and the volume percentage of different blood compartments are all relatively stable, $SctO_2$ can be regarded as a surrogate of cerebral perfusion [5].

3. Clinical Scenarios:
   Cardiac Surgery

   Multiple clinical outcome studies [3, 6, 7] support the concept that CO may allow clinicians to use the brain as an index organ that points to the adequacy of tissue perfusion and oxygenation of other vital organs. Data from the Society of Thoracic Surgeons (STS) National Database strongly suggest that the intraoperative use of CO in cardiac surgery patients frequently (23%) served as a "first alert" indicator of an intraoperative dynamic that could lead to potential adverse clinical outcomes in both adult and pediatric patients. The cerebral frontal cortex is a vulnerable watershed tissue that is sensitive to small decreases in oxygen saturation and therefore can provide an "early warning" about compromised oxygen delivery to the rest of the brain and other major organs [8].

Patients whose saturations fell below 75% of preoperative levels and who were treated spent less time in the ICU and had less morbidity/mortality than the untreated group [6, 9, 10].

Cerebral oximetry has been shown to predict the lower limits of autoregulation during cardiopulmonary bypass [11]. Real-time monitoring of rSO_2 provided more accurate information than routine blood pressure monitoring in identifying the lower limit of autoregulation.

Cerebral Vascular Surgery, Geriatric Surgery, and Thoracic Surgery

Cerebral oximetry preinduction value and/or an intraoperative decrease in rSO_2 value can guide in advance decisions regarding blood pressure manipulation or elective shunting for carotid endarterectomy. For cerebral vascular disease, a cutoff value of 25% or 20% below baseline for prolonged hypoperfusion is used to opt for shunting [12].

Aggressively treating values that fall below 75% of baseline rSO_2 in general surgery and geriatric patients improved or maintained scores on the Mini-Mental State Examination at postoperative day 7 and reduced the length of stay in the postanesthesia care unit [7].

Early cognitive dysfunction after thoracic surgery with single lung ventilation was found to be directly related to intraoperative decline of rSO_2 [13, 14].

Trauma

NIRS cerebral oximetry has been found to correlate with cerebral blood flow in trauma patients with brain injuries [14]. This monitor has found a use in trauma patients on the scene and en route to the hospital providing valuable information [15]. Cerebral oximetry may be a useful technique for predicting mortality and/or adequacy of CPR from cardiac arrest.

Heart Failure and ECMO

In heart failure patients, rSO_2 may be a potential important biomarker and useful monitor of target organ perfusion. When ECMO must be used for a prolonged period of time, brain perfusion in the setting of normal vital signs is undetermined. Sensors measuring rSO_2 can be placed on the forehead and lower extremities to monitor perfusion. When rSO_2 values drop to below 40 or greater than 25% of baseline, interventions such as fluid administration, increase in ECMO flow, vasopressors, or replacement of a functioning distal perfusion catheter can be initiated to reduce the incidence of stroke or limb ischemia [16].

Beach Chair Position

This is an emerging area of cerebral oxygen saturation monitoring. Cerebral malperfusion may be unappreciated in this setting. Blood pressure monitoring may not be optimal, head position may impede cerebral venous drainage thereby decreasing CBF, and positive pressure ventilation impedes an already compromised decreased venous return to the heart because of beach chair positioning [8, 17].

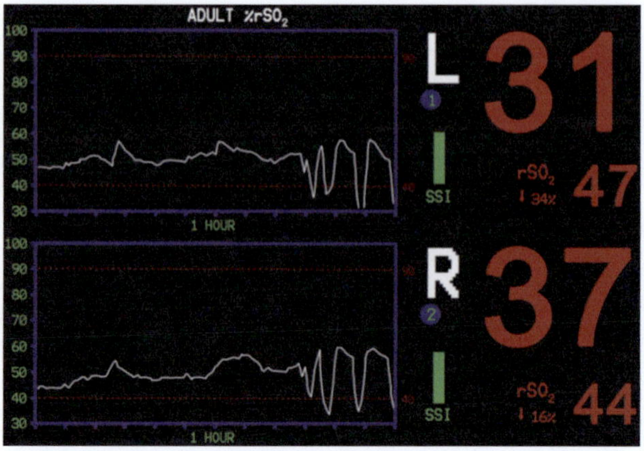

Fig. 10.2 An example of a cerebral oximeter monitor with abnormal values

4. In this technology, near-field photodetection is subtracted from far-field photodetection to provide selective tissue oxygenation measurement beyond a predefined depth [3]. Normal $Sr0_2$ baseline values would be 60–80%. Generally speaking, greater than 25% decrease or 20% decrease from baseline or a SrO_2 value less than 40% is considered a trigger for intervention.

5. The guiding principle in the treatment of cerebral desaturation (Fig. 10.2) is to increase oxygen delivery to the brain and/or decrease cerebral metabolic rate of oxygen utilization. Ways to augment CBF include:

   (a) Increasing cerebral perfusion pressure if it is below the lower limit of cerebral autoregulation and autoregulation is intact
   (b) Increasing cerebral perfusion pressure irrespective of the lower limit if autoregulation is impaired
   (c) Augmenting cardiac output
   (d) Avoiding hyperventilation and hypocapnia, maintaining $PaCO_2$ greater than or equal to 40 mmHg
   (e) Administering a cerebral vasodilator
   (f) Using inhalational anesthetic agents based on their intrinsic cerebral vasodilating properties at less than 1 MAC
   (g) Checking head position to assure optimal cerebral venous outflow
   (h) Augmenting cerebral venous drainage with 30 degree reverse Trendelenburg position.

   Additionally, interventions capable of improving arterial blood oxygen content such as increased inspired oxygen fraction and red blood cell transfusion should be considered to boost oxygen delivery to the brain.

   On the consumption side, deepening anesthesia causes a progressive decline in cerebral metabolic rate of oxygen until EEG becomes isoelectric. Too deep of an anesthetic though causes hypotension and abolishes autoregulation which would be counterproductive [5].

Interventions depending on the clinical scenario but would include:

Cardiac Surgery: correction of patient or cannula positioning, increasing blood pressure, increasing cardiac output or CPB flow to greater than 2.5 L/m2/min, increasing $FI0_2$, increasing $PaC0_2$ to >40 mmHg by decreasing minute ventilation or decreasing oxygenator fresh gas sweep flows during CPB, administering anesthesia and/or muscle relaxants as indicated, and administering a red blood cell transfusion if the hematocrit is <20%.

Carotid Endarterectomy: all of the above maneuvers aside from those related to CPB would be appropriate. Additionally, if rSO_2 values are particularly low on the one side or the other, elective shunting would be indicated for the procedure rather than just clamping the vessel.

6. Essentially any pharmacologic or anatomic abnormality which might involve blood flow, hemoglobin abnormalities affecting light absorption in the same spectra as NIRS, or distance between the near and far-field photodetection. Variations in oximeter design, use of systemic vasoconstrictors, and underlying skin pigmentation may affect the accuracy of cerebral oximetry readings [18]. Deeper anatomical structures such as the skull and frontal sinus may also play a role. Hyperostosis frontalis interna with the resultant shallow frontal sinus may cause unreliable rSO_2 readings. With skull thickness causing low readings, moving the oximeter probes to a more lateral or more cephalad positions where the skull is not as thick or the sinus as superficial might improve readings [19].

   Bilirubin dampens the spectrophotometry determined cerebral saturation at 733 and 809 nm. Normal absorption spectra for this technology are 700 to 1000 nm. A bilirubin level of 370 mmol/L, tissue pigment deposits, or both may render cerebral oxygen saturation impossible [18].

7. Current devices approved by the FDA for CO monitoring include:
   INVOS (Somanetics Corporation, Troy, MI, recently COVIDIEN, Boulder, CO)
   FORE-SIGHT (CAS Medical Systems, Inc., Branford, CT)
   EQUANOX (NONIN Medical, Inc., Minneapolis, Minn.)

References

1. Jobsis FF. Non-invasive monitor of cerebral and myocardial oxygen sufficiency and circulatory parameters. Science. 1977;198(4323):1264–7.
2. McCormick PW, Stewart M, Goetting MG, Balakrishnan G. Regional cerebral vascular oxygen saturation measured by optical spectroscopy in humans. Stroke. 1991;22(5):596–602.
3. Frost E. Cerebral oximetry emerging applications for an established technology. Anesthesiology News Special Edition, October 2012:27–34.
4. Ferari M, Mottola L, Quarisima V. Principles, techniques, and limitations of near infrared spectroscopy. Can J Appl Physiol. 2004;29(4):463–87.
5. Meng L, Gelb A. Cerebral oximetry: Three questions to ask. Rev Col Anesth. 2015;43(Suppl 1):52–6.

6. Murkin JM, Adam SJ, Novick RJ, et al. Monitoring brain oxygen saturation during coronary artery bypass surgery: a randomized prospective study. Anesth Analg. 2007;104(1):51–8.
7. Casati A, Fanelli G, Pietropaoli P, et al. Continuous monitoring of cerebral oxygen saturation in elderly patients undergoing major abdominal surgery minimizes brain exposure to potential hypoxia. Anesth Analg. 2005;101(3):740–77.
8. Trojanos CA. Cerebral oximetry may provide helpful information. ASPF Newsletter. 2009:Spring.
9. Goldman S, Sutter F, Ferdinand F, Trace C. Optimizing intraoperative cerebral oxygen delivery using noninvasive cerebral oximetry decreases the incidence of stroke for cardiac surgical patients. Heart Surg Forum. 2004;7(5):E376–81.
10. Slater JP, Guarino T, Stack J, et al. Cerebral oxygen desaturation predicts cognitive decline and longer hospital stay after cardiac surgery. Ann Thorac Surg. 2009;87:36–45.
11. Joshi B, Ono M, Brown C, et al. Predicting the limits of cerebral autoregulation during cardiopulmonary bypass. Anesth Analg. 2012;114(3):503–10.
12. Pedrini L, Magnoni F, Sensi L, et al. Is near infrared spectroscopy a reliable method to evaluate clamping ischemia during carotid surgery? Stroke Res Treat. 2012;156975:2012.
13. Tang L, Kazan R, Taddei R, Zacuter C, Cyr S, Hemmerling TM. Reduced cerebral oxygen saturation during thoracic surgery predicts early post-operative cognitive dysfunction. Br J Anaesth. 2012;108(4):623–9.
14. Taussky P, Oneal B, Daugherty WP, et al. Validation of frontal near-infrared spectroscopy as noninvasive bedside monitoring for regional cerebral blood flow in brain injured patients. Neurosurg Focus. 2012;32(2):E2.
15. Weatherall A, Skowno J, Lansdown A, Lupton T, Garner A. Feasibility of cerebral near-infrared spectroscopy monitoring in the pre-hospital environment. Acta Anaesthesiol Scand. 2012;56(2):172–7.
16. Wong JK, Smith TN, Picher HT, Hirose H, Cavarocci NC. Cerebral and lower limb near infrared spectroscopy in adults on extracorporeal membrane oxygenation. Artif Organs. 2012;36(8):659–67.
17. Cullin DJ, Kirby RR. Beach chair position may decrease cerebral perfusion: catastrophic outcomes have occurred. APSF Newsletter. 2007;22:25–7.
18. Madsen PL, Skak C, Rasmussen A, Secher N. Interference of cerebral near-infrared oximetry in patients with icterus. Anesth Analg. 2000;90:489–93.
19. Doshi TL, Kangrga I, Vannucci A. Hyperostosis frontalis interna as a potential source of cerebral oximetry signal interference. Eur J Anaesthesiol. 2015;32:439–50.

Chapter 11
EEG

Mehmet S. Ozcan

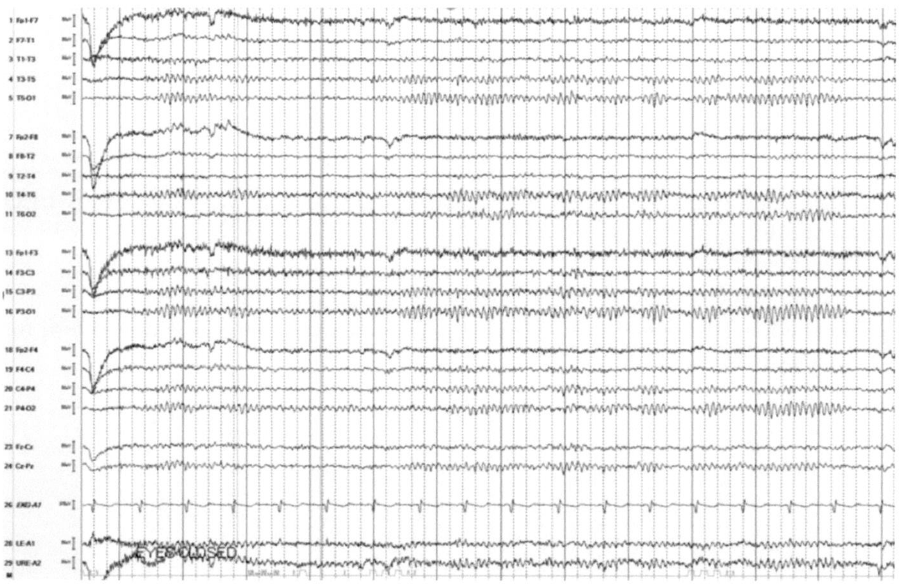

Fig. 11.1

M.S. Ozcan, MD, FCCP
Department of Anesthesiology, The University of Oklahoma Health Sciences Center,
700 NE 13th Street, Suite 200, Oklahoma City, OK 73104, USA
e-mail: Mehmet-Ozcan@ouhsc.edu

T.D. Raj (ed.), *Data Interpretation in Anesthesia*,
DOI 10.1007/978-3-319-55862-2_11

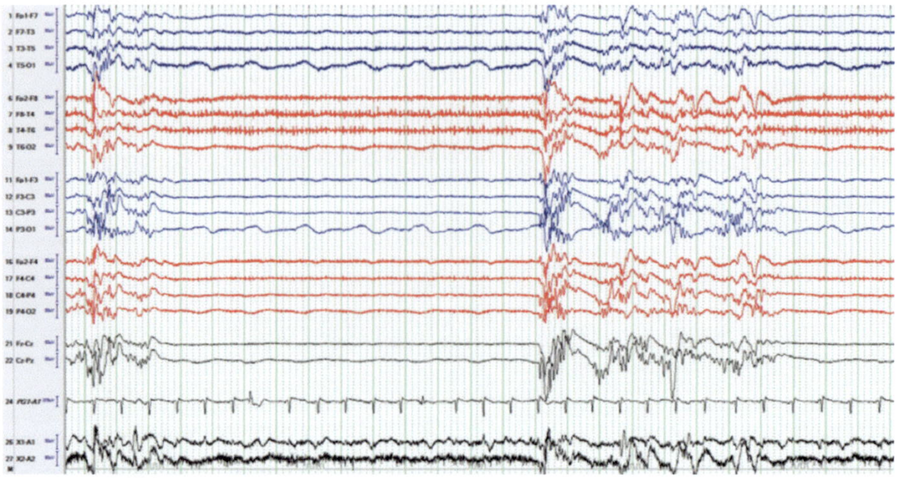

Fig. 11.2

Questions

1. What does Fig. 11.1 represent? Describe the characteristics of various EEG waveforms.
2. Describe the channels and their labels.
3. Identify some of the dominant waveforms seen in Fig. 11.1.
4. What does Fig. 11.2 represent? What is the significance of this EEG pattern for the anesthesia provider?

Answers

1. This is a bilateral, multichannel EEG recording, showing normal (i.e., non-pathologic) waveforms. EEG signals originate from the pyramidal cells of the cerebral cortex. Each EEG electrode can capture the electrical activity of the underlying 1 in square cerebral cortex. For this reason, multiple electrodes simultaneously recording several channels are required to get an overall representation of the electrical activity of the brain. EEG signals are classified in four frequency bands. These are alpha (8–13 Hz), beta (>13 Hz), theta (4–7 Hz), and delta (<4 Hz) [1]. In a nonanesthetized individual, normal EEG can display waveforms that can fall in any one of these categories. However, location of the recording (e.g., posterior vs frontal), age of the individual, and conscious state are all important factors to determine whether a particular frequency band can be regarded as normal or not.

2. EEG electrodes are placed on the scalp at precise locations based on their distance from standard landmarks. Most common method is the International 10–20 system, employing 21 electrodes. Majority of the electrodes are labeled with a letter followed by a number. Letters indicate the region of the scalp: frontal (F), parietal (P), frontal polar (Fp), temporal (T), occipital (O), and central (C). Auricular (A) electrodes are commonly used as reference point. Odd and even numbers that follow the letters indicate left and right sided placement, respectively. The smaller the number, the closer the location of the electrode to the midline. Midline electrodes are labeled with a letter "z" instead of a number (e.g., Fz for the "frontal midline" electrode location). Labels of the individual channels indicate the active (recording) electrode followed by the reference electrode. If both of these are active electrodes, then it is a "bipolar" montage (e.g., Fp1-F7). Alternatively, the reference electrode can be a non-cephalic electrode, which makes the montage "referential" (e.g., Fp1-A1). In the top figure, there are 20 bipolar channels that are arranged in the following fashion: 5 left-hemispheric (starting with Fp1-F7), 5 right-hemispheric (starts with Fp2-F8), 4 right-hemispheric (starts with Fp1-F3), 4 right-hemispheric (starts with Fp2-F4), and 2 midline (Fz-Cz and Cz-Pz) channels. There is also one EKG lead (to assist with artifact rejection) and two ocular electrodes to document eye opening/closure which is an important factor for analysis.

3. There are predominantly beta and alpha frequencies in Fig. 11.1. The solid vertical lines indicate 1 s intervals, which is crucial to determine frequency. In the frontal channels (e.g., Fp1-F7), waveforms have low voltage with a frequency of greater than 13 Hz (i.e., more than 13 small waves between 2 vertical solid lines). These are beta waves. On the other hand, posterior channels (e.g., T5-O1) predominantly display waveforms that have a higher voltage with a frequency in the 8–13 Hz range. The ocular electrodes (last two channels) indicate closed eyes. This is a normal pattern (i.e., alpha dominance in posterior channels) in healthy adults, who are awake with eyes closed. There is symmetry between corresponding channels on the left and right hemispheres. Therefore, this is a normal EEG.

4. Figure 11.2 shows bursts of EEG activity interrupting an isoelectric waveform, commonly known as burst suppression pattern. It can be observed secondary to high doses of certain anesthetic drugs (i.e., iatrogenic) or as a result of a disease process (i.e., pathologic). Certain inhalation anesthetics (e.g., isoflurane, sevoflurane) can cause burst suppression of the EEG in the higher end of their dose range, typically around 1.3 MAC [2]. However, in elderly individuals or patients with severe coexisting severe systemic illness, burst suppression can be observed even around 1 MAC (age adjusted) [3]. Among intravenous anesthetics, barbiturates, propofol, and etomidate can result in burst suppression of the EEG at high plasma concentrations. Short periods of burst suppression can be unintentionally observed during the course of an anesthetic. However, it can be specifically aimed to provide brain protection during procedures in which ischemic brain injury is possible. An example to this is temporary clip application during cerebral aneurysm clipping. This is usually achieved by a continuous infusion of an intravenous agent such as pentobarbital. Burst suppression secondary to underlying pathology is usually an ominous sign and can be seen in critically ill patients with hypoxemia and hypotension [4].

References

1. Purdon PL, Sampson A, Pavone KJ, Brown EN. Clinical electroencephalography for anesthesiologists: part I: background and basic signatures. Anesthesiology. 2015;123(4):937–60. doi:10.1097/ALN.0000000000000841.
2. Pilge S, Jordan D, Kreuzer M, Kochs EF, Schneider G. Burst suppression-MAC and burst suppression-CP_{50} as measures of cerebral effects of anaesthetics. Br J Anaesth. 2014;112(6):1067–74. doi:10.1093/bja/aeu016.
3. Purdon PL, Pavone KJ, Akeju O, et al. The ageing brain: age-dependent changes in the electroencephalogram during propofol and sevoflurane general anaesthesia. Hemmings HC, ed. Br J Anaesth. 2015;115(Suppl 1):i46–57. doi:10.1093/bja/aev213.
4. Myles PS, Daly D, Silvers A, Cairo S. Prediction of neurological outcome using bispectral index monitoring in patients with severe ischemic-hypoxic brain injury undergoing emergency surgery. Anesthesiology. 2009;110(5):1106–15. doi:10.1097/ALN.0b013e31819daef6.

Chapter 12
SSEP's and More

Mehmet S. Ozcan

1. What is the monitoring modality depicted in Figs. 12.1 and 12.2? What do the green and white waveforms correspond to?
2. What are those letters and numbers marked on the waveforms?
3. What types of surgery are suitable for using the above SSEP method?
4. What constitutes a "significant change" from baseline?
5. What are the effects of commonly used anesthetic agents on SSEPs?
6. What are some other physiologic variables known to affect SSEP monitoring?
7. What does Fig. 12.3 represent? What is the advantage of this modality? What are some specific anesthetic concerns with this technique?

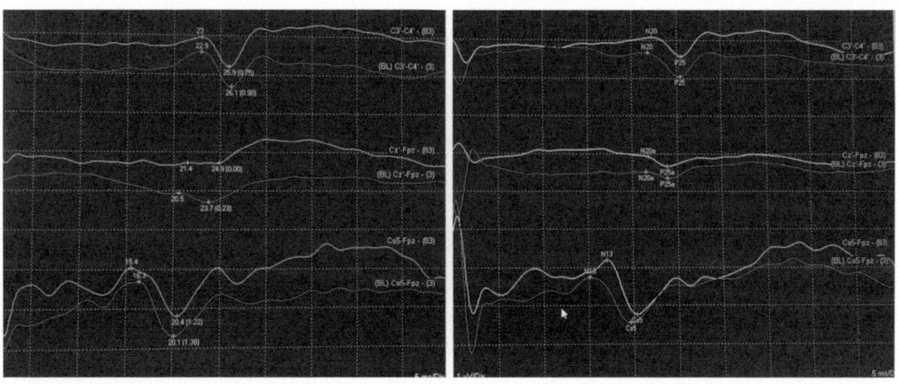

Fig. 12.1

M.S. Ozcan, MD, FCCP
Department of Anesthesiology, The University of Oklahoma Health Sciences Center, 700 NE 13th Street, Suite 200, Oklahoma City, OK 73104, USA
e-mail: Mehmet-Ozcan@ouhsc.edu

T.D. Raj (ed.), *Data Interpretation in Anesthesia*,
DOI 10.1007/978-3-319-55862-2_12

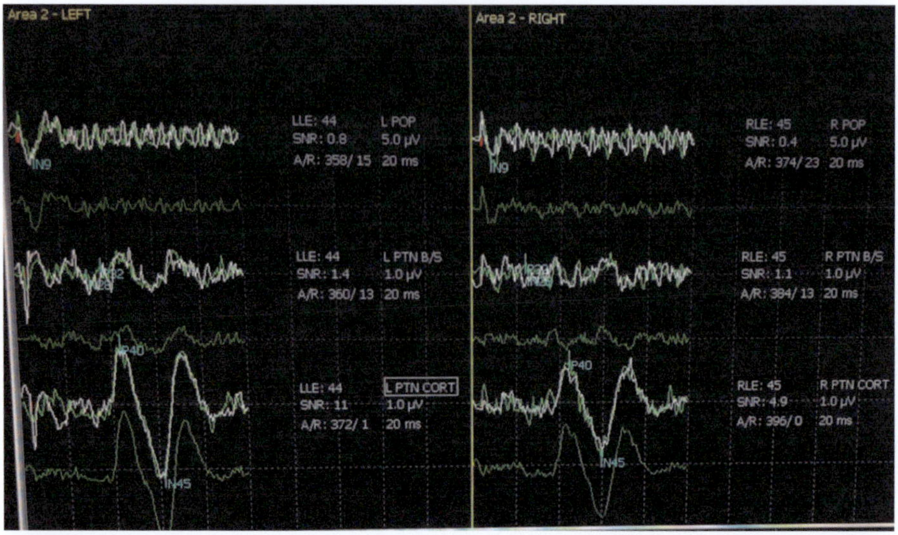

Fig. 12.2

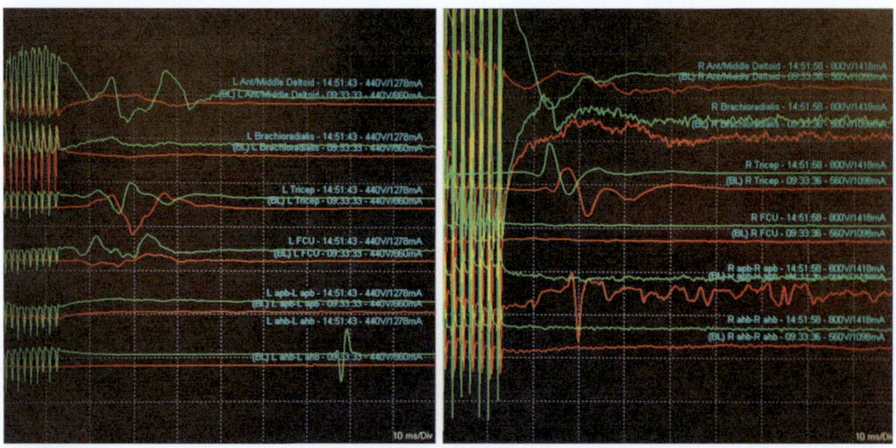

Fig. 12.3

Answers

1. This is an SSEP recording. SSEP is a neuromonitoring technique that involves the repetitive stimulation of peripheral nerves and recording responses at different points along the course of signal propagation [1]. Typically, recordings are obtained at three different points: on the peripheral nerve at a more proximal level, brainstem, and cerebral cortex. In this regard, one can assess the integrity of the peripheral nerve, sensory tracks of the spinal cord, and the sensory cortex by SSEP monitoring. In the Figs. 12.1 and 12.2, median and posterior tibial nerves are stimulated to obtain the tracings, respectively. In the perioperative setting, monitoring is usually performed by comparing the SSEP signals obtained during surgery with the baseline signal obtained immediately before surgery. Therefore, the most current tracings (green and yellow lines) are displayed usually along with the baseline (i.e., control) tracing (red and white) to make the comparison easier.

2. Signals (i.e., peaks and troughs) are typically marked on the tracing with a letter and a number. The letter indicates the direction of the signal: N for negative and P for positive. The height of the signal (in microvolts) is the amplitude. The number shows the duration (in milliseconds) from the delivery of the stimulus until the signal is obtained (i.e., the latency). For example, the median nerve signals labeled on the top panels are N13 (brainstem) and N20 (cerebral cortex). In other words, the signal is detected 13 and 20 ms after its generation at these anatomic locations. For the tibial nerve (the lower panel), the signals are N9 (popliteal fossa), N28 (brainstem), and N45 (cerebral cortex). Compared to the median nerve, there is significantly more delay (i.e., greater latency) in the detection of the signal from the tibial nerve (e.g., 20 ms vs. 45 ms for cortical signals) simply because there is a greater distance for the signal to propagate.

3. Using SSEPs, any structure in the nervous system from the point of stimulus to the sensory cerebral cortex can be monitored. Therefore, SSEP is commonly used for cerebrovascular surgery (to monitor cerebral cortex), spinal surgery (to monitor the posterior one-third of the spinal cord, i.e., the ascending sensory neurons), as well as surgery on the thoracic aorta where perfusion of the spinal cord could be at stake. Although less commonly employed, peripheral nerves and the plexi they originate from (e.g., median nerve/brachial plexus) can be monitored using SSEPs. For monitoring the cerebral cortex, both the upper and lower extremity nerves can be chosen, and the cortical signals (e.g., N20 in Fig. 12.1) on the ipsilateral side of the surgery are monitored for a significant change with potential insult. For spinal cord monitoring, upper extremity (e.g., median nerve) stimulation can only detect a problem above C6 level (i.e., the level of entry of the sensory pathways of the median nerve). As a result, lower extremity stimulation is usually the norm for spinal surgery since it monitors the whole length of the sensory pathways. For spinal surgery, both the brainstem (e.g., N28 in Fig. 12.2, middle tracing) *and* the cortical (e.g., N45 in Fig. 12.2, lower tracing)

signals are expected to change with insult. In the setting of both cortical and spinal cord monitoring, continued presence of brachial plexus and popliteal fossa signals serves as reassurance that the signal is indeed delivered and detected before the area of concern is reached, ruling out technical problems.

4. A significant change in an SSEP signal is defined as a >50% decrease in amplitude or a >10% increase in latency. As an example, the N45 (cortical) signal in the left tibial nerve SSEPs has an amplitude of 1 μV at baseline and a latency of 45 ms (left lower panel). If the amplitude decreases to less than 0.5 μV or detected later than 49.5 ms following stimulus, it constitutes a significant change from baseline. If a significant change occurs, the surgeon and the anesthesiologist should be immediately notified so that they can review potential causes and agree on an action plan before irreversible damage occurs.

5. Many anesthetic agents have profound effects on SSEP. All halogenated agents decrease the amplitude and increase the latency of the cortical signals in a dose-dependent manner [2]. Nitrous oxide has the same effect, even more profound than halogenated agents at equipotent doses [3]. Opioids as well as many commonly used IV hypnotics (including barbiturates, propofol, and midazolam) may cause a small decrease in amplitude with no effect on latency [4, 5]. Neuromuscular blocking agents (NMBs) do not directly affect SSEPs but indirectly improve signal quality by eliminating artifacts related to EMG activity. Ketamine and etomidate both increase the amplitude of the cortical SSEP signals. In fact, their use could be an asset in improving monitoring when baseline signals have low amplitude to begin with [6]. In summary, a total intravenous anesthesia is the most acceptable technique for facilitating SSEP monitoring. Nitrous oxide should be avoided, and halogenated agents should be used in the smallest possible doses if preferred. Whatever technique is used, concentrations of anesthetic agents should not be changed during critical parts of surgery since their effect on SSEPs may mask (or mimic) changes consistent with surgical insult.

6. Amplitude of SSEP (especially cortical) signals decreases with age, so obtaining good baseline signals may become more challenging in the elderly. Hypothermia and hypotension are two modifiable factors that can be controlled by the anesthesiologist. Every 1 °C decrease in body temperature increases cortical signal latency by 0.75–1 ms. Hypotension decreases amplitudes and increases latency, although the blood pressure threshold below which these changes occur is more variable. In general, systolic blood pressures above 80 mmHg should not be expected to produce changes, but due to variability in limits for cerebral autoregulation, certain individuals may need a higher blood pressure to preserve signals. Similar to the concentrations of anesthetic medications, temperature and blood pressure should be maintained as stable as possible during critical parts of SSEP monitoring.

7. Figure 12.3 represents a motor evoked potential (MEP) tracing. As discussed above, SSEPs only monitor the posterior one-third of the spinal cord. Therefore, in complex spinal surgeries, it is a common practice to monitor MEP along with SSEP for a more complete picture [7]. Besides spinal surgery, MEP is a valuable adjuvant to SSEP in monitoring the cerebral cortex. In one large case series, adding MEP monitoring to SSEP decreased false negatives in CEA surgery in detecting cortical ischemia [8]. MEP monitoring is achieved by transcranial stimulation of the motor cortex and eliciting muscle contraction as the response. Therefore, neuromuscular blocking agents clearly present a challenge. Most providers would avoid NMB altogether when MEP is monitored, although a careful maintenance of a stable, partial neuromuscular block (e.g., three-fourths in a train-of-four stimulation) can be feasible. Other anesthetic agents that affect MEPs are similar to that for SSEPs: volatile agents and nitrous oxide are the worst offenders, whereas TIVA with propofol and opioid remains the least confounding technique [9].

References

1. Toleikis JR. American Society of Neurophysiological Monitoring. Intraoperative monitoring using somatosensory evoked potentials. A position statement by the American Society of Neurophysiological Monitoring. J Clin Monit Comput. 2005;19(3):241–58. doi:10.1007/s10877-005-4397-0.
2. Fletcher JE, Hinn AR, Heard CM, et al. The effects of isoflurane and desflurane titrated to a bispectral index of 60 on the cortical somatosensory evoked potential during pediatric scoliosis surgery. Anesth Analg. 2005;100(6):1797–803. doi:10.1213/01.ANE.0000152193.90756.4E.
3. Lam AM, Sharar SR, Mayberg TS, Eng CC. Isoflurane compared with nitrous oxide anaesthesia for intraoperative monitoring of somatosensory-evoked potentials. Can J Anaesth. 1994;41(4):295–300. doi:10.1007/BF03009907.
4. Kimovec MA, Koht A, Sloan TB. Effects of sufentanil on median nerve somatosensory evoked potentials. Br J Anaesth. 1990;65(2):169–72.
5. Sloan TB, Fugina ML, Toleikis JR. Effects of midazolam on median nerve somatosensory evoked potentials. Br J Anaesth. 1990;64(5):590–3.
6. Stoicea N, Versteeg G, Florescu D, et al. Ketamine-based anesthetic protocols and evoked potential monitoring: a risk/benefit overview. Front Neurosci. 2016;10(89):263. doi:10.3389/fnins.2016.00037.
7. Pajewski TN, Arlet V, Phillips LH. Current approach on spinal cord monitoring: the point of view of the neurologist, the anesthesiologist and the spine surgeon. Eur Spine J. 2007;16(2):115–29. doi:10.1007/s00586-007-0419-6.
8. Malcharek MJ, Ulkatan S, Marinò V, et al. Intraoperative monitoring of carotid endarterectomy by transcranial motor evoked potential: a multicenter study of 600 patients. 2013;124(5):1025–1030. doi:10.1016/j.clinph.2012.10.014.
9. Hans P, Bonhomme V. Why we still use intravenous drugs as the basic regimen for neurosurgical anaesthesia. 2006;19(5):498–503. doi:10.1097/01.aco.0000245274.69292.ad.

Chapter 13
Bispectral Index

Mehmet S. Ozcan

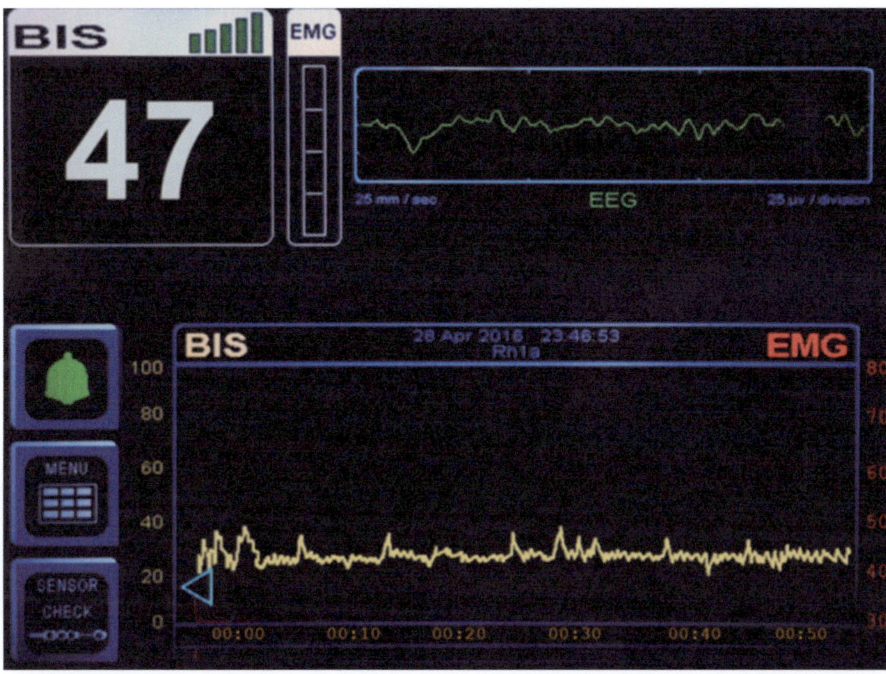

Fig. 13.1

M.S. Ozcan, MD, FCCP
Department of Anesthesiology, The University of Oklahoma Health Sciences Center,
700 NE 13th Street, Suite 200, Oklahoma City, OK 73104, USA
e-mail: Mehmet-Ozcan@ouhsc.edu

T.D. Raj (ed.), *Data Interpretation in Anesthesia*,
DOI 10.1007/978-3-319-55862-2_13

1. What is the monitoring modality seen in Fig. 13.1? Describe the numeric data fields and waveforms displayed on the screen.
2. What are the clinical states that correspond to different BIS ranges?
3. What is an acceptable BIS range for general anesthesia?
4. Which anesthetic drugs are suitable for BIS to be used?
5. List common indications for this monitoring modality in anesthesia practice.
6. Besides anesthetic agents, what are some other conditions that can affect BIS?

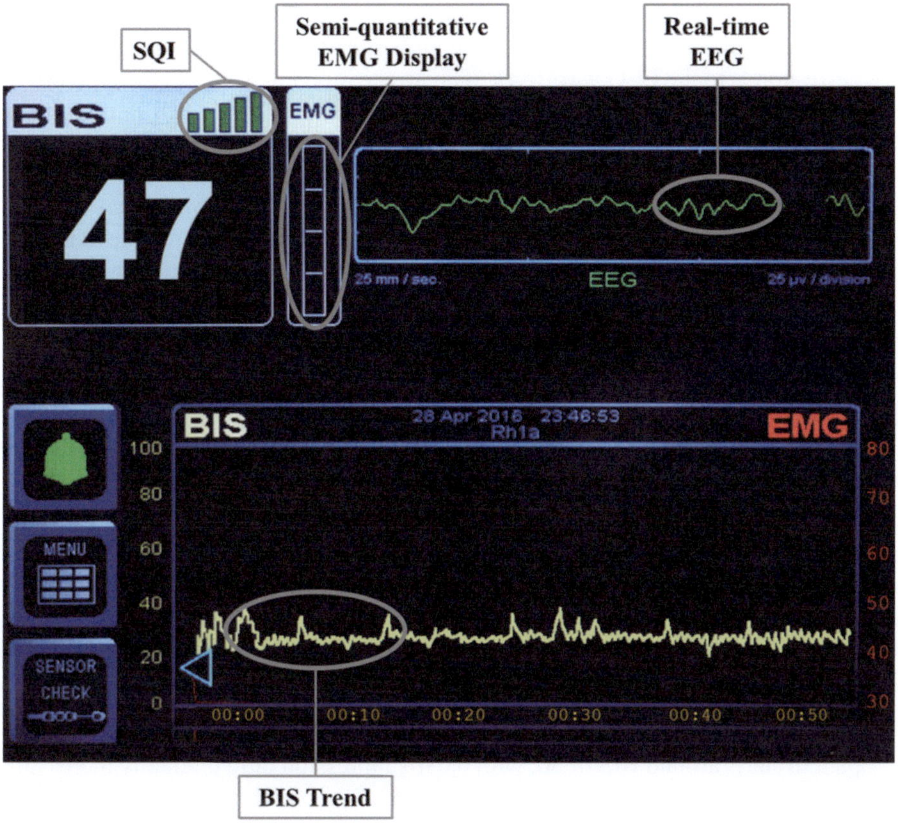

Fig. 13.2

Answers

1. This is a bispectral index (BIS) monitor. BIS is a form of processed EEG that aims to monitor the effect of certain anesthetic medications in an objective fashion. Typically, a single channel of EEG obtained through a strip of skin electrodes over the forehead is acquired by the monitor and analyzed. The process that is used to compute the BIS involves several steps including artifact detection, power spectrum analysis, suppression detection, and fast Fourier transformation [1]. The end result is the "BIS," a unitless number between 0 and 99 (Fig. 13.2). Other information available on the monitor are signal quality index (SQI), a semiquantitative EMG display, and the real-time EEG graph. Suppression ratio (the percentage of isoelectric EEG over a unit time) can also be displayed by turning that variable "on" in the menu. In the lower part of the screen in the picture, a moving trend of BIS is displayed for an overview. Although the algorithm aims to filter the EMG signal from analysis, the presence of EMG can introduce artifact and lead to falsely elevated BIS values.

2. The range of BIS (0–99) can be divided into several zones in terms of clinical state of alertness and sedation [2]. The highest end of the BIS range (i.e., 92–99) corresponds to the EEG waveform of an awake individual. BIS in the high 80s to low 90s is consistent with light sedation. An individual with BIS in mid-80s is likely to fit in a state of "conscious sedation" (i.e., responds after name is called loudly). BIS in the high 70s to low 80s is a state of deep sedation (i.e., responds to shaking) with a potential for airway obstruction. Values lower than mid-70s are usually consistent with an anesthetized state. It is important to note that there is interindividual overlap between BIS ranges and degrees of sedation.

3. BIS range of 45–60 corresponds to a state of general anesthesia. To be more precise, BIS is specifically an index of the hypnotic component of the general anesthetic state, measured through cerebral cortical electrical activity. Since movement to surgical stimulus is mediated largely by the spinal cord, immobility will not be ensured even in the lower end of this range. Equally important is the combination of anesthetics that is producing a certain BIS value: an individual with a BIS value of 50 with propofol alone is more likely to move with noxious stimulus, compared to the same individual with the same BIS value with a combination of propofol and remifentanil. However, explicit recall is highly unlikely with BIS values less than 60 [3], regardless of the anesthetic regimen employed. BIS values below 45 refer to a deep hypnotic state where side effects of anesthetics (e.g., hypotension, prolonged recovery) could be evident without a clear benefit. There have also been reports of increased long-term mortality associated with prolonged periods of BIS values below 45 [4]. Finally, burst suppression pattern starts around BIS of 30, with burst-suppression ratio gradually increasing to 100% as the BIS decreases to 0. In cases where cerebral protection is aimed by inducing burst suppression, BIS can be a useful tool [5].

4. BIS is useful to monitor the hypnotic effect of volatile anesthetics (isoflurane, sevoflurane, desflurane), propofol, and etomidate. The addition of dexmedetomidine to a general anesthetic is also reflected on the BIS [6]. The effects of nitrous oxide or opioids on the hypnotic effect of an anesthetic agent are not reliably reflected on BIS monitoring [7, 8]. Finally, ketamine may lead to a paradoxical increase in BIS, while lower doses of it may not have any effect [9].

5. BIS is not routinely indicated for all patients undergoing general anesthesia [10]. However, it is a useful tool in monitoring the hypnotic component of general anesthesia with volatile anesthetics as well as total intravenous anesthesia (TIVA) with propofol [11]. Compared to standard anesthesia practice, using BIS may decrease the risk of awareness, decrease anesthetic consumption, and modestly improve certain recovery profiles such as time to eye opening, time to extubation, and time to orientation [12].

6. The spectrum of electromyographic (EMG) activity (30–200 Hz) is faster than that of EEG (0.5–30 Hz). The presence of EMG activity of the facial muscles often creates an artifact that results in an erroneously higher BIS value. Therefore, if the BIS readings are higher than what the clinical assessment suggests, reviewing the EMG display is helpful to rule this out. If NMBs are indi-

cated, their administration will easily get rid of this artifact and enable an accurate BIS measurement. Electrocautery unit (ECU) is another common source of artifact. ECU, especially when a unipolar device is used for periods longer than 5 s, usually renders any meaningful measurement impossible. This would be evident in a decreased SQI value, and any interpretation of BIS should be postponed until SQI improves. Drugs that are beta-receptor agonists (e.g., isoproterenol) or antagonists (e.g., esmolol) have also been shown to increase or decrease BIS values, respectively [13, 14]. Clinical implications of these effects have not been established. Hypotension and hypothermia both result in decreases in BIS, probably related to decreased cerebral metabolic rate. Finally, baseline BIS values are often significantly lower (i.e., ranging from 75 to 90) in children with cerebral palsy as well as elderly with dementia. Although administration of anesthetics results in further decreases in BIS values from those baselines, interpretation of absolute values becomes more difficult in these populations since the algorithms have only been validated in individuals without underlying brain pathology.

References

1. Rampil IJ. A primer for EEG signal processing in anesthesia. Anesthesiology. 1998; 89(4):980–1002.
2. Liu J, Singh H, White PF. Electroencephalographic bispectral index correlates with intraoperative recall and depth of propofol-induced sedation. Anesth Analg. 1997;84(1):185.
3. Myles PS, Leslie K, McNeil J, Forbes A, Chan MTV. Bispectral index monitoring to prevent awareness during anaesthesia: the B-Aware randomised controlled trial. Lancet. 2004;363(9423):1757–63. doi:10.1016/S0140-6736(04)16300-9.
4. Monk TG, Saini V, Weldon BC, Sigl JC. Anesthetic management and one-year mortality after noncardiac surgery. Anesth Analg. 2005;100(1):4–10. doi:10.1213/01.ANE.0000147519.82841.5E.
5. Bruhn J, Bouillon TW, Shafer SL. Bispectral index (BIS) and burst suppression: revealing a part of the BIS algorithm. J Clin Monit Comput. 2000;16(8):593–6.
6. Le Guen M, Liu N, Tounou F, et al. Dexmedetomidine reduces propofol and remifentanil requirements during bispectral index-guided closed-loop anesthesia a double-blind, placebo-controlled trial. Anesth Analg. 2014;118(5):946–55. doi:10.1213/ANE.0000000000000185.
7. Ozcan MS, Ozcan MD, Khan QS, Thompson DM, Chetty PK. Does nitrous oxide affect bispectral index and state entropy when added to a propofol versus sevoflurane anesthetic? J Neurosurg Anesthesiol. 2010;22(4):309–15. doi:10.1097/ANA.0b013e3181e4b7c8.
8. Lysakowski C, Dumont L, Pellégrini M, Clergue F, Tassonyi E. Effects of fentanyl, alfentanil, remifentanil and sufentanil on loss of consciousness and bispectral index during propofol induction of anaesthesia. Br J Anaesth. 2001;86(4):523–7. doi:10.1093/bja/86.4.523.
9. Sengupta S, Ghosh S, Rudra A, Kumar P, Maitra G, Das T. Effect of ketamine on bispectral index during propofol – fentanyl anesthesia: a randomized controlled study. Middle East J Anesthesiol. 2011;21(3):391–5.
10. American Society of Anesthesiologists Task Force on Intraoperative Awareness. Practice advisory for intraoperative awareness and brain function monitoring: a report by the American society of anesthesiologists task force on intraoperative awareness. Anesthesiology. 2006;104(4):847–64.
11. Johansen JW. Update on bispectral index monitoring. Best Pract Res Clin Anaesthesiol. 2006;20(1):81–99.

12. Punjasawadwong Y, Boonjeungmonkol N, Phongchiewboon A. Bispectral index for improving anaesthetic delivery and postoperative recovery. Cochrane Database Syst Rev. 2007;(4):CD003843. doi:10.1002/14651858.CD003843.pub2.
13. Gautam NK, Rafique MB, Numan MT. Impact of isoproterenol infusion on BIS and metabolic values in pediatric patients undergoing electrophysiology studies. J Clin Anesth. 2014;26(8):611–5. doi:10.1016/j.jclinane.2014.05.007.
14. Johansen JW. Esmolol promotes electroencephalographic burst suppression during propofol/alfentanil anesthesia. Anesth Analg. 2001;93(6):1526–31–table of contents.

Chapter 14
Fetal Heart Rate Monitoring

Casey Windrix

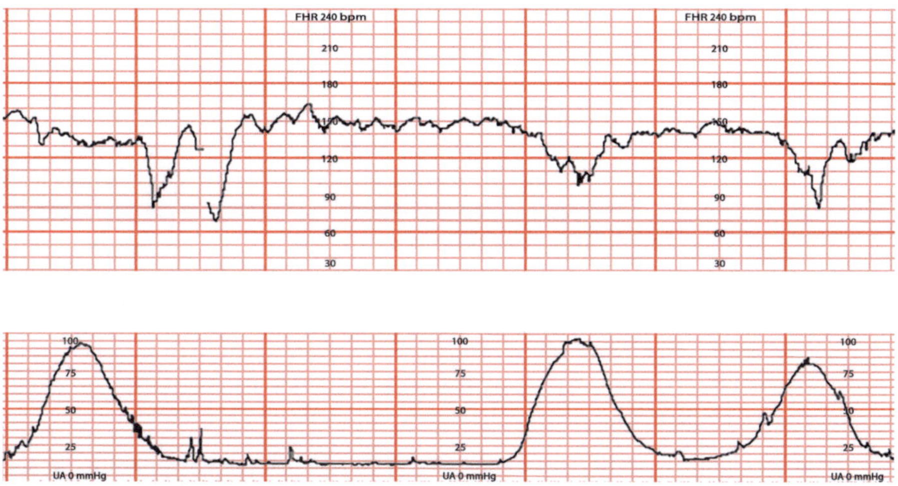

Fig. 14.1 Fetal heart tracing

1. What pattern is this heart rate tracing in Fig. 14.1?
2. What does this tracing tell you about the condition of the fetus?
3. What is the significance of "V"-shaped decelerations in this tracing?
4. How would acidemia present on the fetal heart tracing?
5. What action if any should be taken?
6. What are the characteristics of a normal fetal heart tracing (FHR)?
7. What are the categories of FHR tracings?
8. What are limitations of electronic fetal monitoring (EFM)?

C. Windrix, MD
Department of Anesthesiology, OUHSC, Edmond, Oklahoma, USA
e-mail: Casey-Windrix@ouhsc.edu

T.D. Raj (ed.), *Data Interpretation in Anesthesia*,
DOI 10.1007/978-3-319-55862-2_14

Answers

1. This tracing contains multiple decelerations. Decelerations are characterized by a decrease from baseline of at least 15 beats per minute (BPM), lasting at least 15 s and no longer than 2 min. A deceleration is considered prolonged when it lasts beyond 2 min. Specifically, the tracing above depicts variable decelerations. Variable decelerations have inconsistent shape and timing in relationship to uterine contractions. Variable decelerations are caused by cord compression.

   By contrast early decelerations occur in sync with contractions such that the nadir of the deceleration occurs at the peak of the contraction. Early decelerations relate to fetal head compression during contraction. Late decelerations are also closely associated with contractions with the decrease in heart rate beginning immediately after the peak of the contraction, mirroring the contraction in shape. Late decelerations represent uteroplacental insufficiency and may be due to hypotension or other factors [1].

2. Fetal heart rate is a surrogate measurement for fetal oxygenation and acid/base status. Anytime there is a deceleration, there is presumed to be a decrease in delivery of oxygen to the fetus. This may be mild and of little concern, as in the case of early decelerations, or clinically significant as in the case of late, variable, or prolonged decelerations. With repeated decelerations, hypoxia may lead to acidosis, which could eventually lead to neurologic injury. In particular injury may occur when umbilical artery pH decreases below 7.0 or there is a base deficit of greater than 12 [2].

3. There is no evidence in the literature to support older terms for describing decelerations, such as the presence of "shoulders," variable with late component, or shape of the deceleration. Similarly it is a distraction to categorize the deceleration pattern by severity.

4. The absence of variability is a marker for acidemia. Moderate variability or the presence of accelerations is a very sensitive measure for a normal acid/base status. This strip still has the presence of moderate variability, defined by changes in the baseline heart rate that are nonuniform, which essentially rules out metabolic acidosis.

5. This strip would be defined as a category 2 tracing, which would require careful observation at the least. Further action or intervention would depend on the clinical situation. Recurrent decelerations, in the presence of good variability, usually would be treated by oxygen, repositioning, augmentation of maternal blood pressure, and/or reduction or discontinuation of oxytocin if infusing.

6. A normal fetal heart varies between 110 and 160 beats per minute. It fluctuates irregularly in amplitude and frequency with variability from baseline of at least 6 BPMs. It may include accelerations, which are sudden increases in heart rate with a change from onset to peak in less than 30 s, lasting no longer than 2 min. There may be the presence of early decelerations, which mirror uterine contractions.

7. The American Congress of Obstetricians and Gynecologists has a three-tier interpretation and intervention system that represents a common language and framework to discuss FHTs [3]:
   (a) Category 1 FHR tracings have a normal baseline rate, the presence of at least moderate variability, may lack accelerations, and do not have clinically significant decelerations (anything other than early). These strips are considered normal and do not require any specific action.
   (b) Category 2 tracings lack clear signs of acidemia and are indeterminate. These strips require careful surveillance and may suggest the need for further testing to ensure the health of the fetus.
   (c) Category 3 tracings have absent variability, recurrent late or variable decelerations, or bradycardia, or a sinusoidal pattern. These strips indicate fetal acidemia, are abnormal, and require immediate action.
8. Fetal heart monitoring is prone to many errors and shortfalls. Fetal heart rate may be difficult to consistently observe due to changes in positioning of the mother or fetus. There is significant variability in interobserver interpretation and responses. While the presence of variability may ensure a normal acid/base status, its absence does not assure acidemia, leading to potentially unnecessary action. Finally, continuous fetal heart monitoring alone has not been definitively proven to reduce perinatal mortality; despite its increased use, it has not impacted the rate of cerebral palsy, which has remained constant over decades [4].

References

1. ACOG. Practice Bulletin #106, Intrapartum fetal heart rate monitoring: nomenclature, interpretation, and general management principles. Obstet Gynecol. 2009;114(1):192–202.
2. MacLennan A. A template for defining a causal relation between acute intrapartum events and cerebral palsy: international consensus statement. BMJ. 1999;319:1054–9.
3. Macones GA, Hankins GD, Spong CY, Hauth J, Moore T. The 2008 National Institute of Child Health and Human Development workshop report on electronic fetal monitoring: update on definitions, interpretation, and research guidelines. Obstet Gynecol. 2008;112:661–6.
4. Graham EM, Petersen SM, Christo DK, Fox HE. Intrapartum electronic fetal heart rate monitoring and the prevention of perinatal brain injury. Obstet Gynecol. 2006;108(3 Pt 1):656–66.

Chapter 15
ECG (12 Lead)

Talla A. Rousan

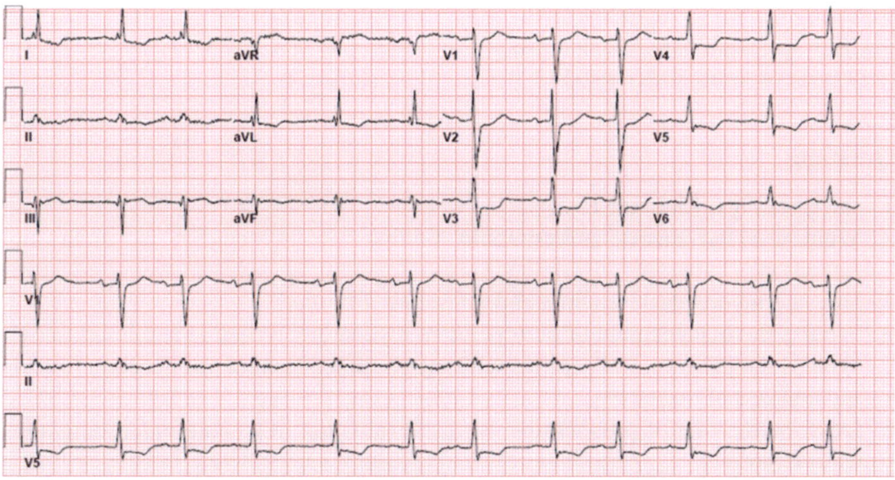

Fig. 15.1 An electrocardiogram illustrating changes suggestive of myocardial ischemia (ST-segment depression in the anterolateral leads I, aVL, and V2–V6)

T.A. Rousan, MD, FACC
Department of Medicine, The University of Oklahoma Health Sciences Center and the Veteran Affairs Medical Center, 800 Stanton L. Young Blvd, COM 5400, Oklahoma City, OK 73104, USA
e-mail: Talla-rousan@ouhsc.edu

T.D. Raj (ed.), *Data Interpretation in Anesthesia*,
DOI 10.1007/978-3-319-55862-2_15

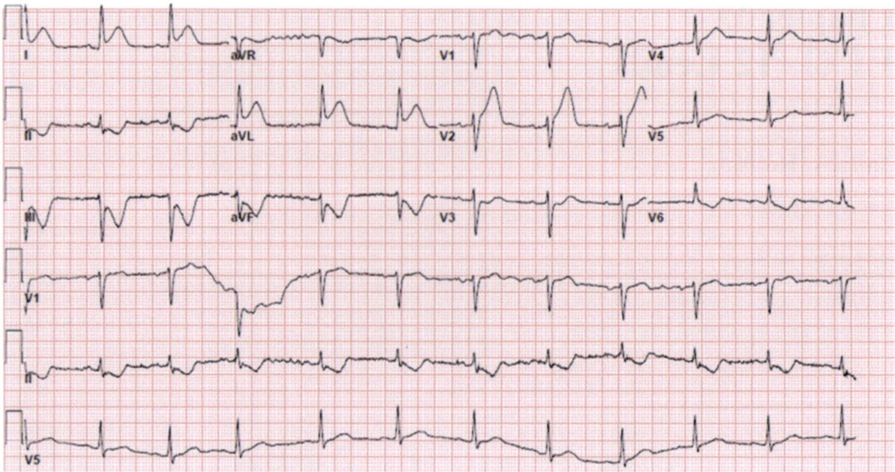

Fig. 15.2 An electrocardiogram illustrating changes suggestive of myocardial injury (ST-segment elevation in the lateral leads I and aVL)

Questions

1. Interpret Figs. 15.1 and 15.2.
2. What are the electrocardiographic findings in myocardial ischemia and infarction?
3. How are myocardial ischemia and infarction different?
4. What is the management of perioperative myocardial ischemia and infarction?
5. What is the prognosis of patients with myocardial ischemia or infarction following noncardiac surgery?
6. Describe the role of preoperative cardiac evaluation in patient undergoing noncardiac surgery.

Answers

1. The figures represent electrocardiograms (ECGs) for patients presenting with chest pain. Figure 15.1 illustrates changes suggestive of myocardial ischemia (ST-segment depression in the anterolateral leads I, aVL, and V2–V6). The ECG shown in Fig. 15.2 depicts changes suggestive of myocardial injury (ST-segment elevation in the lateral leads I and aVL).

2. ECG is considered to be an essential tool in the evaluation for myocardial ischemia or infarction. Changes to indicate myocardial ischemia or infarction include peaked or inverted T waves, ST-segment elevation or depression, and changes in the QRS complex [1]. ST-segment elevations present on the ECG accompanied by symptoms or signs concerning of myocardial infarction (including chest pain, dyspnea, or hemodynamic instability) are an emergency that require immediate attention. The threshold values for significant ST-segment elevation vary based on the gender and age of the individual [1]. For men 40 years of age or older, 2 mm elevation in leads V2 and V3 and 1 mm elevation in all other leads is considered to be significant. For men younger than 40 years old, a significant ST-segment elevation is 2.5 mm in leads V2 and V3. For women of all ages, ST-segment elevation of 1.5 mm in V2 or V3 and 1 mm in all other leads is considered to be significant.

3. Myocardial ischemia results from an imbalance between myocardial oxygen demand and supply [2]. Myocardial oxygen demand is determined by the heart rate, myocardial contractility, preload (end-diastolic pressure or volume), afterload (arterial impedance), and muscle mass. Determinants of myocardial oxygen supply include coronary blood flow and arterial oxygen content [3]. Myocardial infarction (myocardial cell death) occurs if myocardial ischemia is prolonged (as little as 20 min or less). Myocardial infarction is characterized by myocyte necrosis as detected by elevated cardiac biomarkers (troponin-T, troponin-I (preferably), or CKMB) along with ischemia symptoms and ECG changes (as described above) [2].

4. Perioperative management of patients with myocardial ischemia and infarction starts from early detection. Myocardial ischemia or infarction can be detected intraoperatively by ECG changes, ventricular arrhythmias, and hemodynamic instability [4, 5]. If myocardial ischemia or infarction is suspected, a 12-lead unfiltered ECG should be obtained promptly, and cardiac biomarkers should be sent. In addition, a transesophageal echocardiogram can be done (if readily available) to detect the ejection fraction and any new myocardial wall motion abnormalities. The surgeon should be informed to make a decision on completing versus aborting the surgery. If tachycardia along with normo- or hypertension is present, a beta-blocker (intravenous esmolol or metoprolol) or a non-dihydropyridine calcium channel blocker—if left ventricular ejection is normal—(intravenous diltiazem) should be administered [6]. Tachycardia along with hypotension is challenging. Evaluate and treat potential causes (e.g., hypovolemia or anemia).

Vasopressors should be added to maintain mean adequate perfusion pressure (mean arterial blood pressure 65 mmHg or more). In cases of tachyarrhythmias (atrial flutter or fibrillation), direct current cardioversion may be necessary. If ST-segment elevations are present, an emergent cardiology consultation should be obtained to consider coronary angiography and revascularization. The management of patient with suspected myocardial infarction or ischemia in the postoperative period is as challenging given the limitations for the use of anticoagulants and antiplatelet agents. If based on symptoms, acute coronary syndrome is suspected, an ECG should be promptly obtained to assess for changes suggestive of ischemia or infarction. Oxygen should be administered if oxygen saturation is below 90%. Short-acting nitroglycerin (sublingual tablets or oral spray) should be administered to alleviate angina (avoid in hypotension). If there are no contraindications for antiplatelet agents, administer aspirin 162–324 mg oral [7]. Cardiology consult should be sought to direct further management. If changes suggestive of acute ST-segment myocardial infarction are present, cardiology should be contacted emergently. The decision to proceed with invasive coronary angiography should be decided based on the risk-benefit ratio analysis in any given patient weighing the risk of bleeding and the risk of ongoing myocardial ischemia.

5. Patients experiencing a myocardial infarction following noncardiac surgery (whether symptomatic or asymptomatic) are at increased risk for in-hospital and short-term mortality [8, 9]. Nonfatal myocardial infarction is associated with increased in-hospital mortality reaching 25% in some cohorts. A 30-day mortality in this subset of patients was estimated to be approaching 12% [10]. Patients who experience cardiac arrest perioperatively are at the highest risk for cardiac mortality occurring in up to 65% of the cases. Although silent myocardial infarction is associated with increased adverse outcomes, routine postoperative screening with serum troponin levels is not recommended [11]. The usefulness of screening with troponin levels in patients at high risk for myocardial infarction is uncertain especially in the absence of a well-defined management strategy.

6. Studies have shown that patients undergoing noncardiac surgery are at risk of periprocedural myocardial infarction and increased mortality (up to 2% in some cohorts) [8, 9, 11, 12]. The risk of major cardiovascular and cerebral events increases in patients with prior history of diabetes mellitus, hypertension, coronary artery disease, congestive heart failure, stroke, peripheral artery disease, chronic kidney disease, and advanced age [8, 12]. The risk of adverse outcomes decreases as the length of time following an MI increases. Given those reasons, the need for preoperative evaluation rises especially in patients older than 55 years, with history of coronary artery disease or stroke, or patients with symptoms to suggest myocardial ischemia (angina). One of the best tools to risk-stratify patients is using the algorithm and risk calculators available in the 2014 ACC/AHA Perioperative Clinical Practice Guidelines [11]. Based on those

guidelines, patients undergoing emergent surgery need to proceed with surgery without delay. Patients with acute coronary syndrome require to be treated prior to the planned surgery based on the practice guidelines. In patients with low calculated risk (<1%) and also in those with high risk but with good functional capacity (four metabolic equivalents (METs) or greater), one may proceed with surgery without further testing. The subset of patients with high risk and poor functional capacity may require noninvasive functional study (stress test) if it would alter perioperative management. Routine coronary angiography and revascularization are not recommended prior to noncardiac surgery.

References

1. Wagner GS, et al. AHA/ACCF/HRS recommendations for the standardization and interpretation of the electrocardiogram: part VI: acute ischemia/infarction: a scientific statement from the American Heart Association Electrocardiography and Arrhythmias Committee, Council on Clinical Cardiology; the American College of Cardiology Foundation; and the Heart Rhythm Society. Endorsed by the International Society for Computerized Electrocardiology. J Am Coll Cardiol. 2009;53(11):1003–11.
2. Thygesen K, et al. Third universal definition of myocardial infarction. J Am Coll Cardiol. 2012;60(16):1581–98.
3. Burkhoff D, Naidu SS. The science behind percutaneous hemodynamic support: a review and comparison of support strategies. Catheter Cardiovasc Interv. 2012;80(5):816–29.
4. Ludbrook GL, et al. Crisis management during anaesthesia: myocardial ischaemia and infarction. Qual Saf Health Care. 2005;14(3):e13.
5. Satinder Gombar AKK, Gombar KK. Perioperative myocardial ischaemia and infarction–a review. Indian J Anaesth. 2007;51(4):287–302.
6. Landesberg G, et al. Perioperative myocardial infarction. Circulation. 2009;119(22):2936–44.
7. Amsterdam EA, et al. 2014 AHA/ACC Guideline for the Management of Patients with Non-ST-Elevation Acute Coronary Syndromes: a report of the American College of Cardiology/American Heart Association Task Force on Practice Guidelines. J Am Coll Cardiol. 2014;64(24):e139–228.
8. Botto F, et al. Myocardial injury after noncardiac surgery: a large, international, prospective cohort study establishing diagnostic criteria, characteristics, predictors, and 30-day outcomes. Anesthesiology. 2014;120(3):564–78.
9. Devereaux PJ, et al. Perioperative cardiac events in patients undergoing noncardiac surgery: a review of the magnitude of the problem, the pathophysiology of the events and methods to estimate and communicate risk. CMAJ. 2005;173(6):627–34.
10. Devereaux PJ, et al. Characteristics and short-term prognosis of perioperative myocardial infarction in patients undergoing noncardiac surgery: a cohort study. Ann Intern Med. 2011;154(8):523–8.
11. Fleisher LA, et al. 2014 ACC/AHA guideline on perioperative cardiovascular evaluation and management of patients undergoing noncardiac surgery: executive summary: a report of the American College of Cardiology/American Heart Association Task Force on Practice Guidelines. Circulation. 2014;130(24):2215–45.
12. Lee TH, et al. Derivation and prospective validation of a simple index for prediction of cardiac risk of major noncardiac surgery. Circulation. 1999;100(10):1043–9.

Chapter 16
Minimally Invasive Cardiac Output Monitor

Marcos E. Gomes

During major abdominal surgery, urine output in a 90 kg patient decreases to 20 mL per hour over the prior 2 h. Noninvasive cardiac output is being monitored in this patient with a FloTrac system, and the parameters are depicted in Fig. 16.1. which changes to what is depicted in Fig. 16.2 after a single maneuver by the anesthesiologist.

1. What do the figures show?
2. What is the importance of monitoring cardiac output?
3. What are the advantages of the FloTrac/EV1000 system?
4. How does the FloTrac estimate stroke volume?
5. What are the limitations of the FloTrac?
6. What other minimally invasive monitors are available?
7. What is stroke volume variation?
8. Why is the stroke volume higher during the inspiratory phase of the respiratory cycle?
9. What is the relationship of stroke volume variation and the Frank-Starling curve?

M.E. Gomes, MD
Department of Anesthesiology, University of Oklahoma Health Sciences Center, 750 NE 13th Street, Suite 200, Oklahoma City, OK 73104, USA
e-mail: mewgomes@gmail.com

T.D. Raj (ed.), *Data Interpretation in Anesthesia*,
DOI 10.1007/978-3-319-55862-2_16

Answers

1. The figures above represent the moment before and after a fluid challenge on a patient with low urine output. Notice that the cardiac output/cardiac index increased, while the SVV decreased from 19% to 6%. The patient's urine output responded accordingly, representing improved kidney perfusion with the fluid challenge.

2. Monitoring cardiac output is a common practice in anesthesia and critical care as it provides important information about cardiac function, tissue perfusion, and oxygen delivery. It is utilized as a marker of oxygen delivery to tissues based on the equation below:

   $DO_2 = CO \times (1.39 \times [Hb] \times SaO_2 + (0.003 \times PaO_2))$

   DO_2: Rate of oxygen delivery

   CO: Cardiac output

   Hb: Hemoglobin concentration

   SaO_2: Hemoglobin oxygen saturation expressed as a fraction

   PaO_2: Partial pressure of oxygen in the blood

   Its measurement can identify patients at risk for morbidity and/or mortality. In addition, monitoring cardiac output can be used to guide treatment with both fluid resuscitation and/or vasoactive/inotropic drugs.

3. Among different minimally invasive cardiac output monitors, the FloTrac/EV1000 system has the following advantages: no central line required, any arterial line location can be used, easy to set up, no external calibration required, changes in vascular tone and site of arterial cannulation are corrected by built-in software, correction occurs every 60 s, waveform analysis occurs every 20 s, extrasystoles and small artifacts are eliminated by built-in algorithm, option for attaching central venous pressure with which SVR/SVRI (Fig. 16.1) can be calculated, and option to attach PreSep catheter with which ScvO2 can be continuously monitored. In addition, this monitor is able to calculate stroke volume variation (SVV) which is an extra tool to assess volume status.

4. The FloTrac system uses pulse contour analysis with patient demographics and physical characteristics for arterial impedance estimation and ultimately stroke volume (SV) calculation. The basic principle is the linear relation between the pulse pressure and the SV. The SV is estimated using the following equation: $SV = SDap \times X$. The waveform analysis that occurs every 20 s results in 2000 data points. SDap is the standard deviation of these data points and reflects the pulse pressure. The factor X stands for the conversion factor that depends on arterial compliance, mean arterial pressure, and waveform characteristics. These variables are adjusted by the built-in software, and this process is repeated every 60 s. Once SV is calculated, it is multiplied by the heart rate to result in the cardiac output [1].

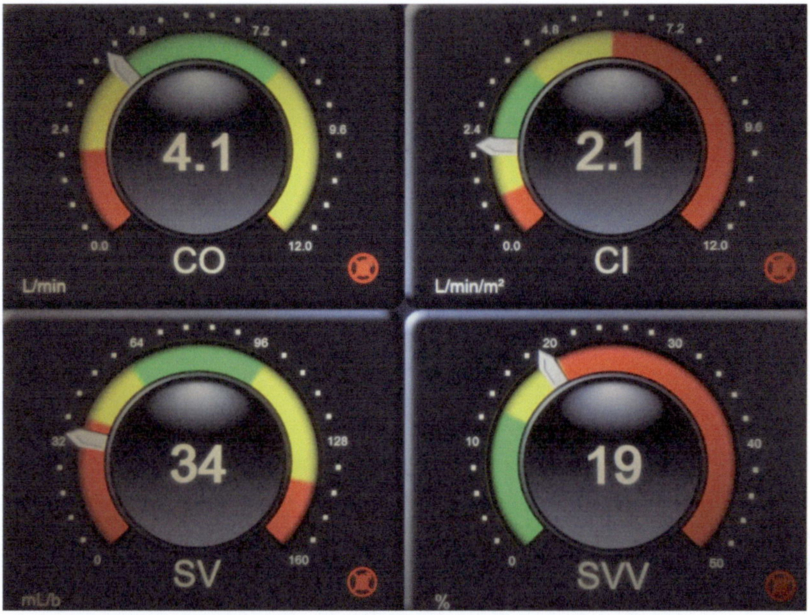

Fig. 16.1 FloTrac monitor showing four different parameters: cardiac output (CO), cardiac index (CI), stroke volume (SV), and stroke volume variation (SVV)

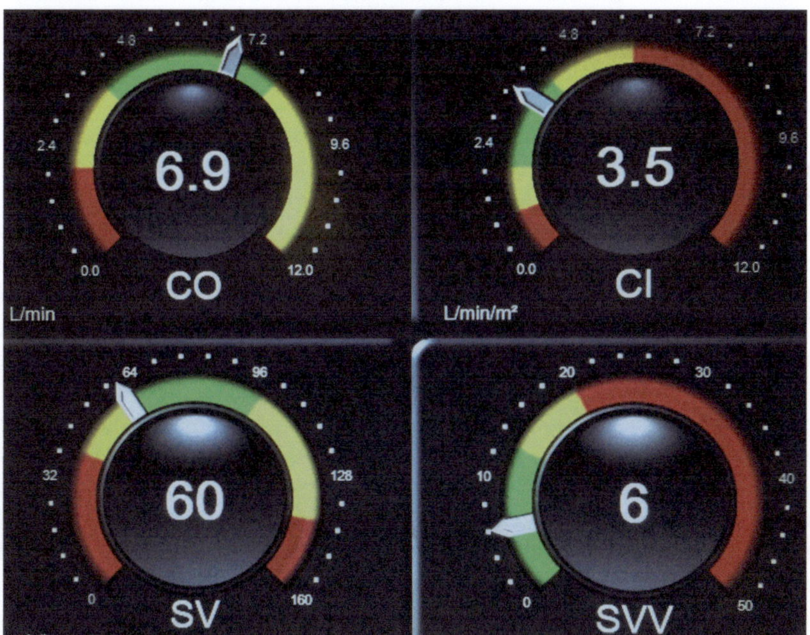

Fig. 16.2 FloTrac monitor showing four different parameters: cardiac output (CO), cardiac index (CI), stroke volume (SV), and stroke volume variation (SVV)

5. The use and accuracy of FloTrac/EV1000, specially for monitoring of SVV, may be compromised in the following scenarios: poor signal, intra-aortic balloon pump, ventricular assist devices, open chest, spontaneous breathing, small tidal volumes, arrhythmia, poor lung compliance, high PEEP, severe obesity (effect of abdominal pressure in lung compliance), and medications (norepinephrine, vasodilators, beta-blockers).

6. Minimally invasive CO monitors using pulse contour analysis can be divided into uncalibrated (or autocalibrated) and calibrated. FloTrac, PulsioFlex, LiDCOrapid, PRAM, Nexfin, and esCCO monitors are examples of uncalibrated monitors, while PiCCO plus and LiDCOplus are examples of calibrated ones. Three other principles support other types of monitors: pulse Doppler technology, applied Fick principle, and bioimpedance/bioreactance [2, 3, 4].

   Calibrated:
   The *PiCCO plus* monitor uses the pulse contour analysis to estimate CO and utilizes the transpulmonary thermodilution method for intermittent calibration. It involves the administration of a cold injectate in the superior vena cava (central venous catheter required) and its detection by a thermistor in the aorta or a major arterial branch (femoral, axillary, or brachial). Other variables measured by this device are global end-diastolic volume (preload estimate), intrathoracic blood volume, extravascular lung water, and pulmonary vascular permeability index. The *LiDCOplus* monitor uses lithium dilution technique to intermittently calibrate the system, generate a curve, and use a built-in equation to calculate CO based on pulse power rather than pulse contour analysis. This system uses a pulse pressure algorithm called PulseCO to obtain such analysis.

   Uncalibrated:
   PulsioFlex is a monitor that uses a *ProAQT* sensor that connects to the peripheral arterial catheter and analyzes the arterial waveform 250 times per second. Patient's characteristics (biometrics) are also inserted into the system. The *LiDCOrapid* system has the same technology as the *LiDCOplus* but instead of thermodilution uses nomograms for the calculation of the CO. *PRAM* (pressure recording analytical method) is based on a mathematical assessment of the pressure signal obtained from an arterial line (pulse contour analysis), without calibration, resulting in estimates of SV and therefore CO. The *Nexfin* monitor does not require an arterial line catheter. It uses an inflatable cuff around the middle phalanx of the finger that is able to generate a pressure waveform. Through a built-in software, the system is able to construct a brachial artery waveform based on the finger version, which is then used as the basis for calculation of continuous CO. The *esCCO* monitor uses a technology that derives the CO using the pulse wave transit time (PWTT), which is obtained by the pulse oximetry and the electrocardiogram signals in each cardiac cycle. It is also completely noninvasive, like the *Nexfin* system.

   Others:
   Pulse Doppler technology uses esophageal or transthoracic Doppler probes to estimate CO by multiplying the cross-sectional area of the aorta by blood flow

velocity. *Applied Fick principle* is used in the *NICO* system, which uses the calculation of carbon dioxide production and elimination every 3 min to estimate CO. Electrical *bioimpedance* uses electric current stimulation to identify thoracic or body impedance variations induced by blood flow changes resulted from each heartbeat. The signal variation is analyzed by built-in algorithms, continuously providing the estimation of the cardiac output. Electrodes can be placed on the skin or endotracheal tubes. Devices that use *bioreactance* technique need further validation studies.

7. Stroke volume variation is a functional hemodynamic variable that estimates fluid responsiveness in ventilated patients with low preload and thus also aids in the guidance of fluid resuscitation therapies. The concept is that cyclic changes in the intrathoracic pressure during positive pressure ventilation induce changes in SV and pulse pressure variation (PPV) secondary to multiple mechanisms. SVV represents the variability of SV during a respiratory cycle, in which it increases during inspiration and decreases during expiration (the opposite occurs during spontaneous ventilation). It is calculated by the following equation: SV max – SV min/SV mean. A result of more than 13% (10–15%) suggests potential preload responsiveness [5].
8. In a given respiratory cycle, during mechanical ventilation, the initial effects of increased intrathoracic pressure cause a preload increase as blood is expelled from the lungs, an afterload decrease, a direct pressure of the expanded lungs on the heart assisting the pump effect, and an improved left ventricular compliance due to the volume decrease in the right chambers of the heart. As the cycle progresses in what is called pulmonary transit time, those effects become overtaken by the gradual decrease on venous return, resulting in a decrease in SV. Such variability is found to be more pronounced in under-resuscitated patients.
9. In the zone of the ascending limb of the Frank-Starling curve, SVV is pronounced indicating low preload (fluid responsiveness). In the shallow part of the curve, SVV is small, indicating no fluid responsiveness.

References

1. Argueta E. Flotrac monitoring system: what are its uses in critically ill medical patients? Am J Med Sci. 2015;349(4):352–6.
2. Marik PE. Noninvasive cardiac output monitors: a state-of the-art review. J Cardiothorac Vasc Anesth. 2012;27:1–13.
3. Alhashemi JA, Cecconi M, Hofer CK. Cardiac output monitoring: an integrative perspective. Crit Care. 2011;15:214.
4. Chamos C, et al. Less invasive methods of advanced hemodynamic monitoring: principles, devices, and their role in the perioperative hemodynamic optimization. Perioper Med. 2013;2:19.
5. Cannesson M, et al. Pulse pressure variation; where are we today? J Clin Monit Comput. 2010;25(1):45–56.

Chapter 17
ECG I

Edward Kosik

A 76-year-old female patient is in the postanesthesia care unit after an ORIF of an acetabular fracture. She underwent general anesthesia with an uneventful surgical procedure. You have been called to evaluate the rhythm above (Fig. 17.1).

Pulse 136, BP 110/50, and SpO_2 97% on 2 L O_2 via nasal cannula

NKDA

Medical history: hypertension (takes amlodipine for it).

Preoperative vital signs

SpO_2 98%, blood pressure 140/90, HR 96, temp 36.4, EKG normal sinus rhythm, normal transthoracic echocardiogram.

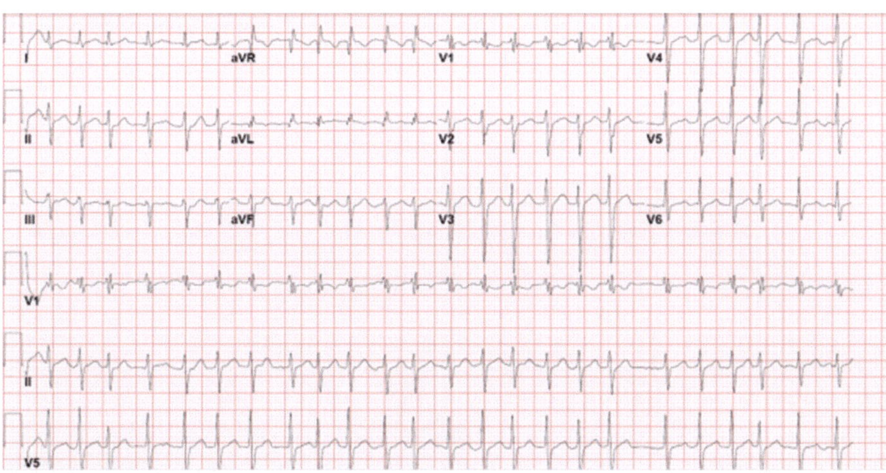

Fig. 17.1 EKG obtained in the postoperative period

E. Kosik, DO
Department of Anesthesiology, University of Oklahoma Health Sciences Center, 750 NE 13th Street, Suite 200, Oklahoma City, OK 73104, USA
e-mail: Edward-kosik@ouhsc.edu

T.D. Raj (ed.), *Data Interpretation in Anesthesia*,
DOI 10.1007/978-3-319-55862-2_17

1. How would you describe this rhythm?
2. Name and define different types (based on occurrence and duration) of the arrhythmia shown above.
3. What is the incidence in the general population? What is the incidence after cardiothoracic surgery and after non-cardiac surgery?
4. How would you treat this patient?
5. What concerns are there whenever a patient with persistent AF is cardioverted?
6. What are precipitants of postoperative atrial fibrillation?
7. What are the $CHADS_2$ and CHA_2DS_2-VASc scores?
8. Is there any relation between neuraxial anesthesia and atrial fibrillation?
9. How does the treatment for Wolff-Parkinson-White syndrome with preexcitation AF differ from atrial fibrillation alone?

Answers

1. This rhythm is atrial fibrillation (AF) with a rapid ventricular response. The pattern is irregularly irregular. The rhythm strip has no distinct p wave but instead many f waves (also known as fibrillary waves) followed intermittently by narrow QRS complexes.

2. **Lone atrial fibrillation**—An outdated term also known as idiopathic atrial fibrillation. It originally meant atrial fibrillation that occurs in a person 40 years or younger without intrinsic cardiac disease [1].
   Paroxysmal atrial fibrillation—AF that occurs spontaneously, lasts less than a week, and occurs at variable frequency [2].
   Persistent atrial fibrillation—Atrial fibrillation that lasts longer than 7 days. It may go away on its own or resolve with treatment [2].
   Long-standing persistent atrial fibrillation—AF lasting longer than 12 months [2].
   Permanent atrial fibrillation—more of a therapeutic decision between the patient and clinician to stop attempting to treat AF for conversion to sinus rhythm [2].

3. Atrial fibrillation is the most common heart arrhythmia. It affects an estimated 2.7–6.1 million people in the United States. About 2% of people over the age of 45 have atrial fibrillation, while 9% of people greater than age 65 have it. It is more likely after cardiac surgery and can affect from 10% to 65% of patients after cardiac surgery. AF is rare after non-cardiac surgery and can affect about 1–3% of the patients. Patients who develop postoperative atrial fibrillation have higher morbidity and mortality rates and have higher costs of care.

4. Complete discussion of the treatment of atrial fibrillation is extensive, but some basic tenets can be kept for this patient's new-onset AF.

   (a) Correct manageable causes
   (b) Rate and/or rhythm control
   (c) Anticoagulation if $CHADS_2$ and CHA_2DS_2-VASc (see description below) scores indicate a benefit

   Acute treatment of atrial fibrillation focuses on keeping the patient hemodynamically stable. Rate and rhythm control are of paramount importance. Symptomatic and unstable patients with mental status changes, chest pain, congestive heart failure, or hypotension should be treated with electrical cardioversion if rate control cannot be accomplished with intravenous medications.

   A history and physical exam should be conducted. Special attention should be paid to cardiac and pulmonary comorbidities. Electrolytes, complete blood count, cardiac enzymes (troponin), thyroid studies (TSH and free T4), renal function, and chest radiograph should be obtained. A transthoracic echocardiogram should be performed to assess for causes of AF and to rule out a thrombus in the left atrial appendage. Consultation of a cardiologist may be necessary.

Rate control could be achieved using intravenous medications such as beta-blockers (BBs) like esmolol, metoprolol, or propranolol and nondihydropyridine calcium channel antagonists (CCAs) such as diltiazem and verapamil. The effect of these medications is slowing of AV node conduction. Digoxin is not typically used for acute rate control and is more often reserved for chronic AF caused by heart failure (do not use beta-blockers in decompensated heart failure) or in patients who do not respond to BBs or CCAs. Amiodarone may be used for patients whose atrial fibrillation is unresponsive to beta-blockers or the calcium antagonists.

Rhythm control strategies use electrical and chemical cardioversion. Medications include amiodarone, flecainide, dofetilide, propafenone, ibutilide, and others.

Additionally, anticoagulation may be warranted in several different situations. Some of these include (1) when the patient remains in AF even after pharmacologic or electrical cardioversion attempts, (2) if there are plans of cardioversion and the AF had an onset of >48 h, and (3) to decrease the risk of stroke by providing antithrombotics 4 weeks after cardioversion.

5. There is a concern that a thrombus could be located in the left atrial appendage which could embolize to the brain and cause a stroke. A transthoracic echocardiogram or transesophageal echocardiogram is usually performed to rule out the existence of a thrombus.

6. Congestive heart failure
   Dilated chambers on the left side of the heart
   Ischemic heart disease
   Age >65
   Hypomagnesemia
   Hyperkalemia
   Hypokalemia
   Anemia
   Hypovolemia
   Hypervolemia
   Hypertension
   Obesity
   European ancestry
   Diabetes
   Hyperthyroidism
   Chronic kidney disease
   ETOH use [3, 4]

7. The $CHADS_2$ and CHA_2DS_2-VASc scores are (Fig. 17.2) clinical tools used to assess the risk of stroke in patients with or without atrial fibrillation. Ultimately, the scores help determine the need for anticoagulation to prevent stroke.
   The $CHADS_2$ score is an acronym tool that assigns one or two points for each stroke risk factor (congestive heart failure, hypertension, age >75 years, diabetes, stroke/transient ischemic attack/thromboembolism).

Fig. 17.2 Annual adjusted stroke risk. The sum of the risk factors equals the CHA_2DS_2 score. Scores are matched to associated annual adjusted rate of stroke. 0 = 0%, 1 = 1.3%, 2 = 2.2%, 3 = 3.2%, 4 = 4.0%, 5 = 6.7%, 6 = 9.8%, 7 = 9.6%, 8 = 6.7%, 9 = 15.2% [2, 5]

CHA_2DS_2 - VASc score		
Acronym	Risk factor	Point
C	Congestive Heart failure or left ventricular systolic dysfunction	1
H	HTN	1
A_2	Age ≥ 75 years	2
D	Diabetes mellitus	1
S_2	Prior stroke/TIA/thromboembolism	2
V	Vascular disease (PVD, Mi, aortic plaque)	1
A_2	Age between 65 and 74	1
Sc	Sex/female gender	1

Annual adjusted stroke risk
CHA_2DS_2 Score = Associated stroke risk
0 = 0%, 1 = 1.3%, 2 = 2.2%, 3 = 3.2%, 4 = 4.0%, 5 = 6.7%, 6 = 9.8%, 7 = 9.6%, 8 = 6.7%, 9 = 15.20%

The CHA_2DS_2-VASc is an updated version of the $CHADS_2$ score. It gives two points for a patient >75 years of age and adds other risk factors such as vascular disease (such as previous myocardial infarction, age 65–75, or female sex). CHA_2DS_2-VASc also includes heart failure with or without preserved ejection fraction under the C listing [2, 5].

8. There are case reports that have documented the onset of atrial fibrillation with the placement of an epidural. This is a rare occurrence and does not necessarily mean that the patient has underlying heart pathology. However, it would be prudent to perform a cardiac workup if atrial fibrillation is encountered in these patients.

   A meta-analysis showed no clear benefit of reducing supraventricular tachyarrhythmias after placement of thoracic epidurals for cardiac surgery [6, 7].

9. Treatment with amiodarone, adenosine, digoxin, or nondihydropyridine calcium channel antagonists (diltiazem, verapamil) in patients with Wolff-Parkinson-White syndrome who have preexcitement AF can cause an accelerated ventricular rate that leads to ventricular fibrillation.

   Because of this danger, treatment with electrical cardioversion is usually a better choice for rate and rhythm control [8].

References

1. Wyse DG, Van Gelder IC, Ellinor PT, Go AS, Kalman JM, et al. Lone atrial fibrillation. Does it exist? J Am Coll Cardiol. 2014;63(17):1715–23. doi:10.1016/j.jacc.2014.01.023.
2. January CT, Wann LS, Alpert JS, MD CH, Cigarroa JE, et al. 2014 AHA/ACC/HRS guideline for the management of patients with atrial fibrillation: executive summary. A report of the American College of Cardiology/American Heart Association Task Force on Practice Guidelines and the Heart Rhythm Society. J Am Coll Cardiol. 2014;64(21):2246–80. doi:10.1016/j.jacc.2014.03.021.
3. Sohn GH, Shin DH, Byunetal KM, Han HJ, Cho SJ, et al. The incidence and predictors of postoperative atrial fibrillation after noncardiothoracic surgery. Korean Circ J. 2009;39(3):100–4.

4. Vaporciyan AA, Correa AM, Rice DC, Roth JA, Smythe WR, et al. Risk factors associated with atrial fibrillation after noncardiac thoracic surgery: analysis of 2588 patients. J Thorac Cardiovasc Surg. 2004;127(3):779–86. http://www.cdc.gov/dhdsp/data_statistics/fact_sheets/fs_atrial_fibrillation.htm. Accessed 30 Mar 2016.
5. Lip GH, Lane DA. Stroke prevention in atrial fibrillation: a systematic review. JAMA. 2015;313(19):1950–62. doi:10.1001/jama.2015.4369.
6. Rogers WK, Schroeder KM. Perioperative atrial fibrillation and epidural anesthesia. J Clin Anesth. 2012;24:329–33. Accessed 30 Mar 2016.
7. Stedman RB, Prejean MA, Russo M. Onset of lone atrial fibrillation during labor under epidural analgesia. Ochsner J. 2013;13(4):544–6. PMCID: PMC3865834. Accessed 04 Apr 2016.
8. Weigner MJ, Caulfield TA, Danias PG, Silverman DI, Manning WJ. Risk for clinical thromboembolism associated with conversion to sinus rhythm in patients with atrial fibrillation lasting less than 48 hours. Ann Intern Med. 1997;126(8):615.

Chapter 18
ECG II

Edward Kosik

You are on the obstetrics ward. You are answering an "Anesthesia Stat" call to the operating room. As you walk into the operating theater, this is the rhythm that is present on the vitals monitor:

A parturient, gravida 7 para 6 at 38 weeks gestation, was placed under general anesthesia for an emergent C-section secondary to fetal bradycardia (Category III fetal heart rate tracings).

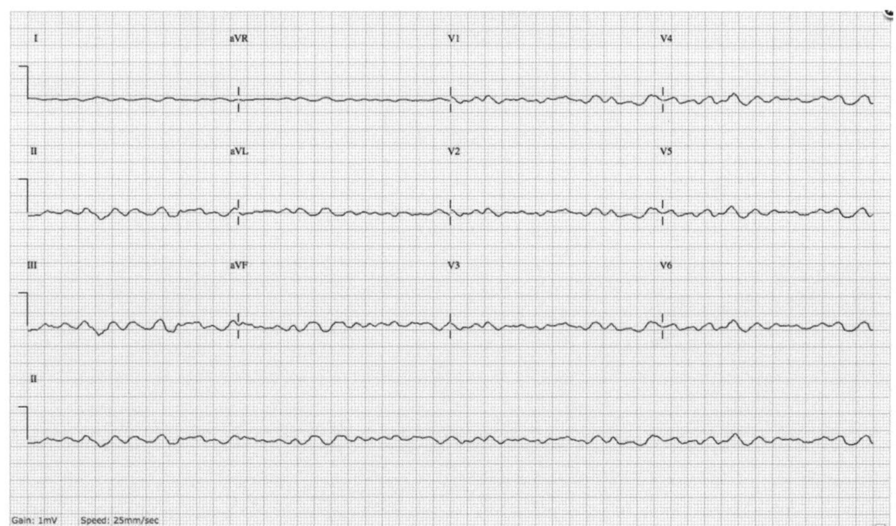

Fig. 18.1 Observed EKG in obstetrics operating theater

E. Kosik, DO
Department of Anesthesiology, University of Oklahoma Health Sciences Center, 750 NE 13th Street, Suite 200, Oklahoma City, OK 73104, USA
e-mail: Edward-kosik@ouhsc.edu

T.D. Raj (ed.), *Data Interpretation in Anesthesia*,
DOI 10.1007/978-3-319-55862-2_18

The anesthesiologist who performed the induction briefs you that a rapid sequence induction included cricoid pressure, 100 μg of fentanyl, 120 mg of propofol, and 100 mg of succinylcholine administered intravenously. A grade I view of the airway was obtained with laryngoscopy and a #7 oral endotracheal tube placed without difficulty. Initially, $ETCO_2$ was positive and auscultation of the lungs revealed bilateral breath sounds.

Preinduction vital signs were SpO_2 100%, pulse 88, BP 110/56, temp 36.6, and weight 55 kg.

1. How would you describe this arrhythmia?
2. In general, what are the potential causes of this arrhythmia in parturients?
3. What are the common causes and prevalence of maternal cardiac arrest?
4. What are your next steps in managing this case?
5. What laboratory tests would you order to help in your management?
6. When should perimortem C-section start?

An OR team member identifies an empty 250 mL bag of 0.25% ropivacaine and 2 μg of fentanyl per mL. With more investigation, the team realizes that this bag was accidentally brought into the OR and administered as "antibiotics."

7. Knowing this information how would you manage the case?
8. Which medications would you avoid in treating this disorder?
9. Is there an upper limit to the amount of medicine/treatment that you would give in this situation?

Answers

1. If the EKG leads are attached and accurate, this is cardiac arrest presenting as pulseless fine ventricular fibrillation.

2. In 2015, the American Heart Association released its first statement regarding maternal cardiac arrest. In that statement they listed common etiologies of maternal arrest and mortality. This list is a mnemonic of the letters A through H, most of which are listed below.

   Anesthetic complications - (neura xial, hypoxia, hypotension) and accidents/trauma (trauma and suicide)

   Bleeding—coagulopathy, placental causes, uterine atony and/or rupture, surgical causes

   Cardiovascular causes—myocardial infarction, cardiomyopathy, pulmonary hypertension, valvular disease, aortic dissection

   Drugs—oxytocin, magnesium, drug error (local anesthetic), illicit drugs, opioids, insulin, and anaphylaxis

*Note that many anesthetic drugs may cause prolonging of the QT interval (volatile anesthetic agents, ondansetron, antibiotics such as ciprofloxacin, erythromycin, etc.) which may result in ventricular fibrillation.

   Embolic causes—pulmonary embolism, amniotic fluid embolism, cerebrovascular event

   Fever—sepsis and infections

   General—Hs and Ts (hypoxemia, hypovolemia, hypo-/hyperkalemia, hydrogen ion (acidosis), hypothermia, tension PTX, tamponade—cardiac, toxins, thrombosis—coronary, thrombosis, pulmonary)

   Hypertension—preeclampsia, eclampsia, HELLP syndrome, intracranial bleed

3. According to Suresh and colleagues, the major causes of maternal cardiac arrest are:

   Pulmonary embolism 29%
   Hemorrhage 17%
   Sepsis 13%
   Peripartum cardiomyopathy 8%
   Stroke 5%
   Preeclampsia-eclampsia 2.8%
   Anesthesia complications (failed intubation, LAST, aspiration) 2% [1]
   Mhyre et al. reported different findings for the Nationwide Inpatient Sample (NIS) from 1998 to 2011:
   Postpartum hemorrhage 27.9%.
   Antepartum hemorrhage 16.8%.
   Heart failure 13.3%.
   Amniotic fluid embolism 13.3%.
   Sepsis 11.2%.
   Anesthesia complications 7.8%.
   Maternal cardiac arrest occurs in 1 in 12,000 hospitalizations for delivery [2].

4. Help should be summoned by announcing maternal code blue. In this cardiac arrest scenario, it is vital to start immediate cardiopulmonary resuscitation (chest compressions of 100–120 per minute, 2 inches in depth with full recoil, and the person doing compressions should switch every 2 min). For a parturient with a uterus located at or above the umbilicus, a left uterine tilt of 15° should be instituted, or if enough help is available, a manual lateral tilt might provide better resuscitation results [1, 3]. Maintaining the airway and avoiding hyperventilation is paramount. ACLS guidelines should be followed.

   An AED or defibrillator should be obtained as quickly as possible, pads placed, and the patient defibrillated with the manufacturer recommended joules, 360 J if it is monophasic or the maximum amount of energy if the recommended energy is unknown. Internal fetal monitors should be removed before defibrillation to reduce chances of team member electrocution [1]. Anesthetic gases should be discontinued and 100% oxygen administered. For the anesthesiologist, it is imperative to verify that the endotracheal tube is secured despite an easily placed airway. Effective chest compressions should show $EtCO_2$ of >10 mmHg. A backboard may not be necessary on a minimally cushioned OR table but should be considered.

   A person should be assigned to document the event. Epinephrine 1 mg IV should be given after the second defibrillation and repeated every 3–5 min. Amiodarone 300 mg IV may be administered for ventricular fibrillation resistant to defibrillation (after three shocks) [4, 5].

   Intravenous access should be present above the diaphragm. A crisis checklist should be used if available and team members are trained in using one.

5. If time permits an arterial blood gas or venous blood gas will permit quick assessment of electrolyte abnormalities, blood status, oxygenation, and ventilation status. A transthoracic echocardiogram or transesophageal echocardiogram will allow quick assessment of the cardiac function. A chest X-ray may help with assessment of the thorax.

6. Perimortem C-section should start at 4 min and the baby delivered by 5 min. However, the obstetric team should prepare for Cesarean section before this time [6].

7. Local anesthetic toxicity treatment requires Intralipid 20% administered in an initial dose of 1.5 mL/kg infused intravenously with simultaneous high-quality CPR maintained. A continuous infusion of 0.25–0.5 mL/kg/min is recommended. Dosages of epinephrine should be decreased to 1 μg/kg. Notify appropriate personnel for cardiac bypass [7].

8. Medications to avoid in local anesthetic toxicity would be lidocaine (once a treatment for ventricular tachycardia or PVCs), calcium channel blockers, vasopressin, and beta-blockers. Propofol should not be substituted for Intralipid [7].

9. ASRA recommends an upper level of 10 mL/kg of lipid emulsion infused over 30 min. Infusion longer than this may indicate other causes of cardiac collapse [7].

Acknowledgment Special acknowledgment to Scott Tatum, R.N., and CAE for EKG image.

References

1. Suresh MS, Mason LC, Munnur U. Cardiopulmonary resuscitation and the parturient. Best Pract Res Clin Obstet Gynaecol. 2010;24(3):383.
2. Mhyre JM, Tsen LC, Einav S, Kuklina EV, Leffert LR, Bateman BT. Cardiac Arrest during Hospitalization for Delivery in the United States, 1998–2011. Anesthesiology. 2014;120:810–8. doi:10.1097/ALN.0000000000000159.
3. Kundra P, Khanna S, Habeebullah S, Ravishankar M. Manual displacement of the uterus during Caesarean section. Anaesthesia. 2007;62(5):460.
4. Jeejeebhoy FM, et al. Cardiac arrest in pregnancy a scientific statement from the American Heart Association. Circulation. 2015;132:1747–73. doi:10.1161/CIR.0000000000000300.
5. Adamson DL, Nelson-Piercy C. Managing palpitations and arrhythmias during pregnancy. Heart. 2007;93(12):1630–6. doi:10.1136/hrt.2006.098822.
6. Katz VL, Dotters DJ, Droegemueller W. Perimortem cesarean delivery. Obstet Gynecol. 1986;68(4):571.
7. Neal JM, Bernards CM, Butterworth JF, et al. https://www.asra.com/advisory-guidelines/article/3/checklist-for-treatment-of-local-anesthetic-systemic-toxicity. Accessed 30 Mar 2016.

Chapter 19
ECG III

Tanmay Shah

A 71-year-old male with no known past medical history was admitted to the hospital with a chief complaint of dyspnea on exertion, swollen legs, and frequent falls since the last 3 weeks. On admission the patient had leukocytosis, bradycardia, and hyponatremia, and an EKG showed second-degree AV block with 2:1 AV conduction. An EKG taken a few hours later is shown below.

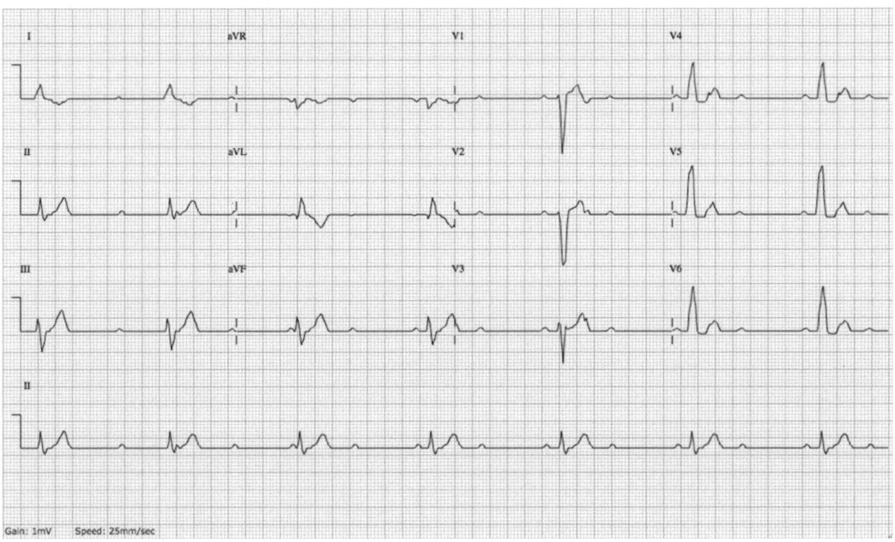

Fig 19.1 EKG showing dissociated pattern for P waves and QRS pattern

T. Shah, MD, MBBS
Department of Anesthesiology, University of Oklahoma Health Sciences Center, 750 NE 13th Street, Suite 200, Oklahoma City, OK 73104, USA
e-mail: Tanmay-Shah@ouhsc.edu

T.D. Raj (ed.), *Data Interpretation in Anesthesia*,
DOI 10.1007/978-3-319-55862-2_19

1. How will you interpret this EKG? (Fig. 19.1)
2. Can you determine the site of block in the AV conduction system by looking at the EKG?
3. Does this patient require any urgent intervention?
4. What are the causes of this condition?
5. How will you decide whether this patient needs permanent pacemaker before proceeding to surgery or not?
6. If this patient has to go for urgent/emergent surgery, is there any preoperative preparation required?
7. What monitors will you use intraoperatively for this patient?

Answers

1. This EKG shows atrial (P waves) and ventricular (QRS complexes) activity which are independent of each other, and there is no association between P waves and QRS complexes. That confirms that our patient has sinus rhythm with complete heart block (CHB).

2. Ventricular rate can help determine the site of block in conduction system. Junctional rhythm tends to have a ventricular rate between 40 and 60 beats per minutes (bpm), while ventricular escape rhythm will have rates of 40 beats per minute or less, and they are often unstable, requiring immediate cardiology intervention [1]. In most cases, the atrial rate will be faster than the ventricular escape rate, and as a general rule, the more distal the level of block in AV conduction and His-Purkinje system, the slower the ventricular rate will be.
   If EKG shows:

   (a) Narrow QRS complex with junctional or AV nodal rhythm, then the AV block has occurred within the AV node or at the level of the bundle of His.
   (b) Wide QRS complex with subjunctional escape rhythm, then the AV block is distal to the His conduction system.

3. Our patient has ventricular rate of 46 beats per minute with narrow QRS complexes which indicate that blockade is around AV node or at the His bundle. Even though our patient has frequent falls, currently he is hemodynamically stable. This patient needs to be admitted to a telemetry bed for continuous EKG monitoring along with serial 12-lead EKG. Cardiology consultation should take place as early as possible to determine the need for pacemaker placement, although an immediate intervention may be needed if ventricular rate stays less than 40 bpm along with any of the following signs/symptoms:

   (a) Hypotension
   (b) Altered mental status
   (c) Signs of shock
   (d) Ischemic chest discomfort
   (e) Acute heart failure

4. Major causes of CHB can be divided into two categories:

   (a) Pathologic causes:

   - Myocardial ischemia involving the conduction system
   - Cardiomyopathy
   - Fibrosis and sclerosis of conduction system (e.g., amyloidosis, sarcoidosis)
   - Myocarditis (e.g., Lyme disease)
   - Congenital heart disease
   - Endocarditis with abscess formation
   - Hyperkalemia
   - Increased vagal tone

(b) Iatrogenic causes:

- AV nodal blocking medications (e.g., digitalis, calcium channel blockers, amiodarone, adenosine)
- Post-cardiac surgery
- Post-catheter ablation
- Transcatheter aortic valve implantation
- Transcatheter ablation of ventricular septal defect (VSD)
- Alcohol septal ablation of hypertrophic obstructive cardiomyopathy (HOCM)

5. After excluding all reversible causes of CHB, if surgery is not urgent, then an intracardiac His bundle study can be done in order to determine the need for permanent pacemaker placement (PPP) [2, 3]. If HV interval (the interval from the His bundle to the right ventricle) is greater than 100 ms, then PPP is required prior to surgery, but if HV interval is normal or 60–100 ms, then PPP may not be needed; however, central venous access (internal jugular) is recommended before proceeding to surgery for transvenous pacing if needed.

6. A temporary transvenous pacemaker or transcutaneous pacemaker should be placed and checked before proceeding with urgent surgery [4]. All drugs and equipment, necessary for cardiopulmonary resuscitation, should be readily available in the operating room. It is also recommended that defibrillator pads are applied to the patient.
7. In addition to standard ASA monitors, an arterial line will be helpful in a patient with poor ventricular function. The EKG monitor should be set to diagnostic mode. In order to minimize interference from electrocautery, if patient has permanent pacemaker in situ, then the grounding plate should be placed as far from the pacemaker generator as possible. Bipolar cautery should be used, limiting its power output in those cases.

References

1. Morgan GE, Mikhail MS, Murray MJ. Clinical anesthesiology. 4th ed. New York: Lange Medical Books/McGraw-Hill; 2006.
2. Guimond C, Puech P. Intra-His bundle blocks (102 cases). Eur J Cardiol. 1976;4:481.
3. Narula OS, Scherlag BJ, Javier RP, et al. Analysis of the A–V conduction defect in complete heart block utilizing His bundle electrograms. Circulation. 1970;41:437.
4. Yao FSF. Yao & Artusio's anesthesiology problem-oriented patient management. 7th ed. Philadelphia: Wolters Kluwer; 2012.

Chapter 20
ECG IV

Ranganathan Govindaraj and Talla A. Rousan

A 65-year-old female presents for emergency laparotomy in the middle of the night. Her ECG is presented below.

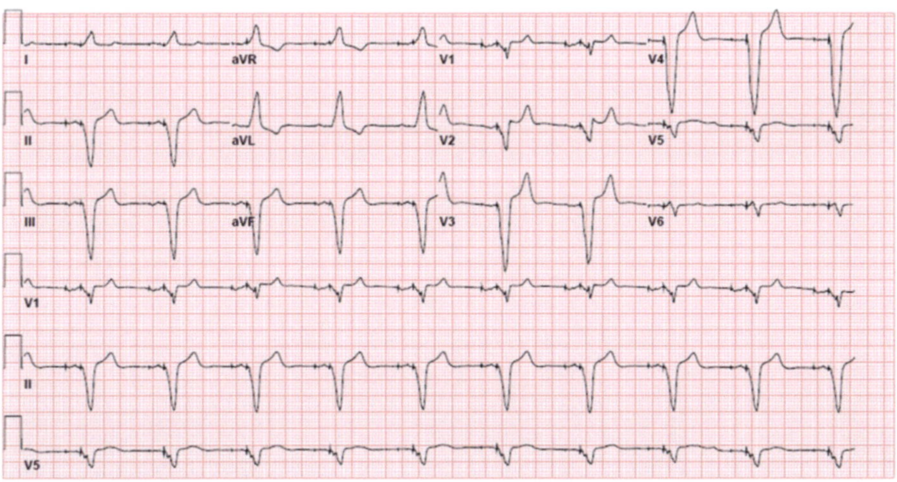

Fig. 20.1

R. Govindaraj, MD, FRCA (✉)
Associate Professor for Anesthesia and Pain, Department of Anesthesiology, UTMB, Galveston, Texas, USA

Director for Ultrasound Guided Regional Anesthesia, Galveston, TX 77555, USA
e-mail: gorangan@utmb.edu

T.A. Rousan, MD, FACC
Department of Medicine, The University of Oklahoma Health Sciences Center and the Veteran Affairs Medical Center,
800 Stanton L. Young Blvd, COM 5400, Oklahoma City, OK 73104, USA
e-mail: Talla-rousan@ouhsc.edu

T.D. Raj (ed.), *Data Interpretation in Anesthesia*,
DOI 10.1007/978-3-319-55862-2_20

1. What is shown in the above image?
2. How do we know if the patient is pacemaker dependent or not?
3. What do the letters before a pacemaker signify?
4. What is a rate modulating pacemaker?
5. What is pacemaker syndrome?
6. What is biventricular pacing? What are its indications and advantages?
7. Why do we place a magnet over a pacemaker?
8. How does the type of cautery affect the pacemaker?
9. How should this device be managed perioperatively?

Answers

1. The image shows a 12-lead ECG with pacing spikes before P waves (**a** spike) and QRS complexes (**v** spike), at a rate of 60/min indicating a dual chamber pacemaker.

2. The definition of pacemaker dependency varies in the literature. It can be defined as the absence of an intrinsic (or escape) rhythm for 30 s during temporary pacing at 30 beats per minute with the pacemaker switched off [1]. To determine if the patient is pacemaker dependent, it is essential to identify the indication for the pacemaker implantation (complete heart block and syncope, for instance, would infer dependency) [1]. In addition, pacemaker interrogation in pacemaker-dependent patients would reveal pacing 100% of the time.

3. This is nomenclature describing the pacemaker therapy modes. Permanent pacemaker nomenclature is based on recommendations by the North American Society of Pacing and Electrophysiology (NASPE) and by the British Pacing and Electrophysiology Group (BPEG).

   AAI pacemaker is useful for sinus bradycardia if the AV node function is normal.

   VVI pacemaker is useful in atrial fibrillation with slow ventricular response.

   DDD is useful if there is complete AV block with a normal sinus node.

   Pacing modes with AV synchrony are AAI, DVI, DDI, and DDD.

   Pacing modes that sense atrial activity and trigger ventricular activity are VAT, VDD, and DDD. They are used during slow ventricular rates or AV nodal block. These modes are synchronous modes.

   Asynchronous modes AOO, VOO, and DOO are not inhibited by the electrical activity of the heart or other exogenous electrical activities (cautery) in contrast to synchronous modes like DDD or VVI which are inhibited. Asynchronous mode is used in emergency situations like in the operating rooms by converting AAI to AOO, VVI to VOO, or DDD to DOO.

Table 20.1 NASPE/BPEG pacemaker code

I Chamber paced	II Chamber sensed	III Response to sensing	IV Rate responsiveness	VI Multisite pacing
0 = none	0 = none	0 = none	0 = none	0 = none
A = atrium	A = atrium	T = triggered	R = rate modulation	A = atrium
V = ventricle	V = ventricle	I = inhibited		V = ventricle
D = dual (A+V)	D = dual (A+V)	D = dual (T+I)		D = dual (A+V)
S = single (A or V)	S = single (A or V)			

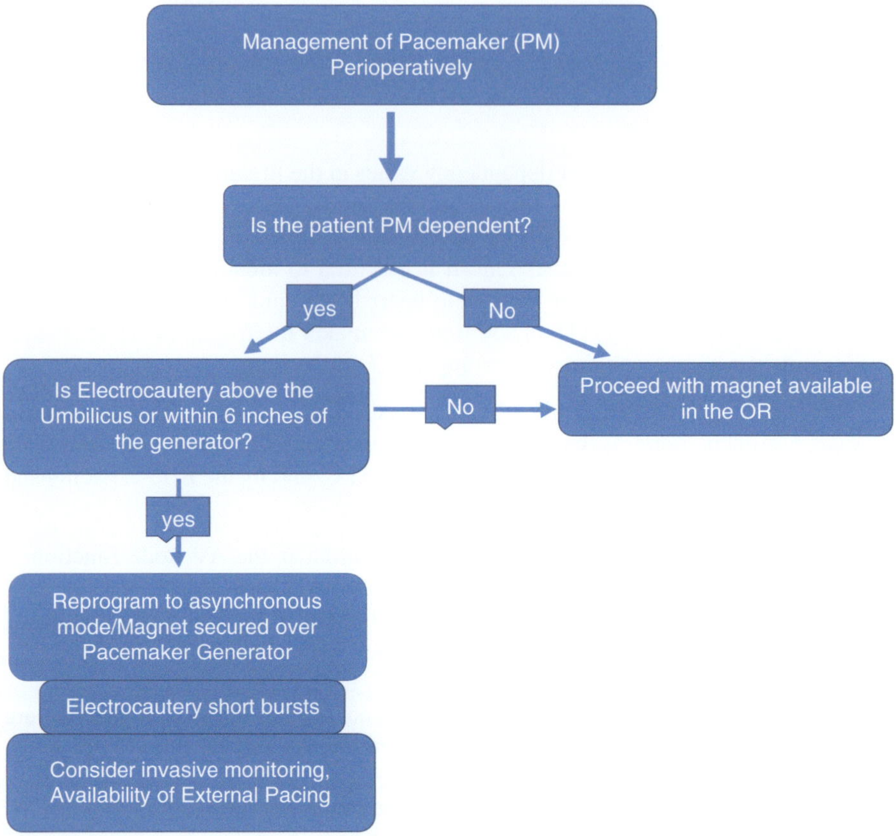

Fig. 20.2 Perioperative management algorithm for pacemaker

4. Rate modulation comes into play when metabolic demands are to be met during conditions such as exercise where physical activity increases. With conventional pacemakers, heart rate functions at a set rate, but pacemakers with rate modulating function adjust the paced rate based on the patient's activity. This is achieved by using sensors like accelerometer to sense motion or by using sensors to calculate thoracic impedance or minute ventilation.

5. The pacemaker syndrome is an iatrogenic condition that occurs as a sequel of ventricular pacing (e.g., VVI) [2, 3]. One postulated mechanism is loss of atrioventricular synchrony [3]. Symptoms of this syndrome include lethargy, palpitations, hypotension, and syncope [2]. The symptoms of this syndrome overlap with those encountered with pacemaker malfunction; thus excluding pacemaker malfunction is the first step when this syndrome is suspected [2]. Restoration of atrioventricular synchrony results in remission of the symptoms [3].

6. Biventricular pacemaker is used when the right ventricular and the left ventricular activities are asynchronous. It is achieved by three leads (right atrium, right ventricle, and coronary sinus (to pace the left ventricle)). The indication for Bi-V pacing (cardiac resynchronization therapy) with the highest level of evidence is EF $\leq$ 35% and sinus rhythm with LBBB and QRS duration 150 ms or more and NYHA II–III or ambulatory IV (class I indication) [4]. Other indications with lower level of evidence also exist, but a full discussion of the guidelines is beyond the scope of this chapter. It is not indicated (no benefit) for patients with NYHA I–II symptoms, non-LBBB pattern with QRS duration less than 150 ms [4].

7. Cautery current or other external electrical signals are inappropriately recognized as native cardiac activity, and pacing is inhibited (**oversensing**). Magnets are placed over pacemaker generator to turn off sensing and hence convert them from synchronous to asynchronous or fixed-rate (usually 70–90/min depending on programming and battery life) mode [5–7].

8. In unipolar cautery the current flows from the generator to the coagulation or cutting end of the cautery tip to the tissues and then through the body to the cautery plate and back to the generator.

   In bipolar cautery the current flows from the generator to the tip of the bipolar cautery holding the tissues and back to the generator via the opposite tip. As the distribution of current is limited to the cautery tips and tissue held within, electrical interference is restricted minimizing potential pacemaker malfunction [5–7].

9. Emergency surgery in the middle of the night does not provide much time or access to the CIED team to interrogate and ascertain pacemaker function or dependency. For the purpose of this emergency laparotomy where the top of the incision will probably extend to within 6 inches of the pacemaker generator, it would be safe to assume pacemaker dependency and proceed with the following plan—an arterial line, a magnet over the generator, communication with the surgeon regarding the need for short bursts with the electrocautery, and having external pacing equipment available nearby [6, 7].

References

1. Lelakowski J, et al. Pacemaker dependency after pacemaker implantation. Cardiol J. 2007;14(1): 83–6.
2. Travill CM, Sutton R. Pacemaker syndrome: an iatrogenic condition. Br Heart J. 1992;68(2): 163–6.
3. Ausubel K, Boal BH, Furman S. Pacemaker syndrome: definition and evaluation. Cardiol Clin. 1985;3(4):587–94.
4. Epstein AE, et al. 2012 ACCF/AHA/HRS focused update incorporated into the ACCF/AHA/HRS 2008 guidelines for device-based therapy of cardiac rhythm abnormalities: a report of the

American College of Cardiology Foundation/American Heart Association Task Force on Practice Guidelines and the Heart Rhythm Society. Circulation. 2013;127(3):e283–352.
5. Stone ME, Salter B, Fischer A. Perioperative management of patients with cardiac implantable electronic devices. Br J Anaesth. 2011;107(Suppl 1):i16–26.
6. Crossley GH, Poole JE, Rozner MA, et al. The Heart Rhythm Society (HRS)/American Society of Anesthesiologists (ASA) Expert Consensus Statement on the perioperative management of patients with implantable defibrillators, pacemakers and arrhythmia monitors: facilities and patient management this document was developed as a joint project with the American Society of Anesthesiologists (ASA), and in collaboration with the American Heart Association (AHA), and the Society of Thoracic Surgeons (STS). Heart Rhythm. 2011;8:1114–54.
7. American Society of Anesthesiologists. Practice advisory for the perioperative management of patients with cardiac implantable electronic devices: pacemakers and implantable cardioverter-defibrillators: an updated report by the American society of anesthesiologists task force on perioperative management of patients with cardiac implantable electronic devices. Anesthesiology. 2011;114:247–61.

Chapter 21
ECG V

Madhumani Rupasinghe

A 68-year-old man with hypertension and diabetes on an ACE inhibitor and insulin presents for an AV fistula placement. He appears lethargic and complaints of nausea. His ECG shows the following rhythm.

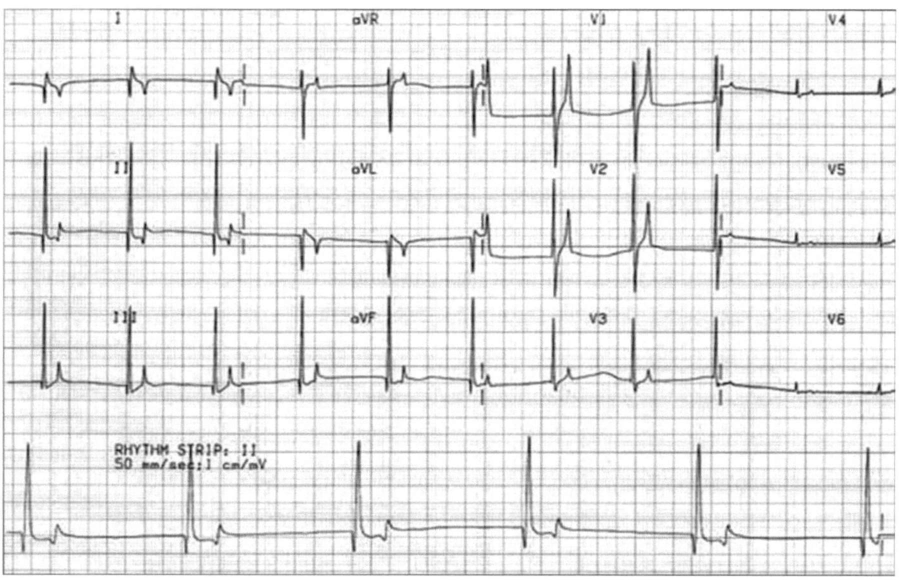

Fig. 21.1 12-lead ECG

M. Rupasinghe, MBBS, FRCA
Department of Anesthesiology, University of Texas Health Science Center at Houston, 6431 Fannin Street, MSB 5.020, Houston, TX 77030, USA
e-mail: Madhumani.Rupasinghe@uth.tmc.edu

T.D. Raj (ed.), *Data Interpretation in Anesthesia*,
DOI 10.1007/978-3-319-55862-2_21

1. What is concerning about this ECG?
2. What factors contribute toward this presentation?
3. How do you emergently correct this abnormality?
4. What are the risks of anesthetizing a patient with this ECG?

Answers

1. The clinical scenario and presentation along with the ECG suggests hyperkalemia.Hyperkalemia is defined as a potassium level >5.5 mEq/L. Moderate hyperkalemia is a serum potassium >6.0 mEq/L, and severe hyperkaliemia is a serum potassium >7.0 mE/L. Easily distinguished ECG signs of hyperkalemia are: Serum potassium >5.5 mEq/L [1]
   - Peaked T waves
   - Serum potassium >6.0 mEq/L
     - P wave widening and disappearance
     - Prolongation of the PR interval
     - QT interval shortening
   - Serum potassium >7.0 mEq/L
     - ST changes (which may mimic myocardial infarction)
     - Conduction block
     - Wide QRS, which may progress to a sine wave pattern and asystole
2. The common reasons that bring about hyperkalemia are:Excessive intake: oral or intravenous supplementation, salt substitute, and blood transfusionsDecreased excretion: diabetic nephropathy, renal failure, congestive heart failure, hypoaldosteronism, systemic lupus erythematosis, and medications, e.g., ACE inhibitors, NSAIDs, and diureticsShift from intra- to extracellular space: hyper osmolality, rhabdomyolysis, malignant hyperthermia (MH), tumor lysis, succinylcholine administration, insulin deficiency, or acute acidosisPseudohyperkalemia: improper blood collection and lab error [2]
3. Stabilize myocardial membrane with the administration of calcium.Drive extracellular potassium into the cells with insulin and glucose, beta-adrenergic agonists (albuterol), or sodium.Eliminate potassium from the body with loop diuretics or dialysis.Sodium polystyrene sulfonate (kayexalate) may be used for non-emergent management [3].
4. Hyperkalemia alters cardiac conduction, increasing automaticity and enhancing repolarization. The use of succinylcholine can dangerously aggravate hyperkalemia. As the effects of hyperkalemia are aggravated by hypoventilation and acidosis, potassium must be lowered preoperatively; otherwise, the patients are at risk of developing ventricular premature contractions, ventricular tachycardia, fibrillation, and cardiac arrest.

References

1. Montague BT, Ouellette JR, Buller GK. Retrospective review of the frequency of ECG changes in hyperkalemia. Clin J Am Soc Nephrol. 2008;3(2):324–30. doi:10.2215/CJN.04611007.
2. Evans KJ, Greenberg A. Hyperkalemia: a review. J Intensive Care Med. 2005;20(5):272–90. PMID:16145218.
3. Hollander-Rodriguez JC, Calvert JF Jr. Hyperkalemia. Am Fam Physician. 2006;73(2):283–90. PMID: 16445274

Chapter 22
ECG Exercise

Tilak D. Raj and Aneesh Venkat Pakala

For each of the ECGs below, what is the diagnosis/abnormality?

1. A 68-year-old male with type II diabetes mellitus being evaluated for inguinal hernia surgery.

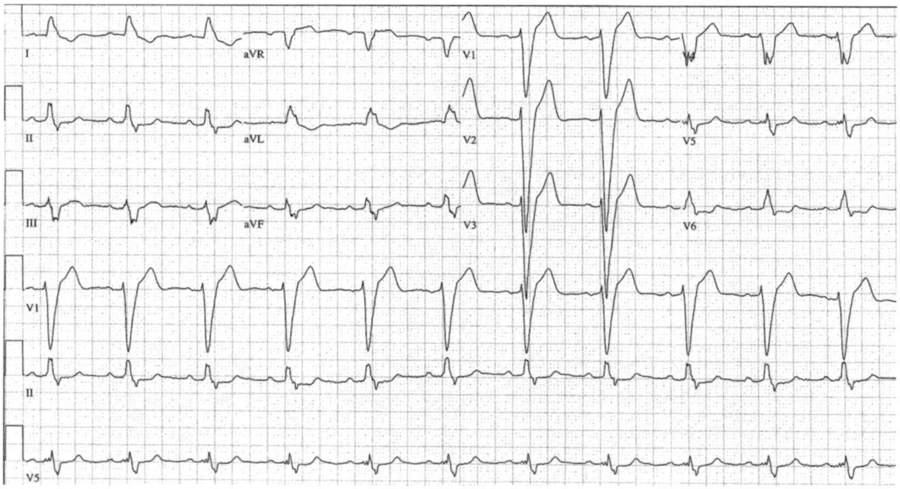

Fig. 22.1

T.D. Raj, MD, MRCP, FRCA (✉)
Department of Anesthesiology, Alliance Health Midwest, Midwest City, OK, USA
e-mail: tilakdraj@gmail.com

A.V. Pakala, MD
Section of Cardiovascular Disease, Department of Medicine, University of Oklahoma College of Medicine, Oklahoma City, OK, USA
e-mail: aneeshpakala@yahoo.com; Aneesh-Pakala@ouhsc.edu

T.D. Raj (ed.), *Data Interpretation in Anesthesia*,
DOI 10.1007/978-3-319-55862-2_22

2. A 65-year-old asymptomatic male with hypertension and COPD awaiting total knee replacement.

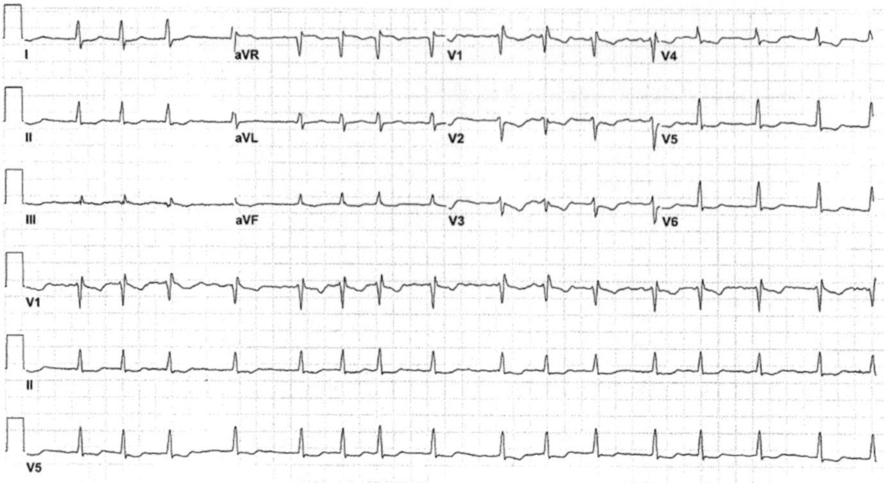

Fig. 22.2

3. A 45-year-old asymptomatic female awaiting cholecystectomy.

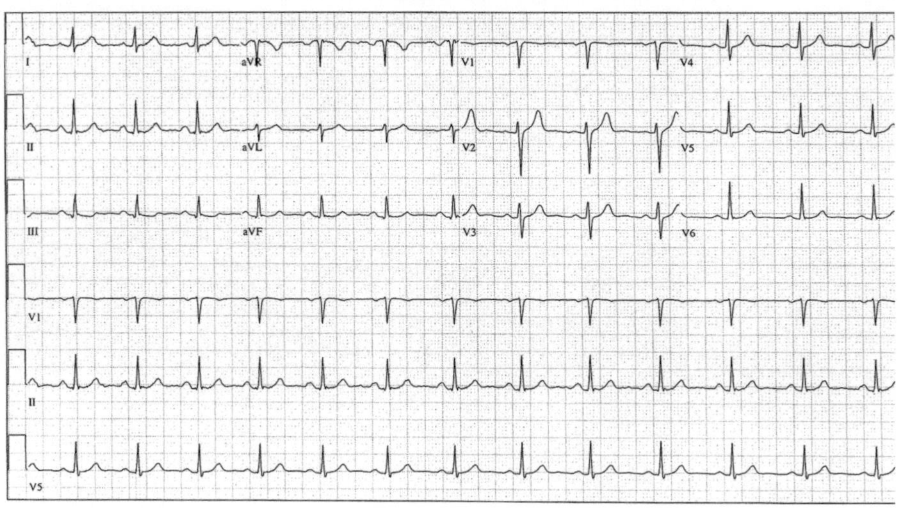

Fig. 22.3

4. A 68-year-old male with ischemic heart disease and diabetes mellitus type II and presents with syncope.

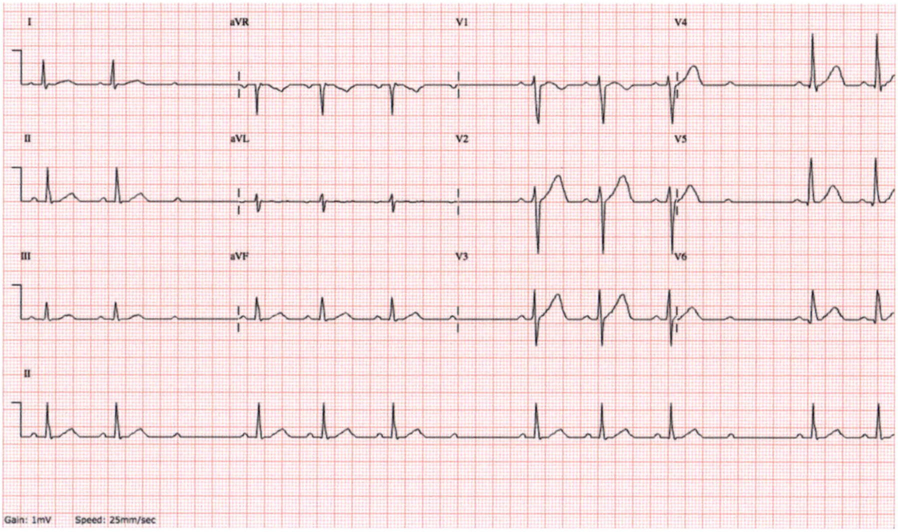

Fig. 22.4

5. A 55-year-old asymptomatic male with chronic obstructive pulmonary disease.

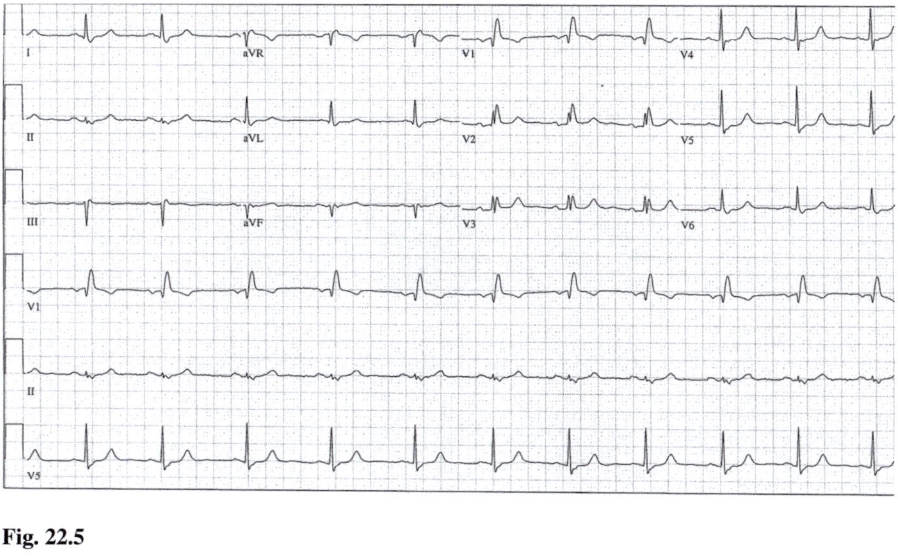

Fig. 22.5

6. A 40-year-old asymptomatic male with hypertension being treated with beta-blockers.

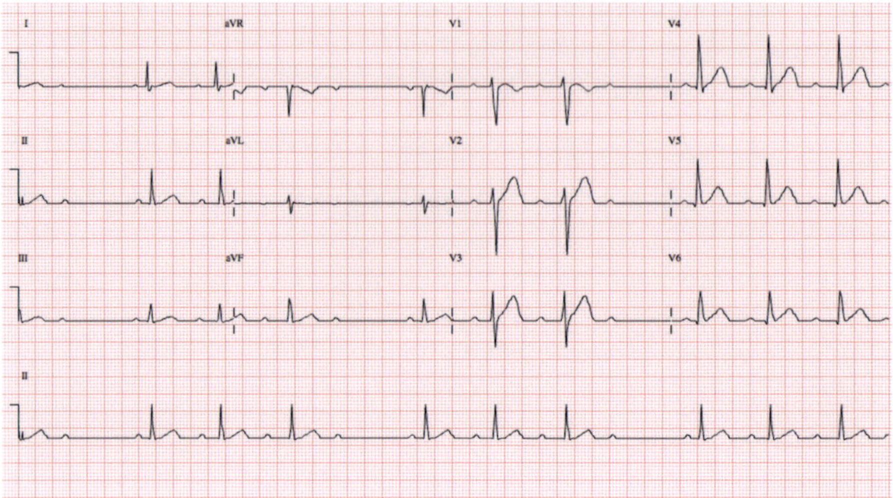

Fig. 22.6

7. A 24-year-old female with palpitations.

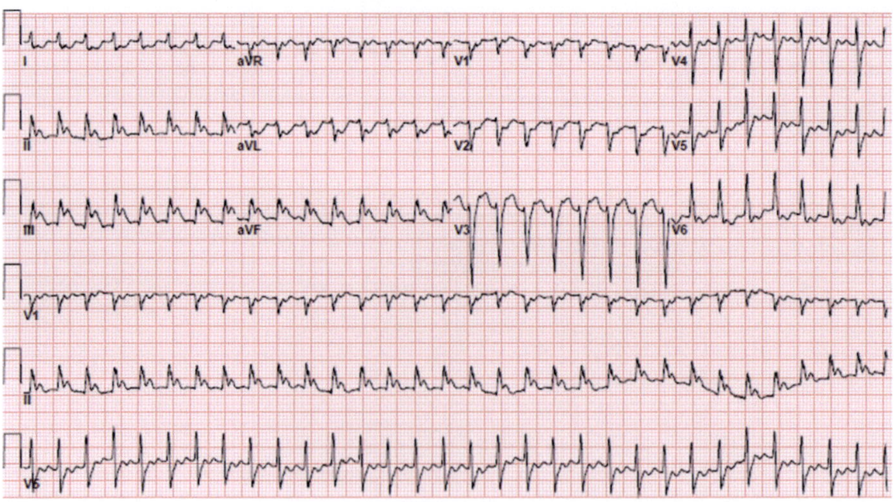

Fig. 22.7

8. A 78-year-old male with type II diabetes mellitus and hypertension admitted with facial trauma and complains of extreme fatigue and dizziness.

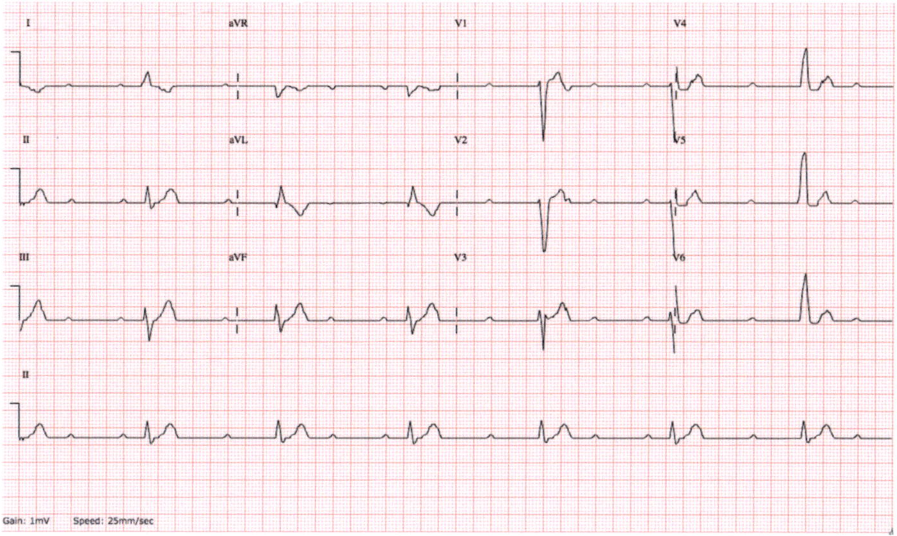

Fig. 22.8

9. A 60-year-old male with heart failure and reduced systolic function (EF 30%) and history of syncope.

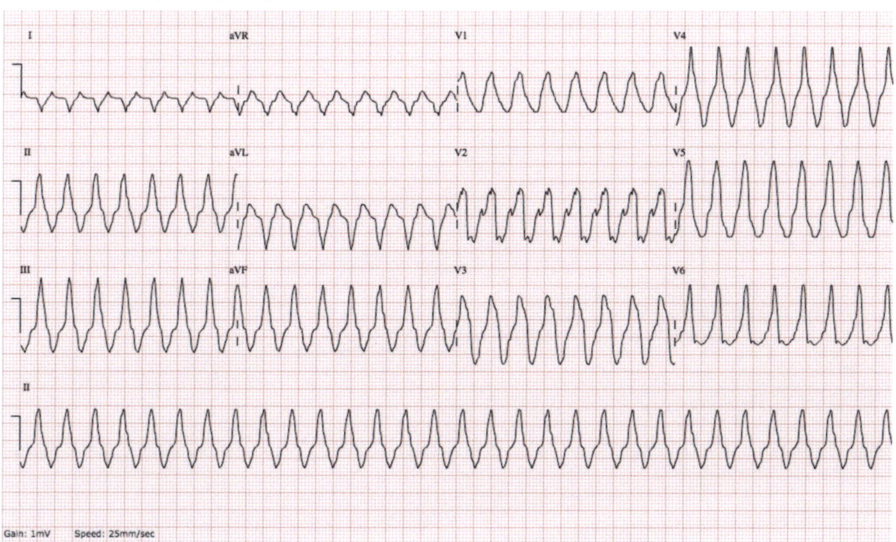

Fig. 22.9

10. A 45-year-old asymptomatic male on diltiazem for hypertension.

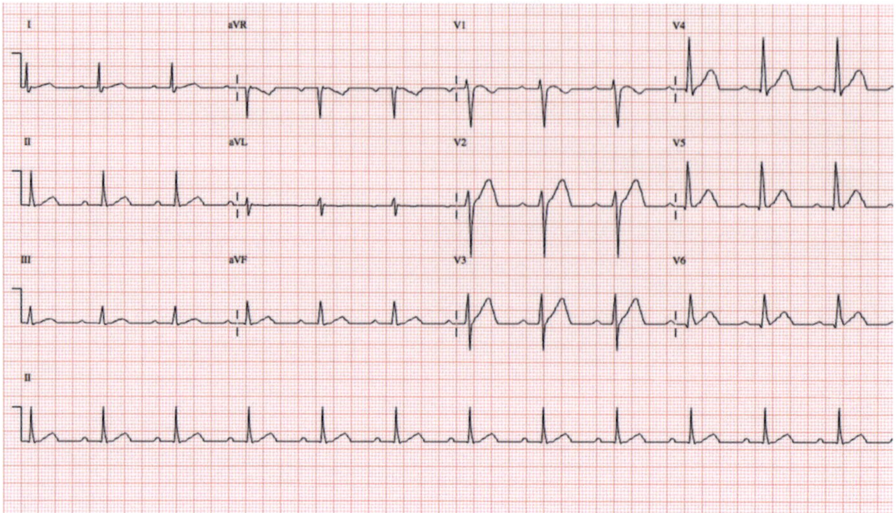

Fig. 22.10

11. A 60-year-old male awaiting routine screening colonoscopy.

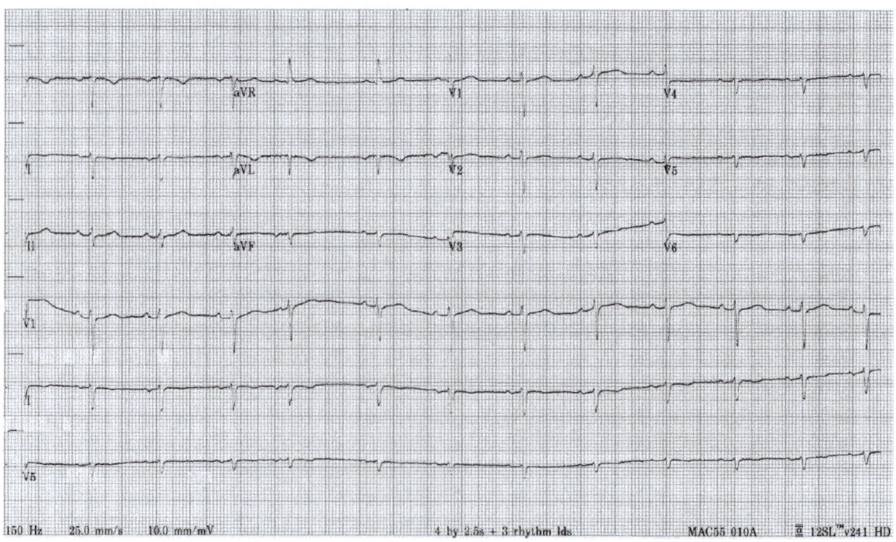

Fig. 22.11

12. A 45-year-old male awaiting ventral hernia repair. He was recently prescribed azithromycin for acute bronchitis.

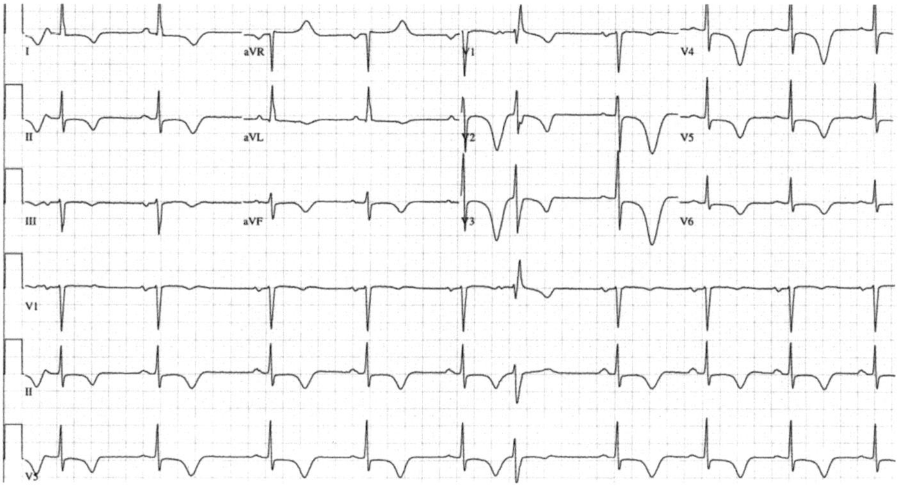

Fig. 22.12

13. A 60-year-old female with end-stage renal disease on dialysis awaiting AV fistula repair.

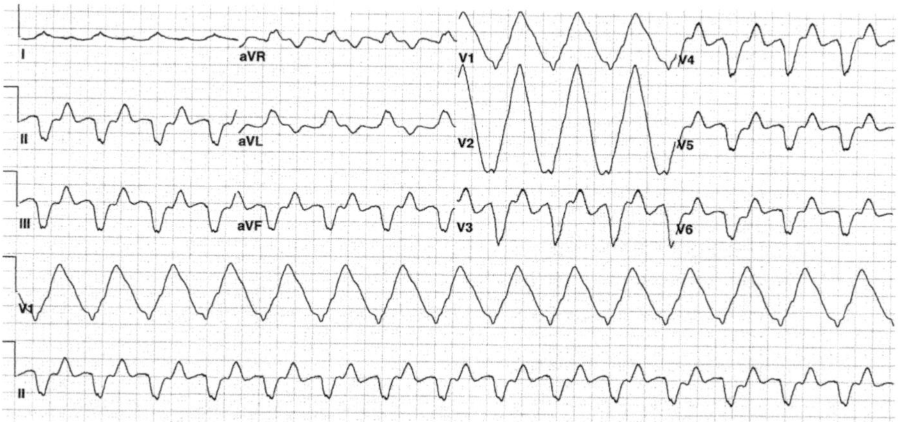

Fig. 22.13

Answers

1. Left bundle branch block (LBBB) [1].
2. Atrial fibrillation.
3. Normal sinus rhythm. Normal ECG.
4. Mobitz type II second-degree AV block. PR intervals constant. P waves blocked intermittently, PR intervals normal.
5. Right bundle branch block (RBBB).
6. Mobitz type I second-degree AV block. PR intervals progressively prolonged until P wave is blocked.
7. Narrow complex tachycardia (SVT) at a rate of about 150 per minute.

   Management: If the patient is stable, then vagal maneuvers followed (if unsuccessful) by adenosine 6 and 12 mg IV push (repeated twice if needed) followed by beta-blocker and an expert consult. Unstable (chest pain, hypotension, altered mental status) patients require synchronized cardioversion [2, 3].
8. Complete heart block. P-P intervals constant, R-R intervals constant but no relationship.
9. Wide complex tachycardia. Rate 188 per minute. Is it VT or SVT with aberrancy? Chapters have been written and there are algorithms for differentiating the two. Generally, VT occurs in people over 35 years of age with heart disease or a family history of sudden cardiac death. VT is generally regular (maybe polymorphic—Torsades) and demonstrates AV dissociation with occasional P waves showing capture (SA node "captures" the ventricles producing a normal QRS) or fusion beats (sinus and a ventricular complex fuse to produce a hybrid complex) [4].

   Brugada's sign: Onset of QRS to the nadir of the S wave >100 ms.

   Ultrasimple Brugada criterion: Onset of QRS to S nadir or peak R if greater than 50 ms in lead II favors VT.

   Management: If the patient is stable, then expert help can be sought or amiodarone 150 mg over 10 min.

   An unstable patient requires synchronized cardioversion.
10. First-degree AV Block. PR interval >0.2 s.
11. Dextrocardia. Occurs in 1:12,000 people. QRS negative in leads I and II (is it northwest axis?). aVR and aVL are reversed meaning the complexes are positive in aVR and negative in aVL. In the chest leads the R waves regress from V1 to V6. The differential diagnosis is reversed arm leads which would show similar features, but the chest leads show normal R wave progression.

12. Normal sinus rhythm, prolonged QT. Normal QT interval is 350–430 ms; prolonged QT is usually >440 ms. QT interval varies with heart rate and several formulae exist for determining corrected QT (QTc). Bazett's formula is the most widely used QTc=QT/ $\sqrt{RR}$interval [5, 3].

    QT prolongation can be inherited as in Romano-Ward or Jervell and Lange-Nielsen syndromes or acquired in a variety of clinical settings including electrolyte abnormalities, medications, acute intracranial event, or hypothermia. Prolonged QT is a risk factor for developing polymorphic ventricular tachycardia (Torsades de pointes).

13. ST and T wave changes secondary to hyperkalemia.

Acknowledgment Scott Tatum RN, BSIT, for the ECGs.

References

1. Eriksson P, Hansson PO. Bundle branch block in a general male population. Circulation. 1998;98:2494–500.
2. Walraven G. Basic arrhythmias. 7th ed. Boston: Pearson Education; 2011.
3. Neumar RW, Shuster M, Callaway CW, et al. Part 1: executive summary: 2015 American Heart Association guidelines update for cardiopulmonary resuscitation and emergency cardiovascular care. Circulation. 2015;132(suppl 2):S315–67.
4. Pava LF, Perafán P, Badiel M, Arango JJ, Mont L, Morillo CA, Brugada J. R-wave peak time at DII: a new criterion for differentiating between wide complex QRS tachycardias. Heart Rhythm. 2010 Jul;7(7):922–6.
5. Goldberger AL, Goldberger ZD, SHvilkin A. Goldberger's clinical electrocardiography: a simplified approach. 8th ed. Philadelphia, PA: Elsevier; 2013.

Chapter 23
Intra-aortic Balloon Pump (IABP)

Mohammad A. Helwani and John David Srinivasan

A 65-year-old male presented with progressing chest pain and dyspnea over the last 3 days. He was diagnosed with acute anteroseptal myocardial infarction. Transthoracic echocardiography revealed akinetic anterior and lateral wall and moderate mitral regurgitation. Coronary angiogram revealed three-vessel disease including severe left main stenosis. An intra-aortic balloon counterpulsation pump (IABP) catheter was inserted, and the patient was taken to the operating room for coronary artery bypass graft surgery.

1. Describe the parts of the IABP device.
2. What are the hemodynamic effects of IABP augmentation?
3. What are the triggers used for balloon counterpulsation?
4. What is the advantage of IABP in this patient?
5. What gas is used for the inflation and why?
6. What is the ideal position of balloon and how can we verify that?
7. Complications of IABP?
8. Contraindication of IABP?
9. What is the IABP-SHOCK II study and the final results?
10. Give some examples of abnormal timing of the balloon and consequences.

M.A. Helwani, MD, MSPH
Assistant Professor, Divisions of Critical Care and Cardiothoracic Anesthesiology, Washington University in St. Louis, School of Medicine, 660 South Euclid Ave., Campus Box 8054, St. Louis, MO 63110, USA
e-mail: helwanim@wustl.edu

J.D. Srinivasan, MD (✉)
Assistant Professor, Department of Anesthesiology and Critical Care, Saint Louis University, School of Medicine, 3635 Vista Ave., PO Box 15250, St. Louis, MO 63110-0250, USA
e-mail: srinivjd@slu.edu

T.D. Raj (ed.), *Data Interpretation in Anesthesia*,
DOI 10.1007/978-3-319-55862-2_23

Answers

1. The IABP device is composed of two main parts:
   (a) A flexible catheter with two lumens, one that allows pressure monitoring and the second that permits the periodic delivery and removal of gas to a closed balloon (2.5–50 mL in volume to fit any age and size of patients).
   (b) A console that contains the system for gas transfer as well as computer control of the inflation and deflation cycle.

2. Intra-aortic balloon pump (IABP) is the most common form of mechanical support for the failing heart, and it is useful as a bridge to definitive therapy. Inflation and deflation of the balloon has two major consequences:
   (a) Inflation occurs immediately after aortic valve closure displacing blood from the thoracic aorta and increasing diastolic pressure and therefore increasing coronary perfusion pressure and coronary perfusion (↑ O_2 supply). Systemic perfusion is also improved. This is brought about by augmentation of the intrinsic **Windkessel effect** whereby potential energy stored in the aortic root during systole is converted to kinetic energy with its elastic recoil (Fig. 23.1) [1].
   (b) Rapid deflation just before aortic valve opening reduces left ventricular diastolic pressure (afterload) and therefore wall tension and ↓ MVO_2 demand) [2].

   The cardiac output is augmented by about 40%, and the left ventricular stroke work is decreased and therefore the myocardial oxygen demand. These effects may be quite variable, and they depend upon the volume of the balloon, its position in the aorta, heart rate and rhythm, the compliance of the aorta, and synchronization with the cardiac cycle [2, 3].

3. The most commonly used triggers are the ECG and arterial waveform.

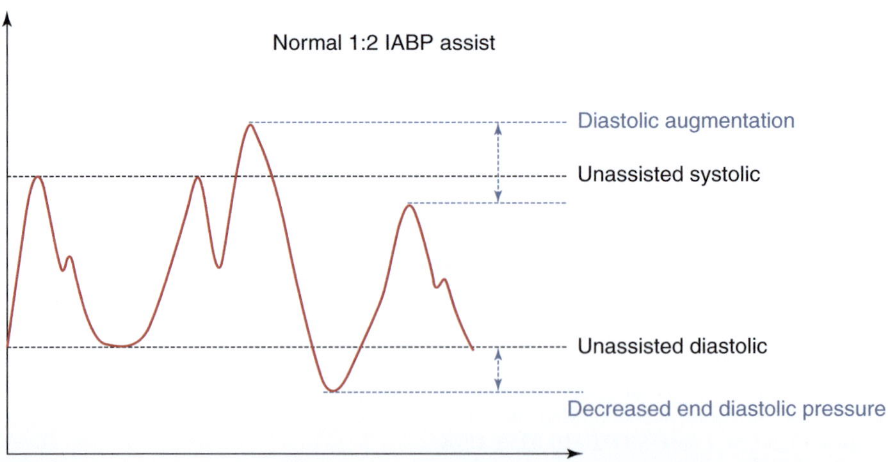

Fig. 23.1 Normal IABP 1:2 assist: diastolic augmentation and decreased end-diastolic pressure

Balloon inflation (onset of diastole after aortic valve closure): middle of T wave on the ECG and the dicrotic notch on the arterial waveform.
Balloon deflation (onset of systole just before aortic valve opening): peak of R wave or just before the systolic upstroke on the arterial waveform [1].

4. Augmentation of diastolic pressure during balloon inflation improves coronary circulation, and the presystolic deflation of the balloon reduces the resistance to systolic output and decreases myocardial work. The overall effects of the IABP therapy in this patient are an increase in the myocardial oxygen supply/demand ratio and improved forward flow and decreased mitral regurgitation.

5. Both helium and carbon dioxide have been used as driving gases; however the use of helium has theoretical advantages because it is less dense facilitating rapid transfer to and from the console. Both helium and carbon dioxide are easily absorbed into the bloodstream (compared to nitrogen and oxygen) in case of rupture of the balloon [1].

6. The closer the balloon is to the aortic valve, the greater the diastolic pressure elevation. It is obvious that local anatomical factors limit the position of the balloon within the aortic arch; therefore the optimal balloon position is situated distal to the left subclavian artery take off. Incorrect balloon position results in reduced diastolic augmentation and increases vascular morbidity.

   With optimal IABP position, on CXR, the tip is seen just below the aortic knob or at 2 cm above the carina. The position can also be confirmed by transesophageal echocardiography [4].

7. Complication of IABP:
   (a) Vascular complications: including limb (and visceral) ischemia, vascular laceration, major hemorrhage, and arterial dissection
   (b) Position complications including obstruction of arterial flow causing visceral ischemia
   (c) Air or plaque embolism
   (d) Thrombosis
   (e) Sepsis and groin infection
   (f) Hemolysis and thrombocytopenia [5]

8. Contraindications to IABP placement [5]
   (a) Moderate or severe aortic regurgitation since the degree of aortic regurgitation will be increased by counterpulsation
   (b) Aortic dissection or clinically significant aortic aneurysm
   (c) Uncontrolled sepsis
   (d) Uncontrolled bleeding disorder
   (e) Severe peripheral artery disease

9. The IABP-SHOCK II trial was a randomized, open-label, multicenter trial. Patients with cardiogenic shock complicating acute myocardial infarction who were undergoing early revascularization and optimum medical therapy were randomly assigned (1:1) to IABP versus control. IABP did not reduce 30-day or 12-month mortality [6].

10. Suboptimal timing of counterpulsation has hemodynamic consequences.
    (a) **Early inflation**: Balloon inflation before aortic valve closure (before dicrotic notch) (Fig. 23.2).
        Effects include reduced stroke volume/CO, potential increase in LVEDV and LVEDP, increased LV wall stress and afterload, and increased MVO_2 demand.
    (b) **Late inflation**: Inflation occurs markedly after aortic valve closure (after the dicrotic notch) (Fig. 23.3).
        Effects include suboptimal coronary perfusion.

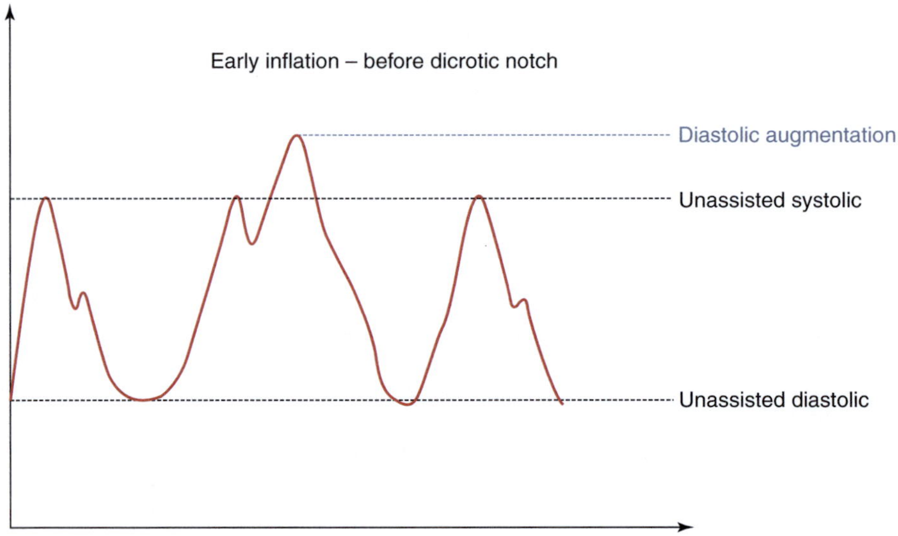

Fig. 23.2 Early inflation: before dicrotic notch—increased afterload

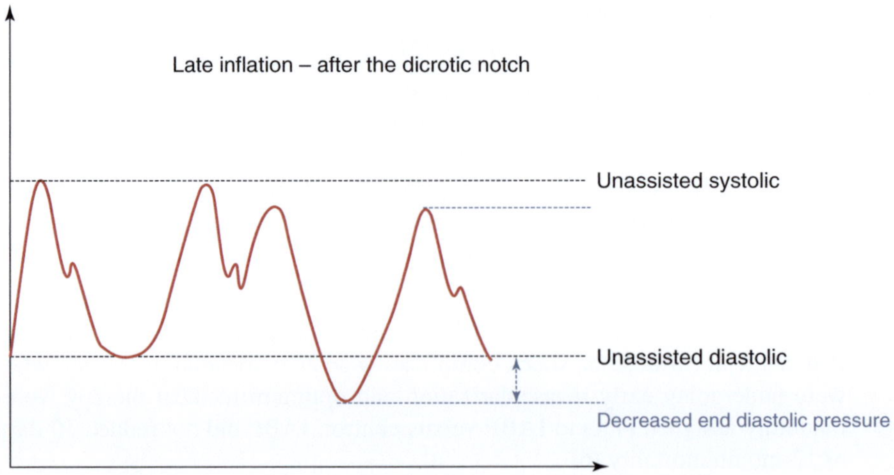

Fig. 23.3 Late inflation: after dicrotic notch—suboptimal diastolic pressure augmentation

(c) **Early deflation**: sharp decrease in waveform after diastolic augmentation. Assisted aortic end-diastolic BP may be equal to or lower than the unassisted aortic end-diastolic pressure (Fig. 23.4).

Assisted systolic pressure may increase. Effect may be suboptimal coronary perfusion, suboptimal afterload reduction and increased MVO_2 demand.

(d) **Late deflation**: IABP may impede LV ejection, afterload reduction is essentially absent, and as the LV ejects against greater resistance, the workload of the LV is increased and the MVO_2 consumption is increased. CO is decreased (Fig. 23.5).

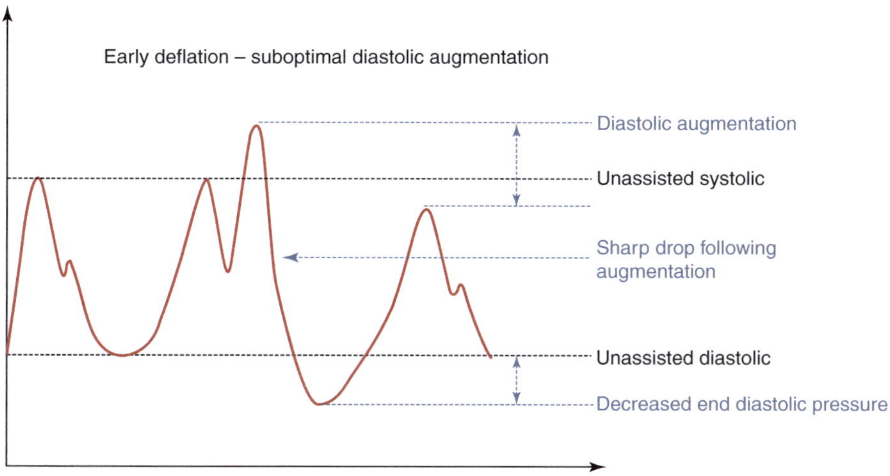

Fig. 23.4 Early deflation: suboptimal diastolic augmentation

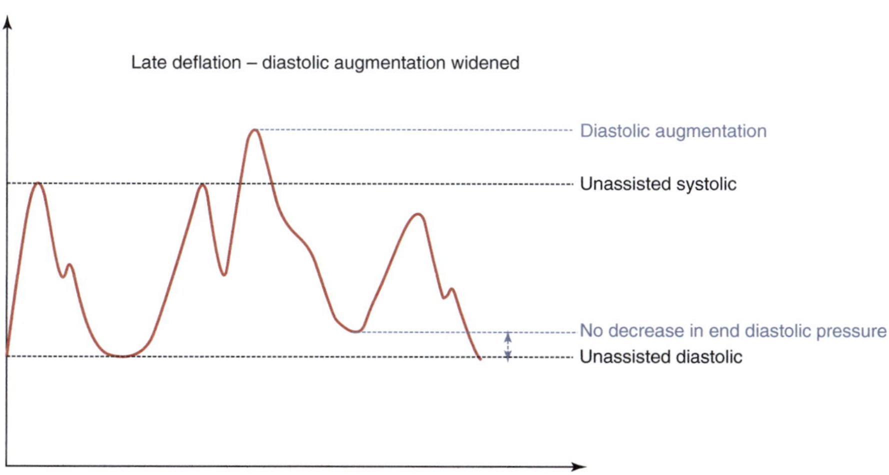

Fig. 23.5 Late deflation: widened diastolic augmentation

References

1. Parissis H, Graham V, Lampridis S, Lau M, Hooks G, Mhandu PC. IABP: history-evolution-pathophysiology-indications: what we need to know. J Cardiothorac Surg. 2016;11:122.
2. Krishna M, Zacharowski K. Principles of intra-aortic balloon pump counterpulsation. Continuing education in anaesthesia. Crit Care Pain. 2009;9(1):24–8.
3. Trost JC, Hillis LD. Intra-aortic balloon counterpulsation. Am J Cardiol. 2006;97(9):1391–8.
4. Kim JT, Lee JR, Kim JK, Yoon SZ, Jeon Y, et al. The carina as a useful radiographic landmark for positioning the intraaortic balloon pump. Anesth Analg. 2007;105(3):735–8.
5. Gilotra NA, Stevens GR. Temporary mechanical circulatory support: a review of the options, indications, and outcomes. Clin Med Insights Cardiol. 2014;8:75–85.
6. Thiele H, Zeymer U, Neumann FJ, Ferenc M, Olbrich HG, et al. Intra-aortic balloon counter-pulsation in acute myocardial infarction complicated by cardiogenic shock (IABP-SHOCK II): final 12 month results of a randomised, open-label trial. Lancet. 2013;382:1638–45.

Chapter 24
Peripheral Nerve Stimulator

Gulshan Doulatram

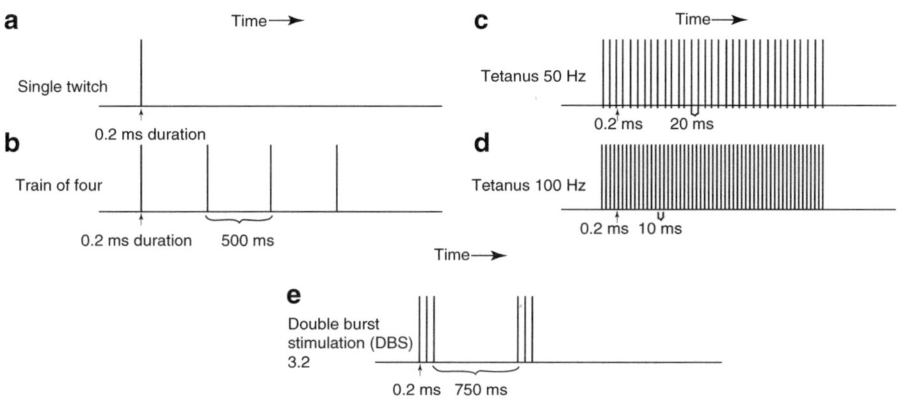

Fig. 24.1 Different patterns of nerve stimulation

Questions

1. What does the above figure depict?
2. Are there different types of peripheral nerve stimulation?
3. What is the principle behind a peripheral nerve stimulator? Describe its use.
4. Describe the commonly used patterns of stimulation.
5. What sites are used to monitor peripheral nerve stimulation?
6. How do different muscles vary in their response to neuromuscular blockade?
7. What are the quantitative measures of neuromuscular monitoring?

G. Doulatram, MD
Department of Anesthesiology, University of Texas Medical Branch,
301 University Blvd, Galveston, TX, USA
e-mail: gdoulatr@utmb.edu

T.D. Raj (ed.), *Data Interpretation in Anesthesia*,
DOI 10.1007/978-3-319-55862-2_24

Answers

1. Figure 24.1 illustrates the different patterns of stimulation obtained when monitoring peripheral neuromuscular function. The responses recorded serve as a guide during critical periods including intubation and recovery from a general anesthetic. Neuromuscular monitoring should be always used as an adjunct to other clinical signs of muscle recovery, including grip strength, sustained head lift maneuver, and respiratory mechanics.

2. Neuromuscular function is monitored intraoperatively by evaluating the muscular response to supramaximal stimulation of a peripheral motor nerve [1]. There are two kinds of stimulation: electrical and magnetic. Electrical nerve stimulation is used most commonly clinically. Magnetic stimulation has a theoretical advantage of not being painful and not requiring body contact. However, the bulk of the equipment and difficulty monitoring the train-of-four responses to stimulation preclude its practical use in the operating room.

3. The reaction of a single muscle fiber to an electrical stimulus is an all-or-none occurrence. The response of the muscle will decrease depending on the number of muscle fibers blocked in response to a neuromuscular blocking agent. The electrical stimulus applied should be 20% to 25% above that necessary for a maximal response to obtain a consistent response. This supramaximal stimulation, although painful, is possible during anesthesia [2]. A current of uniform amplitude (20–60 mA) at a short duration (0.1–0.2 ms) is applied to a peripheral nerve and the motor response is observed. Common sites include facial nerve (facial twitch) and ulnar nerve (thumb abduction). A current of greater than 0.5 ms will cause direct muscle stimulation which is not optimal. Assessment is most commonly by tactile or visual method of elicited muscle twitches. While this is the most practical method, it is subjective and not accurate. Objective methods including electromyography, acceleromyography, and mechanomyography will give a more accurate assessment compared to tactile responses [3]. The peripheral nerve stimulator should be able to generate 60 to 70 mA, be battery operated, and alarm if the current is not being delivered. The stimulator should be able to deliver single-twitch stimulation, TOF, and double-burst, tetanic stimulation and have a time constant to facilitate a posttetanic count [2].

4. There are five patterns of stimulation:

   (a) **Single-twitch stimulation**: A single supramaximal electric current is applied at a frequency ranging from 1.0 Hz (one every second) to 0.1 Hz (one every 10 s) (Fig. 24.1A).

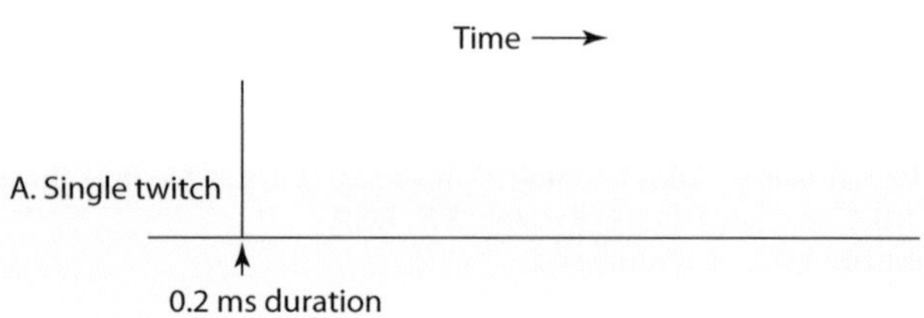

Fig. 24.1A Single-twitch stimulation

(b) **Train-of-four stimulation**: Four stimuli at 2 Hz are applied (four stimuli in 2 s) that are repeated every 10 to 12 s if needed. The ratio of the fourth response to the first response ($T4/T_1$ ratio) is used to assess the presence of neuromuscular blockade and its degree. In the absence of neuromuscular block, the ratio is 1. During a nondepolarizing block, the ratio decreases in proportion to the degree of the block. A depolarizing block, on the other hand, decreases all the four responses equally with TOF ratio of 1. A decrease in the TOF ratio after the administration of succinylcholine is indicative of phase II block. TOF value of 0.70 is associated with impaired respiratory muscle function, hypoxia, and aspiration in the immediate postoperative phase. Neostigmine is given only when the TOF count has returned spontaneously to three and preferably four responses. The availability of sugammadex as a reversal agent does not obviate the need for monitoring. The appropriate dose of sugammadex is adjusted according to the TOF and posttetanic stimulation responses (Fig. 24.1B).

(c) **Tetanic stimulation**: A stimulus of 30, 50, 100, or 200 Hz is applied for 5 s and the response of the muscle is recorded. The response of the muscle to this stimulus is sustained both in normal neuromuscular transmission and in a depolarizing block. The response however is not sustained in a nondepolarizing block and a phase II depolarizing block. The decrease in the response is called fade and is caused by depletion of acetylcholine stores over time and is directly proportional to the degree of neuromuscular blockade. Posttetanic facilitation is caused by an increase in the muscle response when stimulated right after tetanic stimulation. This is caused by mobilization and synthesis of acetylcholine to give a stronger response. The degree of posttetanic potentiation is also dependent on the degree of neuromuscular block. The major disadvantage of tetanic stimulation is that is it painful and only applicable in an anesthetized patient (Fig. 24.1C and D).

(d) **Posttetanic count stimulation**: When response to TOF and single-twitch stimulation is absent due to high degree of neuromuscular block, posttetanic count stimulation can be used to determine the degree of blockade. A tetanic stimulation (50 Hz for 5 s) is applied, and the posttetanic response to single-twitch stimulation given at 1 Hz starting 3 s after the end of tetanic stimulation is observed. During very intense blockade, there is no response to either tetanic or posttetanic stimulation. The first response to posttetanic twitch stimulation occurs as the block begins to dissipate. The time until the return

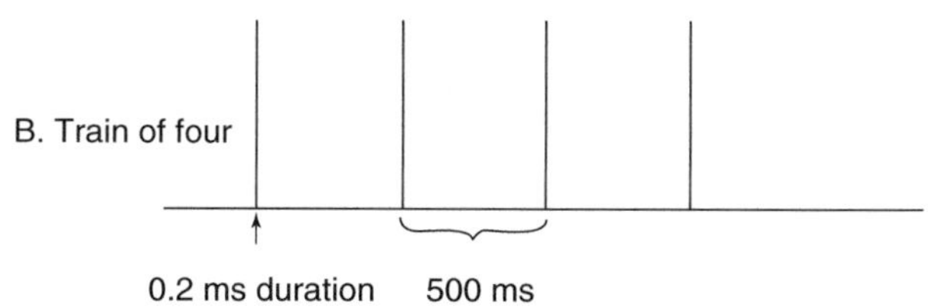

Fig. 24.1B Train-of-four stimulation

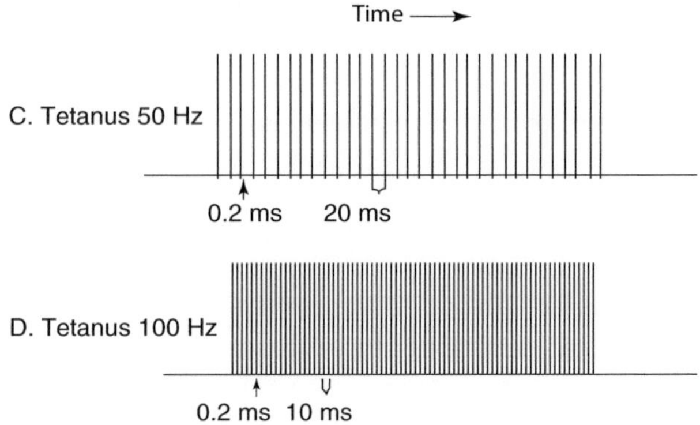

Fig. 24.1C and D Tetanic stimulation

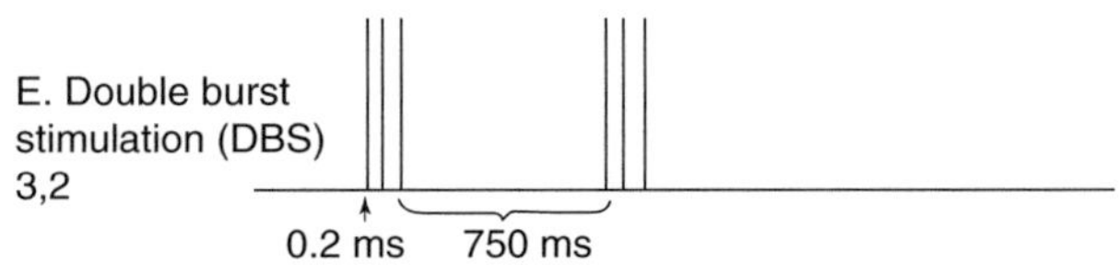

Fig. 24.1E Double-burst stimulation

of the first response to TOF stimulation is related to the number of posttetanic twitch responses present at a given time (the posttetanic count).

(e) **Double-burst stimulation**: DBS consists of two short bursts of 50-Hz tetanic stimulation separated by 750 ms. The duration of each square wave impulse in the burst is 0.2 ms. The most commonly used is DBS with three impulses in each of the two tetanic bursts. In the absence of neuromuscular blockade, the response to DBS is two short muscle contractions of equal strength. In nondepolarizing block, the second response is weaker than the first. DBS allows for detection of small amounts of residual blockade during emergence and in the postoperative period. The DBS response is more easily felt than TOF making it a superior option. As with all modalities of testing, the frequency and duration should be kept constant for the entire operative time (Fig. 24.1E).

5. The ulnar and fascial nerves are the most common sites used for peripheral nerve stimulation. Other sites include common peroneal and posterior tibial nerves. In the case of ulnar nerve, the electrodes are placed on the volar surface of the wrist with the negative electrode 1 cm proximal to the wrist on the ulnar nerve and the positive electrode 2–5 cm proximal to it, and the response to adductor pollicis is recorded [4]. In the case of fascial nerve, the negative electrode is placed directly over the fascial nerve and the positive electrode is placed over the forehead and response of orbicularis oris and corrugator supercilii muscles is recorded.

6. The diaphragm is the most resistant muscle to neuromuscular blockade; however, it recovers the fastest compared to the hand muscles. The most sensitive muscles include the abdominals, the muscles of the extremities, and upper airway. The response to facial nerve stimulation mimics the response of laryngeal

muscles; however, an adequate response might not be an indicator for extubation as the peripheral muscles might still be blocked. Reliance on facial muscles is associated with an increased incidence of postoperative residual neuromuscular block in the PACU. A normal response from the ulnar nerve would ensure that the muscles of the diaphragm and larynx have completely recovered. On the other hand, an absent response during intubation may not ensure appropriate intubating conditions.

7. The tactile and visual responses are subject to human error especially when the TOF ratio is greater than 0.4 [5]. Quantitative monitoring techniques give a more precise assessment of neuromuscular blockade especially during emergence, before, and after neostigmine administration. There is good emerging evidence that objective monitoring performed perioperatively ensures both a TOF greater than 0.9 and a subsequent decrease in the incidence of postoperative residual paralysis [2]. The techniques include mechanomyography (MMG), electromyography (EMG), acceleromyography (AMG), and phonomyography (PMG). AMG measures the isotonic acceleration of the stimulated muscle. It uses a small piezoelectric transducer, which is attached to the stimulated muscle. The movement of muscle generates voltage in the piezoelectric crystal, which is proportionate to the acceleration of that muscle. The signals are analyzed and recorded. The monitors are small, portable, and easy to use [6]. PMG measures low-frequency sounds that are generated by the contraction of skeletal muscles, and MMG measures force of the contraction to indicate the degree of neuromuscular blockade. While all these techniques give you quantitative measures, they cannot be reliably compared to each other.

References

1. Viby-Mogensen J. Neuromuscular monitoring. Curr Opin Anaesthesiol. 2001;14(6):655–9.
2. Lien CA, Kopman AF. Current recommendations for monitoring depth of neuromuscular blockade. Curr Opin Anaesthesiol. 2014;27:616–22.
3. Viby-Mogensen J, Casper C. Evidence-based management of neuromuscular block. Anesth Analg. 2010;111(1):1–2.
4. Ghai B, Makkar JK, Wig J. Neuromuscular monitoring: a review. J Anaesth Clin Pharmacol. 2006;22(4):347–56.
5. Jensen E, Viby-Mogensen J, Bang U. The accelograph: a new neuromuscular transmission monitor. Acta Anaesthesiol Scand. 1988;32:49.
6. Miller RD, Pardo MC. Basics of anesthesia. 6th ed. Philadelphia, PA: Elsevier Saunders; 2011.

Part II
Laboratory Testing

Chapter 25
Complete Blood Count (CBC)

John David Srinivasan and Mohammed A. Helwani

A 25-year-old man is brought to the emergency department after a motor vehicle accident in which he was an unrestrained passenger. He is otherwise healthy. Clinically he was alert but confused and in pain. BP on arrival was 88/60 mmHg, HR 124/min, and RR 24/min. He weighed 70 kg. His skin was cool and clammy to touch. X-rays showed right thigh and pelvic fracture. CT scans of the head, chest, and abdomen were normal. CT scan of the pelvis showed a complex fracture of pelvis.

Labs on admission were hemoglobin 9.1 gm/dL, platelets 118,000/mL, prothrombin time (PT) and partial thromboplastin time (PTT) mildly elevated, and lactate 4.2 mmol/L. The patient had received 1500 cc of normal saline from the time of injury to admission.

Questions

1. Is the patient in hemorrhagic shock?
2. What is the estimated blood volume in this patient?
3. Does this patient need blood transfusion with hemoglobin of 9.1 gm/dL?
4. Was this patient coagulopathic on admission?
5. How is ATC initiated?
6. What other factors exacerbate ATC?
7. What are the current guidelines regarding transfusion of blood and blood products in massive trauma?

J.D. Srinivasan, MD (✉)
Assistant Professor, Department of Anesthesiology and Critical Care, Saint Louis University, School of Medicine, 3635 Vista Ave., PO Box 15250, St. Louis, MO 63110-0250, USA
e-mail: srinivjd@slu.edu

M.A. Helwani, MD, MSPH
Assistant Professor, Divisions of Critical Care and Cardiothoracic Anesthesiology, Washington University in St. Louis, School of Medicine, 660 South Euclid Ave., Campus Box 8054, St. Louis, MO 63110, USA
e-mail: helwnaim@wutl.edu

T.D. Raj (ed.), *Data Interpretation in Anesthesia*,
DOI 10.1007/978-3-319-55862-2_25

Table 25.1 Classification of stages of hemorrhagic shock

Hemorrhagic shock class	I	II	III	IV
Blood loss (mL) (% blood volume)	<750 (15%)	750–1500 (15–30%)	1500–2000 (30–40%)	>2000 (>40%)
HR	<100	>100	>120	>140
BP	Normal	Normal	Decreased	Decreased
PP	Normal	Decreased	Decreased	Decreased
RR	14–20	20–30	30–40	>35
UOP	>30	20–30	5–15	Negligible
CNS	Slightly anxious	Mildly anxious	Anxious, confused	Confused, lethargic

HR heart rate, *BP* blood pressure, *PP* pulse pressure, *UOP* urine output, *CNS* central nervous system

Answers

1. The patient is in hemorrhagic shock—a condition produced by rapid and significant loss of intravascular volume, which may lead sequentially to hemodynamic instability and decreased tissue perfusion. The injuries this patient suffered are associated with significant amount of bleeding. Fractures of the pelvis and femurs can hide massive amounts of bleeding with little external evidence and potentially put the patient at risk for hemorrhagic shock. Signs of shock in this patient are decrease in BP, tachycardia, tachypnea, confusion, cool and clammy skin, and elevated lactate. Other signs that could be present in shock state include oliguria and metabolic acidosis. This patient most likely has class III hemorrhagic shock (Table 25.1) [1].

2. The average adult blood volume represents 7% of body weight (or 70 mL/kg of body weight) [2]. Estimated blood volume for a 70 kg person is approximately 5 L.

3. Yes, maintaining a higher hemoglobin level of 10 g/dL is a reasonable goal in actively bleeding patients and with signs of shock. Hemoglobin concentration in an actively bleeding individual has dubious diagnostic value because it takes time for the various intravascular compartments to equilibrate. Hemoglobin concentration should not be the only therapeutic guide for blood transfusion in actively bleeding patients. Rather, therapy should be guided by the rate of bleeding and changes in hemodynamic parameters.

4. Yes, as evident by the prolongation of the PT and PTT. Many patients with severe injuries seen in the emergency department have an established coagulopathy called trauma-induced coagulopathy or acute traumatic coagulopathy (ATC). ATC is an impairment of hemostasis and activation of fibrinolysis that occurs early after injury and is biochemically evident prior to, and independent of, the development of significant acidosis, hypothermia, or hemodilution. This has driven a change in the early resuscitation of these patients with blood and blood components [3].

5. Acute traumatic coagulopathy (ATC) or trauma-induced coagulopathy (TIC), as stated earlier, is an impairment of hemostasis and activation of fibrinolysis that occurs in response to severe injury and hypoperfusion. TIC can contribute significantly to the bleeding from the injury. It is mediated primarily by activation of the thrombomodulin-protein C system. Activated protein C inhibits coagulation cofactors V and VIII, reducing further thrombin generation. Platelet dysfunction has an important role in the pathophysiology of TIC. When present in excess, activated protein C depletes plasminogen activator inhibitor-1 (PAI-1) thus reducing tissue plasminogen activator (tPA) inhibition and accelerating the conversion of plasminogen to plasmin [3].
6. Acidosis and hypothermia alongside consumption and blood loss and the dilutional effects of resuscitation may worsen ATC/TIC.
7. The recommendations suggest early plasma-based resuscitation, targeting ratios of packed red blood cells, FFP, and platelets approaching 1:1:1 [4]. The PROPPR (Pragmatic Randomized Optimal Platelet and Plasma Ratios) trial randomly assigned 680 severely injured patients identified at risk of requiring massive transfusion from 12 North American level I trauma centers to transfusions of plasma, platelets, and red blood cells in ratios of either 1:1:1 or 1:1:2. There were no significant differences in primary outcomes of 24-h or 30-day mortality between the groups. But, death from hemorrhage was significantly less common in the 1:1:1 cohort at 3 h after injury [5–7].

References

1. Gutierrez G, Reines HD, Wulf-Gutierrez ME. Clinical review: hemorrhagic shock. Crit Care. 2004;8(5):373. doi:10.1186/cc2851.
2. Kasuya H, Onda H, Yoneyama T, Sasaki T, Hori T. Bedside monitoring of circulating blood volume after subarachnoid hemorrhage. Stroke. 2003;34(4):956–60. doi:10.1161/01.str.0000064321.10700.6.
3. Cap A, Hunt BJ. The pathogenesis of traumatic coagulopathy. Anaesthesia. 2014;70:96–e34. doi:10.1111/anae.12914.
4. Helwani MA, Gillihan JR. Mortality and ratio of blood products used in patients with severe trauma. JAMA. 2015;313(20):2078. doi:10.1001/jama.2015.4424.
5. White NJ. Mechanisms of trauma-induced coagulopathy. Hematology Am Soc Hematol Educ Program. 2013;2013(1):660–63. ASH Education Book.
6. Brohi K. Trauma induced coagulopathy—LTC2008 Karim Brohi, London, UK, October 18, 2009. http://www.trauma.org/index.php/main/article/927/
7. Holcomb JB, Tilley BC, Baraniuk S. Transfusion of plasma, platelets, and red blood cells in a 1:1:1 vs a 1:1:2 ratio and mortality in patients with severe trauma: the PROPPR randomized clinical trial. JAMA. 2015;313(5):471–82.

Chapter 26
Basic Metabolic Panel I

Tilak D. Raj

HR 105, BP 155/89, Sats 94%.

Hb 9.9 g/dL, Hct 29.7%, Na 120 mEq/L, K 3.2 mEq/L, Ca 9.1 mg/dL, BUN 7 mg/dL, glucose 100 mg/dL.

Above values are obtained in a patient in PACU 30 min post-TURBT. The patient is extremely drowsy and not arousable. No medications were given in PACU.

Questions

1. What are the causes of postoperative drowsiness and the likely cause in this patient?
2. What is the next step?
3. How do you calculate plasma osmolality?
4. What is the difference between osmolality and osmolarity?
5. How would you manage this condition?
6. What is SIADH?

T.D. Raj, MD, MRCP, FRCA
Department of Anesthesiology, Alliance Health Midwest, MIdwest City, OK, USA
e-mail: Tilak-raj@ouhsc.edu

T.D. Raj (ed.), *Data Interpretation in Anesthesia*,
DOI 10.1007/978-3-319-55862-2_26

Answers

1. (a) Medications including long-acting anesthetics, benzodiazepines, barbiturates, long-acting opiates, or large doses of fentanyl
(b) Timing of the medications—if the medications were given toward the end of the procedure
(c) Profound hypoxemia
(d) hypercarbia—PCO_2 greater than 75 mmHg
(e) Hypothermia and hypotension
(f) Hypoglycemia and hyperglycemia
(g) Cerebral—ischemia, hemorrhage, preexisting causes like tumor, trauma, seizures, and intracranial spread of local anesthetics (associated with apnea)
(h) TURP syndrome—circulatory overload, hyponatremia, glycine, and ammonia toxicity
(i) Hypothyroidism, hepatic or renal failure
Likely cause in this patient is hyponatremia (defined as serum sodium less than 135 mEq/L).

2. At this stage a few things need to be done—clinical assessment of the patient for acuteness (hyponatremia 120 mmol/L and below is severe), volume status, calculation, and measurement of plasma osmolality and measurement of urine sodium to assess the cause of hyponatremia Fig. 26.1.

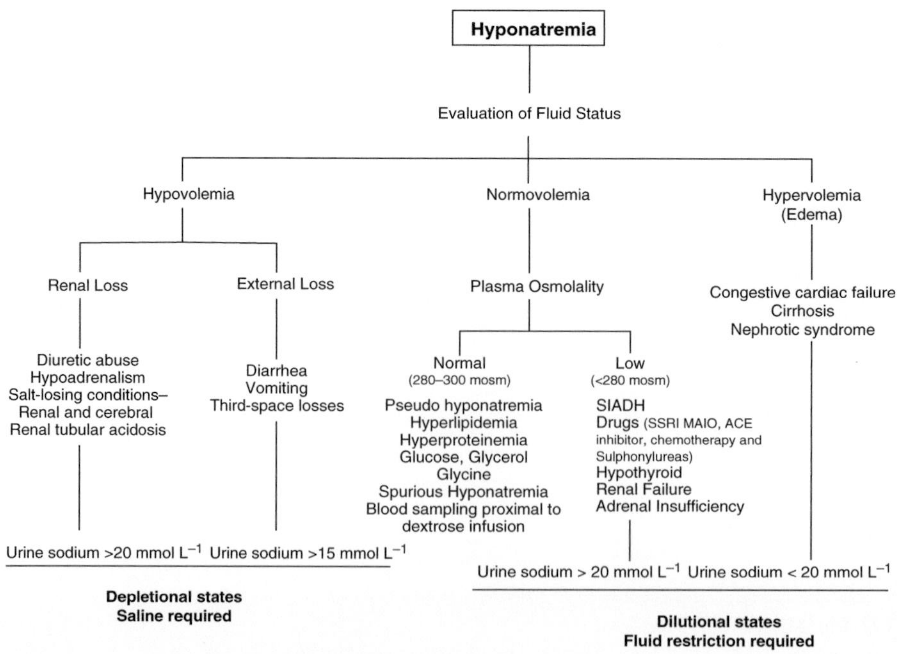

Fig. 26.1 Causes of hyponatremia [1, 2]

Plasma osmolality is calculated with the formula:

(2 × Na + K) + (glucose/18) + (urea/2.8)
Lab values for glucose and urea are reported in conventional units (mg/dL) and need conversion to SI units (mmol/L). An alternate method of conversion is glucose × 0.0555 and urea × 0.357.
Normal = 280–300 mosm/kg.
The difference between the measured and calculated osmolality is the osmolal gap normally less than 10 mosm/kg. Elevated levels are seen in the presence of ethanol, methanol, isopropyl alcohol, and ethylene glycol.

3. Osmolarity is a measure of the osmoles of solute per liter of solution. A capital letter M is used to designate units of mmol/L. Volume of solution changes with the amount of solute added and also with temperature and pressure changes.

   Osmolality is a measure of the osmoles of solute per kilogram of solvent and is reported commercially using mOsm/kg. As the amount of solvent remains constant regardless of temperature and pressure changes, osmolality is preferred and is commonly used.

4. Management [1, 3, 4]:

   (a) Correct underlying cause.
   (b) If severe, expert help should be obtained.
   (c) The magnitude and rapidity of correction is controversial due to observations that rapid correction may lead to central pontine myelinosis with paralysis, coma, and death.
   (d) **Severe cases** may need 3% (hypertonic) saline which contains 514 mmol/L of sodium in aliquots of 3–5 mL/kg over 15 min–1 h to raise the plasma sodium by 2–4 mmol/L and only to return the plasma concentration to 125 mmol/L.
   (e) In less severe cases, management depends on fluid status. Hypovolemia requires 0.9% saline. In normovolemic and hypervolemic states, correction is done by fluid restriction with or without diuretics.

5. The syndrome of inappropriate ADH secretion (SIADH) is characterized by hyponatremia, low plasma osmolality with normovolemia, and an inappropriately high urine osmolality [5]. It may be seen in the presence of malignant tumors which produce ADH-like substances, in neurological disorders (head injury, tumors), and in pneumonia. Some drugs (barbiturates, opioids, chlorpropamide, anticonvulsants, and indomethacin) may also potentiate or increase ADH effect. Treatment is with fluid restriction, and in severe or resistant cases, demeclocycline or lithium may be tried.

References

1. Fourlanos S, Greenberg P. Managing drug-induced hyponatraemia in adults. Aust Prescr. 2003;26:114–7.
2. Aitkenhead AR, Moppett IK, Thompson JP. Smith and Aitkenhead's textbook of anesthesia. 6th ed. London, UK: Churchill Livingstone Elsevier; 2013.
3. Sterns RH, Nigwekar SU, Hix JK. The treatment of hyponatremia. Semin Nephrol. 2009;29(3):282–99.
4. Craig S. Hyponatremia in emergency medicine, Medscape, Apr 2010.
5. Ellison DH, Berl T. Clinical practice. The syndrome of inappropriate antidiuresis. N Engl J Med. 2007;356(20):2064–72.

Chapter 27
Basic Metabolic Panel II

Raghuvender Ganta

A 63-year-old man with hypertension, diabetes, and generalized weakness presents for resection of small bowel. The patient's medications include furosemide, metoprolol, and acetazolamide.

Lab values: HR 90, BP 105/65, Sats 96%, Hb 11 g/dL, Hct 31%, Na 130 mEq/L, K 2.3 mEq/L, and Cr 2.0

His EKG shows the following rhythm.

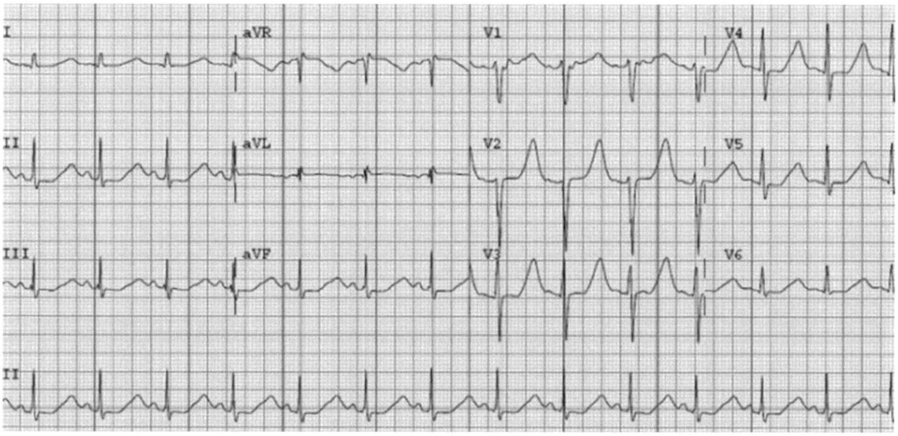

Fig. 27.1 Reproduced with permissions from The Permanente Journal [1]

R. Ganta, MD, FRCA
Department of Anesthesiology, VA Hospital, OUMC,
921 NE 13th Street, Oklahoma City, OK 73104, USA
e-mail: raghuvender-Ganta@ouhsc.edu

T.D. Raj (ed.), *Data Interpretation in Anesthesia*,
DOI 10.1007/978-3-319-55862-2_27

Questions

1. What are your concerns regarding his EKG?
2. What are the causes for this abnormality?
3. How do you emergently correct low potassium preoperatively in this patient?
4. How do you monitor and manage perioperatively?
5. What are the anticipated problems and concerns anesthetizing this patient?

Answers

1. The clinical presentation along with EKG (Fig. 27.1) features (prominent U waves and apparent QT/U prolongation) suggests significant hypokalemia.

   Hypokalemia is defined as plasma potassium of less than 3.5 mEq/L. For every 0.3 mEq/L decrease in plasma potassium, the total body potassium stores decrease by 100 mEq/L.

   Mild hypokalemia is serum potassium >2.0 mEq/L; Severe hypokalemia is serum potassium <2.0 mEq/L.

   The electrocardiographic changes include:

   Early—decrease in T wave.

   Later—ST depression and T inversion. PR interval prolongation. U waves appear in mid precordial leads.

   Severe—U and T fuse-producing giant U waves and apparent prolongation of QT interval which is actually QU interval.

2. Causes:
   (a) Inadequate intake: diet and alcoholism.
   (b) Excessive renal loss: mineralocorticoid excess, Cushing's syndrome, diuretics, hydrochlorothiazide and furosemide therapy, carbonic anhydrase inhibitors, chronic metabolic alkalosis, renal tubular acidosis, and ureterosigmoidostomy.
   (c) Gastrointestinal losses: vomiting and diarrhea, which are commonly implicated as nutritional deficiency causes; nasogastric suctioning; and villous adenoma [2, 3].
   (d) β-Adrenergic agonists, insulin, and alkalosis (respiratory and metabolic) shift potassium to the intracellular space.
   (e) The most common renal cause of hypokalemia is diuretic therapy when loop diuretics and thiazides are co-prescribed. Loop diuretics block the sodium-potassium-chloride cotransporter in the thick ascending limb of the loop of Henle, while thiazides block the sodium-chloride cotransporter in the distal convoluted tubule [4].

3. Hypokalemia treatment consists of oral or intravenous replacement of potassium.

   Mild hypokalemia (>2.0 mEq/L): infuse potassium chloride up to 10 mEq/h iv
   Severe hypokalemia (<2.0 mEq/L, ECG changes, intense skeletal muscle weakness): infuse potassium chloride up to 40 mEq/h iv, with continuous ECG monitor.

   Total KCL required is determined by calculating the K deficit.

   K deficit (mEq/L) = (Goal K – Measured K)/serum Creatinine × 100
   K deficit (mEq/L) = (4.0–2.3)/2 × 100
   = 1.7/2 × 100 = 85 mEq/L
   = 85 mEq/L

4. (a) Monitoring
    - EKG
    - Plasma potassium levels
    - ABG
    - Peripheral nerve stimulator

   (b) Maintenance
    - Avoid hyperventilation.
    - Avoid hyperglycemia.
    - Avoid epinephrine and other beta-2 agonist.
    - Avoid diuretics unless supplemented with potassium chloride.

5. (a) Severe hypokalemia may lead to arrhythmias, ventricular tachycardia, and ventricular fibrillation [5].
   (b) Hypokalemic patients may be sensitive to vasodilators or cardiac-depressant effects of volatile anesthetics.
   (c) Potential for prolonged response to non-depolarizing muscle relaxants.
   (d) Digoxin toxicity can occur with low potassium levels.
   (e) Insulin therapy can lower potassium levels.
   (f) While treating hypokalemia, concurrent hypomagnesemia should also be corrected.

References

1. Lewis JT. ECG diagnosis: hypokalemia. Perm J. 2012;16(2):57.
2. Alasdair R, Gareth J, Chris I. Hypokalaemia: common things occur commonly—a retrospective survey. JRSM Short Rep. 2012;3:80.
3. Faust RJ. Anesthesiology review. 4th ed. New York: Churchill Livingstone; 2014. p. 109–10.
4. Morgan GE, Jr. Clinical anesthesiology. 3rd ed. New York: Lange Medical Books/McGraw-Hill Medical Publishing Division; 2014.
5. Rastergar A, Soleimani M. Hypokalemia and hyperkalemia. Postgrad Med J. 2001;77:759–64.

Chapter 28
Liver Function Testing

Robert C.M. Stephens

A 75-year-old man is scheduled to undergo urgent laparotomy for small bowel obstruction. On preoperative examination he looks jaundiced, and you request a full liver function test profile including total bilirubin, AST, ALT, Alk Phos, gamma-glutamyl transferase (γGT), and glucose. The results show:

Total bilirubin	3.2 mg/dL	(0.2–1.2 mg/dL)
Direct bilirubin	2.8 mg/dL	(0.1–0.4 mg/dL)
AST	14 U/L	(10–40 U/L)
ALT	35 U/L	(7–56 U/L)
Alk phos	260 IU/L	(44–147 IU/L)
γGT	73 IU/L	(0–30 IU/L)
Glucose	81 mg/dL	(79.2 to 110 mg/dL)
Albumin	3.9	(3.4 to 5.4 g/dL)

Questions

1. What are liver function tests, and what are the different ways we can monitor liver function via blood tests?
2. Why might the bilirubin be elevated?
3. What are AST and ALT?
4. Why are alkaline phosphatase and γGT elevated?
5. Why order blood glucose?
6. Are there any other tests that might reflect liver function?
7. What might be the next steps to use or further investigate these results?

R.C.M. Stephens, BA, MBBS, FRCA, MD, FFICM
Department of Anaesthesia, University College London Hospitals, London, UK
e-mail: robcmstephens@googlemail.com

T.D. Raj (ed.), *Data Interpretation in Anesthesia*,
DOI 10.1007/978-3-319-55862-2_28

Answers

1. Liver function tests can [1]:

   - Detect the presence of liver disease and dysfunction
   - Distinguish between different types of liver disorders
   - Monitor the extent of liver damage
   - Monitor responses to treatment

Liver function tests can look at the liver's function in the following ways:

   - Hepatic cell death: transaminases
   - Biliary tree: alkaline phosphatase and γGT
   - Bilirubin manufacture, conjugation, and bile obstruction
   - Synthetic function: albumin, coagulation, and glucose

2. Total bilirubin is made up of unconjugated and conjugated (often called direct) bilirubin. Unconjugated bilirubin is initially formed from heme, mostly from red cell hemoglobin, and is hydrophobic so it is mainly albumin bound. It can also be made from muscle myoglobin, mitochondrial cytochromes, catalase, peroxidase, and nitric oxide synthase. The liver clears the blood of unconjugated bilirubin via hepatocyte conjugation to make it conjugated water-soluble bilirubin. This is secreted into the bile and subsequently the intestine where metabolism of conjugated bilirubin into urobilinogen and its reabsorption accounts for the yellow color of urine. The metabolism of urobilinogen into stercobilin while in the bowels accounts for the brown color of stool; hence having white or clay-colored stool may indicate a blockage in bilirubin processing and thus potential liver dysfunction or obstruction to bile (cholestasis). Raised bilirubin above about 3 mg/dL causes jaundice (from the French "jaune," yellow), the dark yellow pigmentation of the skin, sclerae, and other mucous membranes resulting from excess bilirubin in the extracellular fluid.

   Raised unconjugated bilirubin is caused by pathology prior to the conjugation process: hemolysis, abnormal erythropoiesis, reduced delivery of bilirubin to the liver (cardiac failure, drugs), and defective bilirubin conjugation (congenital syndromes and hyperthyroidism).

   Conjugated hyperbilirubinemia occurs in individuals with hepatocellular damage, biliary obstruction (either intra or extra hepatic), and sepsis.

3. The enzymes aspartate transaminase (AST) (also known as serum glutamic oxaloacetic transaminase, or SGOT) and alanine transaminase (ALT) (formerly called serum glutamic pyruvic transaminase or SGPT) are associated with liver parenchymal cells, and if the liver is damaged, the increased permeability of the hepatocyte membrane causes enzyme leakage out into the systemic circulation. ALT is mainly hepatic, but AST can also be found in cardiac and skeletal muscle. Any liver damage from hepatitis, physical trauma (e.g., surgery), ischemia, or injury from some drugs or toxins may elevate AST and ALT [2].

4. Slightly different forms of the enzyme alkaline phosphatase (Alk Phos) are present in many tissues including the liver, bile ducts, and bones. The enzyme gamma-glutamyl transferase (γGT) is also present in many tissues including the bile duct, pancreas, gallbladder, and kidneys.

Both Alk Phos and γGT are often elevated together in diseases of the biliary tract. Due to γGT's role in drug detoxification, it can be raised by large amounts of alcohol ingestion, although it is not specific to alcohol.

5. If there is severe liver damage, blood glucose can fall as hepatic gluconeogenesis—the liver's ability to produce glucose from noncarbohydrates—goes down, although this is a late feature.

6. Prothrombin time (PT) and its derivative the international normalized ratio (INR) are measures of the extrinsic coagulation pathway. Factors I (fibrinogen), II (prothrombin), V, VII, and X are made in the liver. When liver function is significantly reduced, lowered hepatic production of these factors prolongs the PT and raises the INR.

   Albumin is made in the liver. It transports (hormones, fatty acids, drugs, calcium), buffers plasma pH, and maintains oncotic pressure. Liver disease can result in hypoalbuminemia, although it can also be lost via damaged kidneys, the GI tract (enteropathy), skin (burns), and other conditions. As it is a weak acid, hypoalbuminemia can cause a metabolic alkalosis.

7. After a history and examination, a liver ultrasound or CT abdomen can image the liver, biliary tree, and surrounding structures and identify any hepatic space-occupying lesions. Other tests, for example, for viruses, autoantibodies, or a "fibroscan" (a noninvasive test to quantify liver fibrosis) may be requested as needed.

   Several liver function tests are used as part of risk scoring systems. The Child-Pugh score considers five factors, three of which assess the synthetic function of the liver (total bilirubin level, serum albumin, and INR) along with two more subjective clinical factors (degree of ascites and hepatic encephalopathy). The Model for End-Stage Liver Disease ("MELD") score uses bilirubin, creatinine, and the INR. These scores have been used to predict mortality in patients with hepatic cirrhosis, in patients with cirrhosis undergoing abdominal surgery or hepatic procedures and as part of the assessment for liver transplantation [3, 4].

   The King's College Criteria for transfer to a liver center includes some liver function tests, which differ depending on the cause of the liver disease.

References

1. Limdi JK, Hyde GM. Evaluation of abnormal liver function tests. Postgrad Med J. 2003;79(932):307–12.
2. Giannini ED, Testa R, Savarino V. Liver enzyme alteration: a guide for clinicians. CMAJ. 2005;172(3):367–79.
3. Vaja R, McNicol L, Sisley I. Anaesthesia for patients with liver disease. Contin Educ Anaesth Crit Care Pain. 2010;10(1):15–9.
4. Angermayr B, Cejna M, Karnet F, et al. Child-Pugh versus MELD score in predicting survival in patients undergoing transjugular intrahepatic portosystemic shunt. Gut. 2003;52(6):79–885.

Chapter 29
Coagulation Profile

Abigail Whiteman

A 36-year-old gentleman is admitted to the intensive care unit following major trauma secondary to a road traffic accident. In the course of resuscitation and emergency surgery, he required a 20-unit blood transfusion. Six hours following admission, it is noted that he is bleeding from wound and line puncture sites. The following lab blood tests results are received:

Hemoglobin	73 g/L	(115–145)
Platelets	46×10^9/L	(150–400)
Prothrombin time	33 s	(10–12)
INR	3.3	(0.7–1.3)
Activated partial thromboplastin time	102 s	(25–37)
Fibrinogen	0.6 g/dL	(1.5–4)
D dimer units	1026 ng/mL	(<250)

Questions

1. What is the differential diagnosis of a low platelet count?
2. What is the likely cause of the low platelets in this patient, and how is this condition diagnosed?
3. Which other clinical states are associated with it?
4. Can you describe the pathophysiology behind this condition?
5. What are the principles of management of this condition?
6. Most patients suffering this complication require extensive transfusion of blood products. What are the short- and long-term complications of transfusions of blood products?
7. What is the prothrombin time, and how is it related to the INR?

A. Whiteman, MA(Cantab),MB BChir,FRCA,PGCert
Department of Anaesthesia and Perioperative Medicine,
University College London Hospitals, London, UK
e-mail: abigail.whiteman@doctors.org.uk

T.D. Raj (ed.), *Data Interpretation in Anesthesia*,
DOI 10.1007/978-3-319-55862-2_29

Answers

1 Thrombocytopenia is defined as a platelet count of less than $150 \times 10^9/L^7$. It may be due to:

- A decreased production of platelets:
  - Selective impairment of platelet production: drugs (alcohol, thiazide diuretics, cytotoxic drugs) and viral infections
  - Generalized disease of the bone marrow: aplastic anemia or marrow infiltration in leukemia or dissemination cancer
- Decreased platelet survival
  - With an immune basis: idiopathic thrombocytopenia purpura, systemic lupus erythematosus, drugs (heparin), and infections (infectious mononucleosis, HIV, CMV)
  - Without an immune basis: disseminated intravascular coagulation, thrombotic thrombocytopenic purpura, and cardiopulmonary bypass
- Sequestration
  - Hypersplenism
- Dilutional
  - Following massive transfusion of stored blood

2 The likely diagnosis in this patient is disseminated intravascular coagulation (DIC). The diagnosis of DIC is not made by the examination of a single laboratory marker but based on the combination of clinical history and a number of test results [1, 2].

Features suggestive of DIC in the clinical history include the presence of clinical conditions known to trigger DIC (see below) and also the clinical presentation due to the resultant consumptive coagulopathy: widespread petechiae and ecchymosis and blood oozing from wound sites, intravenous lines, catheters, and surgical drains. When injury to the pulmonary vasculature occurs, hemoptysis and acute respiratory distress syndrome may result. Other serious complications of DIC include acute renal failure, thrombosis, gangrene, and loss of digits, intracerebral hematoma, and cardiac tamponade.

Laboratory features suggestive of DIC include:

- Rapidly declining platelet count
- Prolonged prothrombin (PT) time
- Prolonged activated partial thromboplastin (aPTT) time
- Low fibrinogen levels, although only a clinical feature of approximately 30% of the more severe cases
- Raised fibrin degradation products (FDPs) and elevated D dimer level

3 Disseminated intravascular coagulation is an acquired complication of an underlying illness where systematic activation of the coagulation system occurs when blood is exposed to procoagulants [1, 2]. The process can be classified as either:

- Acute or decompensated DIC, which occurs over a short-time period

- Chronic or compensated DIC, where small amounts of procoagulant are released over longer-time period

Conditions commonly associated with DIC include:

- Sepsis and severe infection
- Trauma: severe tissue injury, head injury, fat embolism
- Cancer: myeloproliferative diseases and solid tumors, e.g. pancreatic or prostate carcinomas
- Obstetric complications: amniotic fluid embolism and placental abruption
- Vascular disorders: aortic aneurysm and giant hemangiomas
- Reaction to toxins: snake venom and drugs
- Immunologic disorders: severe allergic reaction, hemolytic transfusion reaction, and transplant rejection

4 Disseminated intravascular coagulation is characterized by systemic activation of coagulation through the release of tissue thromboplastin or thromboplastic substances into the circulation. This leads to the widespread intravascular deposition of fibrin throughout the microcirculation [1, 2, 3]. As a result of this widespread thrombosis, there is a depletion of coagulation factors and platelets. There is also a secondary pathological activation of fibrinolysis.

Thus DIC may result in microinfarcts and tissue hypoxia caused by microemboli as well as a coagulopathy due to the deletion of factors required for hemostasis (consumption coagulopathy).

5 Management of DIC should involve:

1. Treatment of the underlying cause
2. Supportive therapy and replacement of blood components [4]

The major focus of management of DIC is specific and vigorous treatment of the underlying disorder. This may be an aggressive management of sepsis or an infective source, evacuation of the uterus in the case of intrauterine death or debridement of tissues in the case of severe burns or trauma. Without management of the cause, treatment of DIC is likely to fail.

The decision to transfuse blood products should not be based on the results of coagulation tests alone but on the need to treat an actively bleeding patient. Blood products may also be used as prophylaxis to prevent bleeding but the literature to support this use is limited.

Commonly transfused products to correct coagulopathy:

- Fresh frozen plasma: a standard dose of 10–15 mL/kg should be used during active hemorrhage, aiming for an INR of less than 1.5 and an aPTT ratio of less than 1.5.
- Platelets: the current British Society of Haematology guidelines suggest that platelet counts should be maintained at over 75×10^{-9}/L in patients who are bleeding. The platelet count is expected to rise by $30–50 \times 10^{-9}$/L after the transfusion of a single pooled unit.

- Cryoprecipitate: cryoprecipitate should be used in a bleeding patient when the fibrinogen level is less than 1.5 g/L. A standard transfusion of two bags of cryoprecipitate is expected to increase the fibrinogen concentration by 0.5 to 1 g/L.

The use of anticoagulants, such as heparin, has been proposed to interrupt the systemic activation of coagulation seen in DIC. However, clinical trials have so far failed to show benefit.

6 The transfusion of blood products to support the hemoglobin level and correct coagulation abnormalities can be a life-saving intervention in DIC [7]. However, prior to any transfusion, full consideration should be given to its necessity; transfusion of blood products has been proven to have multiple long- and short-term complications [5, 4].
Early complications of blood product transfusion

- Hemolytic reactions
  - Immediate
  - Delayed
- Acute nonhemolytic transfusion reactions
  - Febrile
  - Allergic
  - Hypotensive
- Transfusion-related acute lung injury (TRALI)
- Transfusion-associated circulatory overload (TACO)
- Reactions secondary to bacterial contamination

Complications specific to massive transfusion (complete replacement of the circulating blood volume in 24 h)

- Hypothermia
- Dilutional coagulopathy if inadequate coagulation factors replaced relative to packed red cells
- Hyperkalemia
- Citrate toxicity resulting in hypocalcemia and hypomagnesemia

Late complications of blood product transfusion

- Transmission of infection
  - Viral (hepatitis A, B, and C, HIV and CMV)
  - Bacterial (*Treponema pallidum*, *Salmonella*)
  - Parasites (malaria, toxoplasma)
- Transfusion-associated graft-versus-host disease
- Immune modulation possibly resulting in worse outcomes in cancer recurrence and metastases
- Immune sensitization (Rhesus D antigen)

7 The prothrombin time is an assay to evaluate factors within the extrinsic pathway of the coagulation cascade: II, V, VII, and X [6]. Tissue thromboplastin (a brain extract) and calcium are added to citrated plasma. Clotting normally takes place in 10 to 12 s.

The prothrombin time has significant interlaboratory variability influenced by the thromboplastin used. In an effort to offset variation in thromboplastin reagent and enhance standardization of PT in patients receiving oral anticoagulants, the World Health Organization (WHO) introduced the international normalized ratio (INR) in 1983.

The INR is a mathematical conversion of a patient's PT that accounts for the sensitivity of the reagent used in a given laboratory, by factoring in the international sensitivity index (ISI). Each manufacturer assigns an ISI value for any tissue factor they manufacture. The ISI value indicates how a particular batch of tissue factor compares to an international reference tissue factor. The ISI is usually between 0.94 and 1.4.

The INR is then calculated using the following formula:

$INR = [\text{Patient PT}/\text{Mean PT}]^{ISI}$

In this formula, patient PT is measured prothrombin time, mean PT is geometric mean PT of at least 20 healthy subjects of both sexes tested at a particular laboratory, and ISI is international sensitivity index that is specific to each reagent-instrument combination.

References

1. Levi M, Ten-Cate H. Disseminated intravascular coagulation. N Engl J Med. 1999;341(8):586–92.
2. Levi M. Disseminated intravascular coagulation. Crit Care Med. 2007;35(9):2191–5.
3. Kumar V, Cotran RS, Robbins SL. Basic pathology. 6th ed. Philadelphia: Saunders; 1997.
4. Maxwell MJ, Wilson MJA. Complications of blood transfusion. Contin Educ Anaesth Crit Care Pain. 2006;6(6):225–9.
5. Clevenger B, Kelleher A. Hazards of blood transfusion in adults and children. Contin Educ Anaesth Crit Care Pain. 2014;14(3):112–8.
6. Levy JH, Szlam F, Wolberg AS, Winkler A. Clinical use of the activated partial thromboplastin time and prothrombin time for screening: a review of the literature and current guidelines for testing. Clin Lab Med. 2014;34(3):453–77.
7. Retter A, Barrett NA. The management of abnormal haemostasis in the ICU. Anaesthesia. 2015;70:121–7.

Chapter 30
Thromboelastogram I

Tilak D. Raj

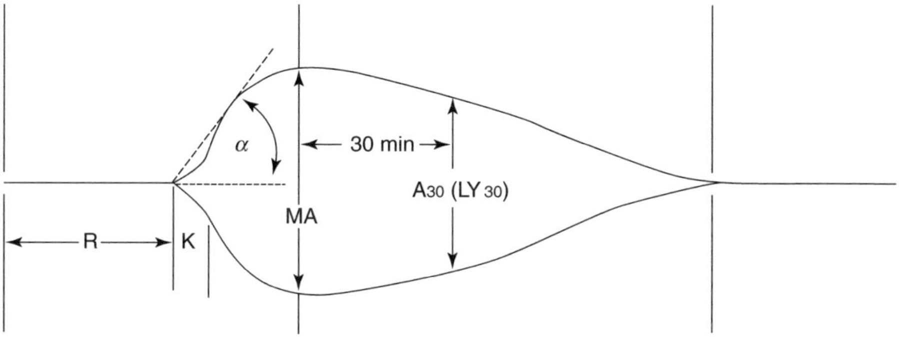

Fig. 30.1

Questions

1. What does the data in Fig. 30.1 show?
2. When can it be used?
3. How is it produced?
4. What do the parameters R, K, α, MA, and A_{30} (LY_{30}) indicate?
5. How can the above parameters be used to guide therapy?
6. What is platelet mapping and how does it help?
7. How does thromboelastography (TEG®) differ from rotational thromboelastometry (ROTEM®)?

T.D. Raj, MD, MRCP, FRCA
Department of Anesthesiology, Alliance Health Midwest, Midwest City, OK, USA
e-mail: tilakdraj@gmail.com

T.D. Raj (ed.), *Data Interpretation in Anesthesia*,
DOI 10.1007/978-3-319-55862-2_30

Answers

1. The data shown represents a typical thromboelastography (TEG) trace. Thromboelastography is a viscoelastic hemostatic assay that measures global properties of whole blood clot formation. It shows the interaction of platelets with the coagulation cascade including aggregation, clot strengthening, fibrin cross-linking, and fibrinolysis. TEG is an effective and convenient means of monitoring whole blood coagulation and provides a global assessment of hemostatic function.

   It can assist in determining if a patient has normal hemostasis or is bleeding due to a coagulopathy or anticoagulant therapy.

2. Conventional coagulation tests like PT and aPTT poorly reflect in vivo hemostasis. As they are performed in plasma, they assess only a portion of the coagulation system and do not provide information on the full balance between coagulation and anticoagulation. In contrast TEG is performed on whole blood and provides information on clot formation, stabilization, and dissolution thus assessing coagulation and fibrinolysis.

   TEG is used to assess hemostasis during liver transplantation, postpartum hemorrhage, cardiac surgery, and in trauma resuscitation. It can also be used in coagulopathy due to other reasons such as sepsis and guide management. TEG can also provide information on the presence and adequacy of platelet inhibition.

   In cardiac surgery during cardiopulmonary bypass, abnormal coagulation can be identified before heparin reversal with the addition of heparinase to the testing. This will be useful in long pump runs, in deep hypothermia, in the presence of ventricular assist devices, and in major vascular procedures. In pinpointing the specific problem, TEG has been shown to reduce blood transfusion in cardiac surgery [1, 2].

3. The test sample is placed in an oscillating cup (4–45° every 5 s) heated to 37 °C. A pin is suspended into the sample by a torsion wire which is attached to a mechanical/electrical transducer. The elasticity and strength of the developing clot changes the motion of the pin which is converted into a graphical and numerical output which is displayed.

4. The above tracing can be looked at in the following phases.
   (a) **Initial clot formation**

   Split point (SP) time = from the start of the test to the split of the trace (first detectable fibrin)

   Reaction (R) time = from the start till the trace reaching 2 mm amplitude (1 mm either side of baseline) and represents continued production of thrombin and conversion of fibrinogen to fibrin (normal 4–9 min kaolin activated). Prolonged R in factor deficiency and anticoagulants.

   R-SP = delta (**Δ**). Thrombin burst. Low delta indicates hypercoagulability and vice versa (normal 0.7–1.1 min). The test can be performed with heparinase (TEG-H), and a difference of more than 2 min between R value of TEG and TEG-H indicates heparin effect.

Fig. 30.2 TEG technology—how it works

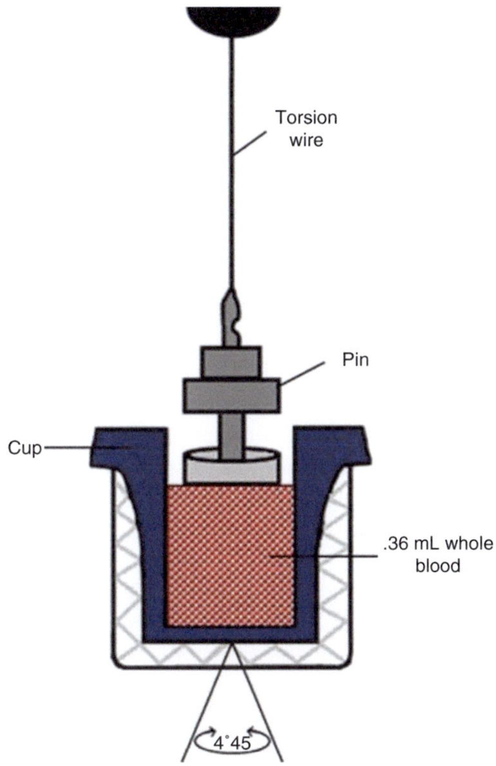

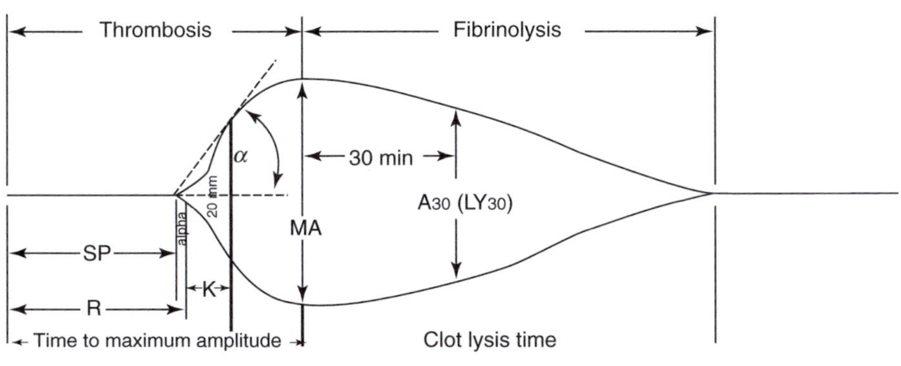

Fig. 30.3 Components of normal TEG tracing

(b) **Conversion of fibrinogen to fibrin**

Kinetics (K) time = time interval between 2 mm and 20 mm on the trace and represents fibrin cross-linkage and rate of bonding between fibrin and platelets and is a measure of fibrinogen function (normal 1–3 min kaolin activated). Prolonged by anticoagulants, hypofibrinogenemia and thrombocytopenia and shortened by increased fibrinogen level and platelet function.

Angle (α) = the angle at which the curve rises from SP to K and is related directly to K time as a measure of fibrin platelet interaction and therefore functional fibrinogen (normal 59–74°)

(c) **Clot strength**

Maximum amplitude in mm (MA) = represents clot strength and platelet function (normal 55–74 mm).

G = this is calculated from platelet performance (MA) and expressed as resistance unit (normal 5.3–13.2 dynes/cm^2).

(d) **Clot lysis**

A_{30}, LY_{30}, EPL_{30} = percentage amplitude at 30 min post-MA (A_{30}). Clot lysis begins a short period after MA is reached and continues for about 15 min. The software estimates the percent lysis during this period (EPL_{30}). After 30 min the EPL_{30} becomes the percent lysis LY_{30} (normal 0–7.5%).

The interpretation of the parameters can be summarized as:

Hypocoagulable	↑ R (min)	↑ K (min) ↓ α (deg)	↓ MA	LY30 > 7.5% EPL > 15%
Hypercoagulable	↓ R (min)	↓ K (min) ↑ α (deg	↑ MA	NA

5. Increased R time—FFP (one unit of FFP will decrease R time by 2.5 min)

   Decreased angle—cryoprecipitate

   Decreased MA—DDAVP for slight decrease and platelets for more significant decrease (one unit of platelets increase MA by 7–9 m)

   Fibrinolysis—tranexamic acid, aminocaproic acid, or aprotinin

	TEG interpretation and treatment protocol—guidelines	
TEG parameter	Cause	Treatment
R and K decreased, MA increased	Hypercoagulability	Anticoagulant
Normal parameters, patient bleeding	Surgical	Reexplore
Difference in R between TEG plain and TEG-H > 2 min	Heparin	Protamine
Delta <1.2, R > 9 min, normal MA and G	Hemodilution	If bleeding reexploration or DDAVP
Prolonged R and delta, normal MA	Factor deficiency	FFP (one unit for every 2.5 min R prolongation)
Angle less than 45°	Low fibrinogen	Cryo 0.06 U/kg
MA 46–54 mm	Low platelet function	DDAVP 0.3 mcg/kg
MA less than 45 mm	Very low platelet function	Platelets one unit for every 8 mm
LY30 7.5% or more, CI < 1	Primary fibrinolysis, e.g., TPA	Antifibrinolytic
LY30 7.5% or more, CI > 3	Secondary fibrinolysis (DIC)	Anticoagulant

6. Platelet mapping provides the degree of inhibition of platelets via the ADP (Plavix) and AA (Aspirin) pathways and thereby the effectiveness of the antiplatelet drugs which cannot be done with routinely available coagulation tests. This involves four separate (channels) analyses.

   (a) Baseline—kaolin activates platelets maximally as in regular TEG.
   (b) Activator—heparin (via heparinized tube to draw the sample) to inhibit thrombin and activator to convert fibrinogen to fibrin. Activator is reptilase and Factor XIIIa (contribution of fibrin to clot).
   (c) ADP—like previous (for fibrin clot) plus ADP added to activate platelets via the GP IIb/IIIa receptor.
   (d) AA—activator for fibrin clot and arachidonic acid to activate thromboxane A2 pathway producing platelet aggregation.

   It is possible to determine the (percent) platelet inhibition by comparing the relative strengths of the clots in the activator, ADP or AA cups with the baseline. The residual function (percent aggregation) is multiplied by the baseline G to get the net G or net clot strength. The goal is to maintain it between 5 and 9 to prevent bleeding or thrombosis [3].

7. While TEG and ROTEM both measure the viscoelastic hemostasis of whole blood ROTEM is a modern modification of TEG. There are differences in the operations of the testing and the nomenclature. In ROTEM, the heated cup with the sample is fixed, but the pin suspended on a ball bearing mechanism rotates through an arc of 4–75° every 6 s, and the clot characteristics are measured by an optical sensor.
   ROTEM can measure four samples, while TEG can measure two samples simultaneously.
   ROTEM utilizes automated pipetting, while TEG requires manual pipetting.
   TEG is sensitive to vibrations, whereas ROTEM is resistant to mechanical shocks.
   Nomenclature (not interchangeable) for ROTEM as compared to TEG:
   Clotting time (CT) = R (reaction) time (time for trace to reach 2 mm in both)

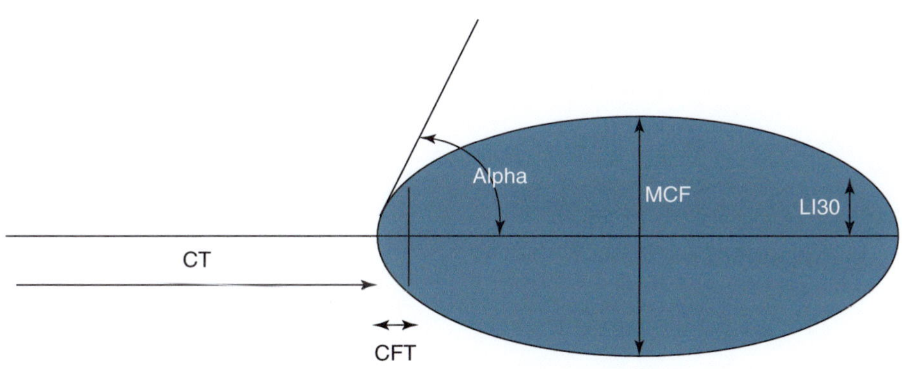

Fig. 30.4 Components of normal ROTEM tracing

Clot formation time (CFT) = K (kinetics) time (time for trace to reach 20 mm in both)
α angle = α angle
Maximum clot firmness (MCF) = maximum amplitude (MA)
Lysis = lysis index 30 (LI30) is the percent reduction in MCF 30 min after CT in ROTEM, whereas in TEG LY30 and LY60 (lysis 30 and lysis 60) are the percent reductions of the curve 30 and 60 min after MA is reached.
Additional ROTEM assays:
INTEM = contact activation, information similar to APTT
EXTEM = tissue factor activation, information similar to PT
HEPTEM = assesses heparin effect
APTEM = in conjunction with EXTEM assesses fibrinolysis
FIBTEM = in conjunction EXTEM allows qualitative analysis of the contribution of fibrinogen to clot strength independent of platelets [4].

References

1. Müller MC, et al. Utility of thromboelastography and/or thromboelastometry in adults with sepsis: a systematic review. Crit Care. 2014;18:R30.
2. Thakur M, Ahmed AB. A review of thromboelastography. Int J Periop Ultrasound Appl Technol. 2012;1(1):25–9.
3. TEG: THEORY AND APPLICATION. http://www.visaliapath.com/tegtheory/. Accessed 2 June 2016.
4. Whiting W, DiNardo JA. TEG and ROTEM: technology and clinical applications. Am J Hematol. 2014;89:228–32.

Chapter 31
Thromboelastogram II

Tilak D. Raj

For each of the TEG tracings below, provide the abnormality and intervention if appropriate.

1.

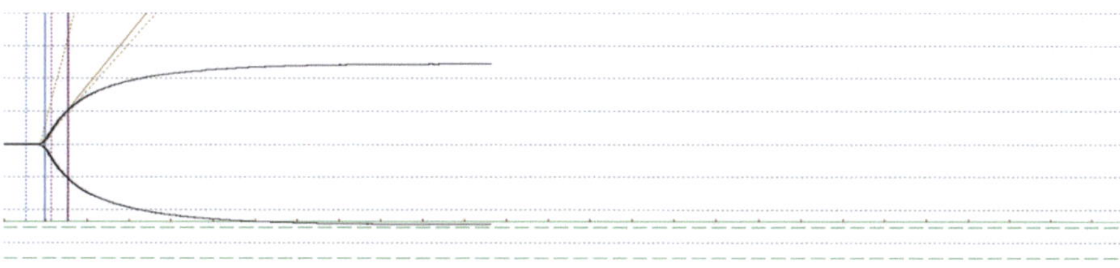

R	K	Angle	MA	PMA	G	EPL	A	CI	LY30
min	min	deg	mm		d/sc	%	mm	−1.8	%
4.8	2.7	57.6	47.0	0.0	4.4K	0.0	49.0	−3—3	0—8
2—8	1—3	55—78	51—69		4.6K—10.9K	0—15			

Fig. 31.1

T.D. Raj, MD, MRCP, FRCA
Department of Anesthesiology, Alliance Health Midwest, Midwest City, OK, USA
e-mail: tilakdraj@gmail.com

T.D. Raj (ed.), *Data Interpretation in Anesthesia*,
DOI 10.1007/978-3-319-55862-2_31

2.

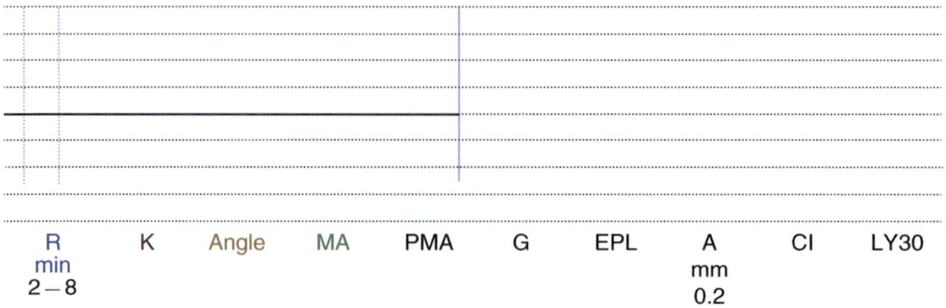

Fig. 31.2

3.

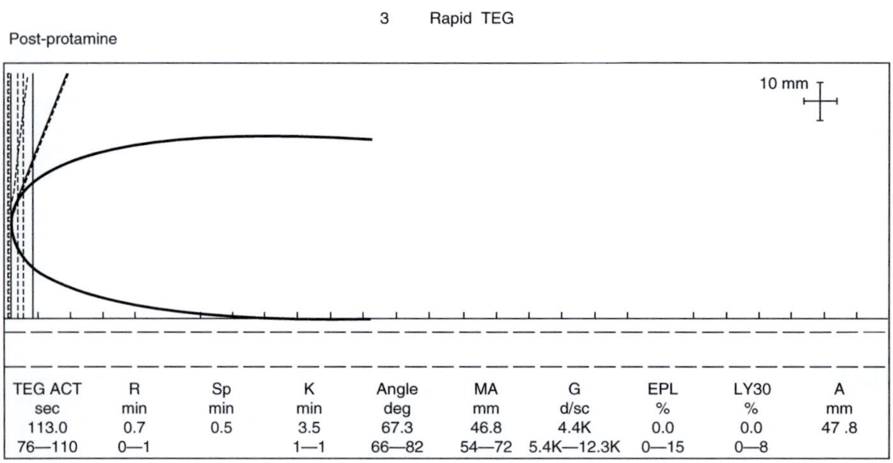

Fig. 31.3

4.

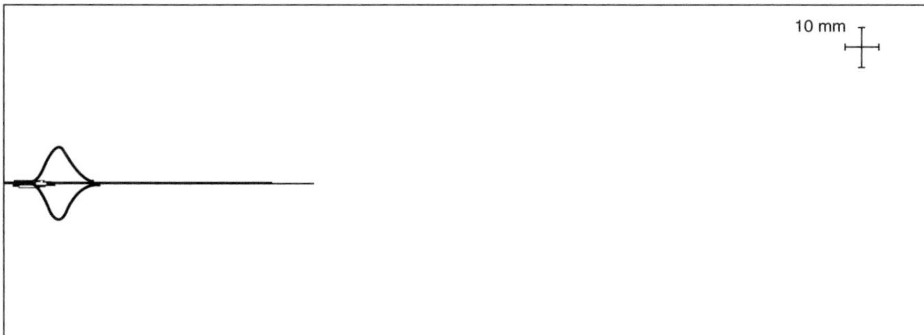

TEG ACT	SP	R	K	Angle	MA	G	EPL	LY30	A
	min	min	min	deg	mm	d/sc	%	%	mm
	4.3	4.9	N\A	53.3	17.5	1.1K	93.0	93.0	0 .2
		5—10	1—3	53—72	50—70	4.5K—11.0K	0—15	0—8	

Fig. 31.4

5.

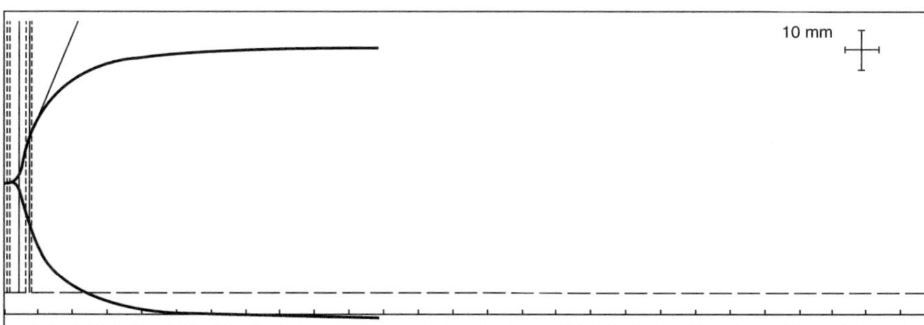

TEG ACT	R	Sp	K	Angle	MA	G	EPL	LY30	A
sec	min	min	min	deg	mm	d/sc	%	%	mm
245.0	2.1	0.5	1.6	66.2	64.6	9.1K	0.0	0.0	66.4
76—110	0—1		1—2	66—82	54—72	5.4K—12.3K	0—15	0—8	

Fig. 31.5

6.

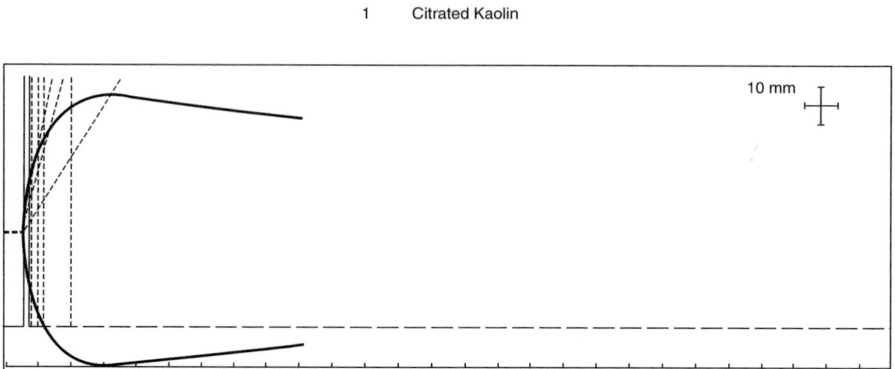

TEG ACT	SP	R	K	Angle	MA	G	EPL	LY30	A
	min	min	min	deg	mm	d/sc	%	%	mm
	2.6	2.9	0.8	77.3	69.9	11.6K	8.2	8.2	58.6
		5—10	1—3	53—72	50—70	4.5K—11.0K	0—15	0—8	

Fig. 31.6

7.

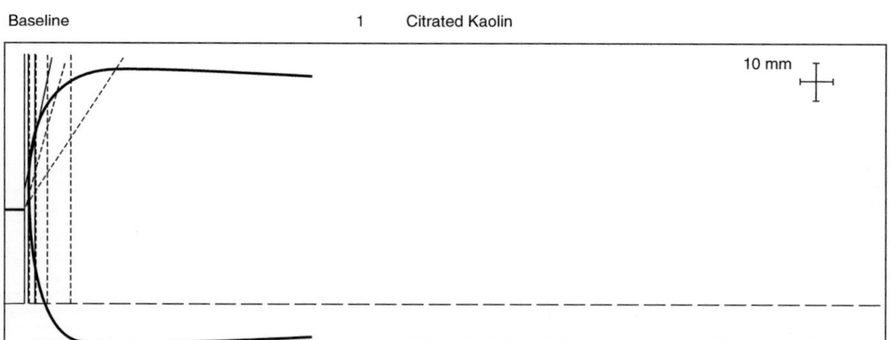

TEG ACT	SP	R	K	Angle	MA	G	EPL	LY30	A
	min	min	min	deg	mm	d/sc	%	%	mm
	3.4	3.7	0.8	78.8	72.3	13.0K	2.5	2.5	68.0
		5—10	1—3	53—72	50—70	4.5K—11.0K	0—15	0—8	

Fig. 31.7

8.

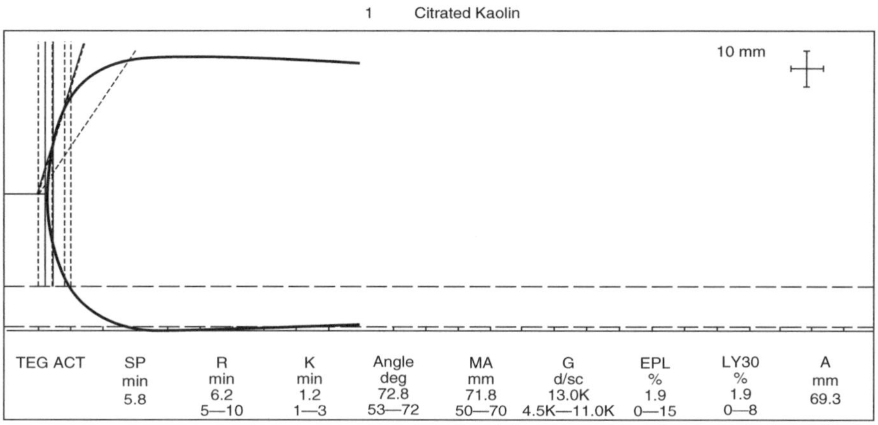

Fig. 31.8

9.

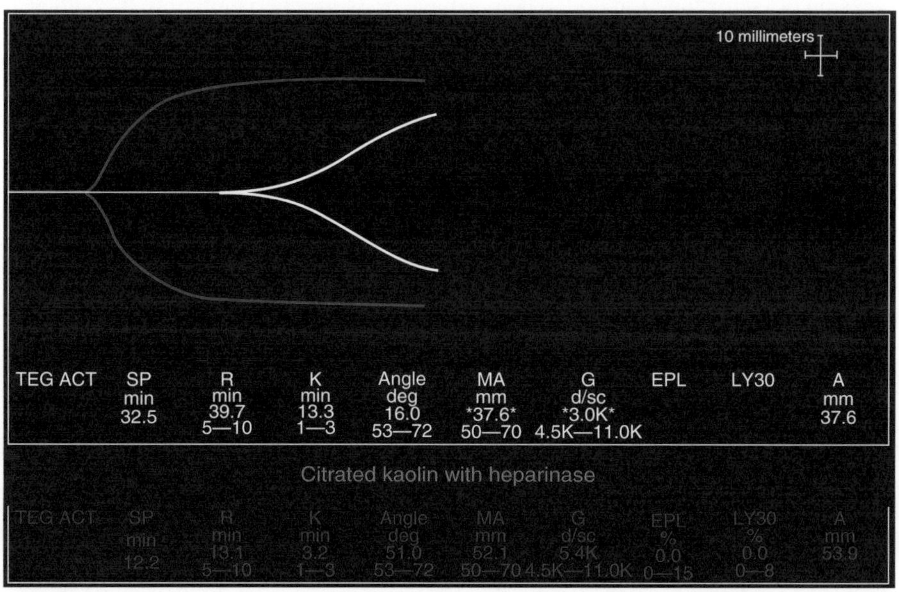

Fig. 31.9

10.

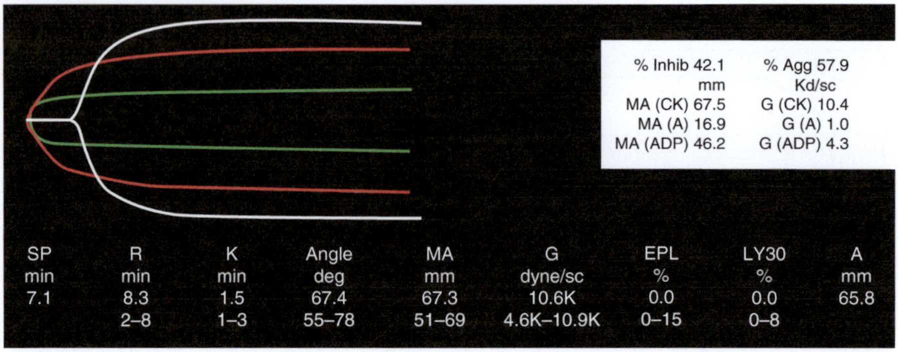

Fig. 31.10

Answers

1. The low MA and G demonstrate hypocoagulable platelet function. If the patient is bleeding, platelets and/or DDAVP may be indicated.

2. This flatline tracing demonstrates a complete inability to form a clot and can be a result of several things. Clinically, it can be an extreme deficiency/suppression of factor function due to hemorrhage or over-anticoagulation. It could also be a technical error in the running of the test (not adding calcium to a citrated sample, or not loading the cup/pin properly). If it is due to any of the clinical reasons mentioned, FFP or reversal of anticoagulation would be indicated.

3. This tracing shows a minor decrease in factor function (TEGACT) and a significant reduction in platelet function with the low MA and G values. Fibrinogen function is also affected slightly (angle and K). If the patient is bleeding, a dose of platelets should not only improves platelet function but contains a unit of thawed plasma and about 400 mg of fibrinogen, which should normalize the TEGACT and K values. DDAAVP may be useful to get the maximum impact from the platelets.

4. This tracing demonstrates primary fibrinolysis. The key criteria are a decreased MA and G and elevated fibrinolysis (LY30). Treatment is an antifibrinolytic like Amicar or tranexamic Acid. Factors demonstrate slightly hypercoagulability with the shortened R value, but no assessment of fibrinogen or platelet function can be made, until the fibrinolysis is corrected. The antifibrinolytic will typically correct the lysis quickly.

5. This tracing shows prolonged TEGACT indicating either factor deficiency or anticoagulant effect. Since this is a post-protamine sample, it may be due to residual heparin still circulating. If the heparinase tracing shows a lower TEGACT value, then additional protamine would be indicated. If the TEGACT does not shorten in the heparinase cup, then FFP would be indicated.

6. This tracing shows hypercoagulability of factors (shortened R); fibrinogen (K and angle), and platelets indicate slight hypercoagulability. Fibrinolysis (LY30)

is also elevated. This could be indicating stage 1 DIC, or a patient with some form of thrombus that is initiating the lytic system. The assessment of the patient should focus on identifying the underlying cause of the hypercoagulability and treating the cause, and possibly treating the hypercoagulability with some form of anticoagulant.

7. This tracing shows hypercoagulability of factors (R), fibrinogen (K and angle), and platelets (MA and G). First priority is to identify the cause of the hypercoagulability. If it is thrombin driven (due to trauma, cancer, or some other inflammatory process), then anticoagulation may be the treatment of choice. If it is likely platelet driven (stents or artificial surfaces exposed to the blood), then antiplatelet agents may be the treatment of choice.

8. Platelet function is hypercoagulable (MA and G), and fibrinogen function (angle) is borderline hypercoagulable. As the angle is indicative of platelet-fibrin interaction, platelets would be the primary target of inhibition.

9. The citrated kaolin tracing (white) shows decreased function of all parameters. This dysfunction significantly improves in the heparinase cup, leaving only milder factor deficiency (R), and slightly hypocoagulable fibrinogen function (K and angle). Treatment would be protamine to treat the heparin effect, and possibly some FFP (depending upon presence or degree of bleeding). The approximately 300 mg of fibrinogen contained within a bag of FFP will likely correct the fibrinogen values.

10. This set of tracings is an ADP study of the PlateletMapping® assay. There is a slight prolongation of the R value (8.3; range: 2–8), but with 42.1% inhibition on the ADP assay, the platelet function is not at the high end of normal, as the basic TEG would suggest. Looking at the MA value of the ADP tracing (46.2 in the popup box), this is a little below the normal range for MA of 51–69 mm. This would indicate decreased platelet function and, if the patient was going for a procedure, an increased risk of bleeding with the procedure. Options would be to delay procedure, if elective, until the inhibition decreases (if due to meds) or, if urgent, to proceed with platelets and/or DDAVP being available.

Further Reading

1. Holcomb JB, Minei KM, Scerbo ML, et al. Admission rapid thromboelastography can replace conventional coagulation tests in the emergency department. Ann Surg. 2012;256(3):476–86.
2. Kashuk JL, Moore EE, Wohlauer H, et al. Initial experiences with point-of-care rapid thromboelastography for management of life threatening postinjury coagulopathy. Transfusion. 2012;52:23–33.
3. McGrath DJ, et al. [Thromboelastography analysis] maximum amplitude predicts postoperative thrombotic complications including myocardial infarction. Anesth Analg. 2005;100:1576–83.
4. Cryer GH, et al. Massive transfusion in trauma guidelines. In American College of Surgeons. Trauma Quality Improvement Program. Best Practice Guidelines. https://www.facs.org/~/media/files/quality%20programs/trauma/tqip/massive%20transfusion%20in%20trauma%20guildelines.ashx. Accessed 9 October 2016.

Chapter 32
Urine Testing

John David Srinivasan

A 55-year-old, 110 kg male with a history of alcoholic cirrhosis was admitted with mental status changes and a decrease in urine output over the last 2 days.

Labs from this admission showed: creatinine 3.4 mg/dL (was 1.1 mg/dL, a month ago), blood urea nitrogen (BUN) 70 mg/dL (18 mg/dL, a month ago), serum bilirubin 3 mg/dL, potassium 5.7 mg/dL, and sodium 125 mEq/L. The patient was diagnosed with acute renal failure.

Questions

1. What is the initial step in the evaluation of this patient?
2. What are the basic diagnostic tests that are used to distinguish prerenal disease from acute tubular necrosis (ATN)?
3. How is FENa estimated? How does it help in diagnosis?
4. What is contrast-induced nephropathy, its risk factors and measures to decrease risk?
5. What is FEUrea? When is it used?
6. What are the causes of ARF in this patient?
7. Is hepatorenal syndrome (HRS) a type of ATN?
8. What is RIFLE criteria and AKIN classification?

J.D. Srinivasan, MD, FRCA
Assistant Professor, Department of Anesthesiology and Critical Care,
Saint Louis Univeristy, School of Medicine, 3635 Vista Ave., PO Box 15250, St. Louis, MO 63110-0250, USA
e-mail: srinivjd@slu.edu

T.D. Raj (ed.), *Data Interpretation in Anesthesia*,
DOI 10.1007/978-3-319-55862-2_32

Answers

1. A careful history and physical examination frequently identify events and/or disease processes that result in decreased tissue perfusion that can lead to prerenal disease (e.g., vomiting, diarrhea, bleeding, or sepsis) or post-ischemic acute tubular necrosis (ATN). Clinical setting may help identify the underlying cause of AKI (e.g., hypotension, sepsis, aminoglycoside therapy, NSAIDS, or the administration of radiocontrast media).

   Physical examination may suggest hypovolemia, such as unexplained tachycardia, dry mucous membranes, decreased skin turgor, cool extremities, and orthostatic hypotension. Other physical exam findings may reveal signs of heart failure or cirrhosis presenting with edema, ascites, and other signs of specific organ dysfunction or may reveal abdominal compartment syndrome.

   Examination should also include ultrasonography of the bladder to rule out obstructive etiology.

2. There are three basic diagnostic tests:
   (a) Urinalysis with sediment examination:
   - Normal or near normal (hyaline and/or fine granular casts) in prerenal disease.
   - Muddy brown granular, epithelial cell casts, and free renal tubular epithelial cells in ATN.
   - RBC/WBC casts could suggest glomerulonephritis.
   - WBC casts with eosinophils could suggest interstitial nephritis.

   (b) Fractional excretion of sodium (FENa), and to a lesser degree, the urine sodium concentration. The fractional excretion of urea may be helpful in patients being treated with diuretics as FENa is increased by diuretics due to the natriuresis.

   (c) Response to fluid repletion: This is the gold standard for the distinction between prerenal disease secondary to volume depletion and post-ischemic or nephrotoxic ATN. Return of the serum creatinine to the previous baseline within 24 to 72 h after volume repletion represents prerenal disease, whereas persistent AKI represents ATN.

3.

$$\text{FENa} = \frac{\text{urinary Na} \times \text{serum Cr} \times 100}{\text{serum Na} \times \text{urinary Cr}}$$

By definition, FENa is the ratio between the quantity of Na excreted in the urine relative to the amount filtered at the glomerulus. Measuring urine sodium concentration alone is not sufficient, as the sodium concentration in urine varies with water reabsorption. It is necessary to plug in the serum and urinary creatinine into the calculation, in order to calculate the amount of fluid and sodium that is filtered through to glomerulus [1, 2].

Prerenal AKI can be due to intrarenal vasoconstriction, systemic vasodilation, and volume depletion. These patients will try to compensate and retain sodium and usually have a FENa of less than 1%. If any of the above insults continue and become intense, the blood supply to the renal tubules is severely reduced leading to acute tubular necrosis. Once the tubules are damaged, they lose their ability to reabsorb sodium, and the FENa will usually be greater than 2–3%.

FENa is often used in the setting of acute renal failure to help distinguish between prerenal (decreased renal perfusion) and intrinsic renal (ATN due to renal hypoperfusion) causes. In general, a FENa of <1% suggests prerenal disease, between 1 and 2% is indeterminate, and >2% suggests ATN. There are some exceptions to this, but overall, the specificity of this test is >80%.

There are **limitations** to FENa. The threshold used to distinguish prerenal and intrinsic renal disease may vary; there are other causes of low FENa and salt-wasting conditions (like diuresis) affect urinary sodium levels.

4. **Contrast-induced nephropathy** (CIN) is either a relative increase in serum creatinine from baseline value by 25% or an absolute increase of 0.5 mg/dL within 48 to 72 h after contrast exposure not attributable to other causes and must persist for 2 to 5 days. FENa may vary widely and in the minority of patients with oliguric CIN, the FENa may be low despite lack of clinical evidence of volume depletion [3].

   Risk factors include pre-existing renal dysfunction, diabetes with renal dysfunction, age >70 years, cardiorespiratory disease, hypotension or dehydration, and nephrotoxic medications (NSAIDs or aminoglycosides). Contrast agent volume, route of administration (intra-arterial), hyperosmolarity, and multiple doses in 72 h also add to the risk.

   Measures to decrease risk of CIN include prehydration with saline, using the lowest dose of low osmolar contrast, IV bicarbonate infusion, N-acetylcysteine (controversial), discontinuation of nephrotoxic drugs for 48 h prior to contrast, and the use of hemofiltration (expensive) pre- and post-contrast use.

5. Fractional excretion of other substances such as urea and uric acid can also be measured to determine their renal clearance to help distinguish prerenal from intrinsic renal causes. The FEUrea may be more accurate in distinguishing ATN from prerenal disease in patients being treated with diuretics since diuretics as mentioned earlier cause natriuresis.

$$\text{FEUrea}\left(\text{percent}\right) = \frac{\text{Urinary urea} \times \text{Serum Creatinine}}{\text{Serum urea} \times \text{Urinary Creatinine}} \times 100$$

   FEUrea is 50 to 65% (>0.5) in acute tubular necrosis (ATN) and usually below 35% in prerenal disease [1, 2].

6. The differential diagnosis of acute kidney injury (AKI) or acute renal failure (ARF) in this patient with cirrhosis includes prerenal azotemia, acute tubular necrosis, and hepatorenal syndrome (HRS). Prerenal azotemia is caused by hypovolemia (e.g., aggressive diuresis, diarrhea, and/or gastrointestinal bleeding) or by other causes of decreased effective blood volume induced by infections or vasodilators. Prerenal azotemia responds to volume expansion, and vasoconstrictors and dialysis are not required.

   Acute tubular necrosis mostly occurs in patients presenting with shock or a history of exposure to nephrotoxins/contrast agents. Acute tubular necrosis is treated with renal replacement therapy if indicated.

HRS occurs in patients with cirrhosis or liver failure when there is a sudden rapid deterioration of liver function due to an insult like gastrointestinal bleed, infection, or excessive diuresis. It is caused by extreme vasodilatation with consequent renal vasoconstriction and is treated with vasoconstrictors and volume expansion with albumin. HRS remains a diagnosis of exclusion. Therefore, the first step in its diagnosis is to exclude the presence of structural kidney injury (acute tubular necrosis, glomerulonephritis, and acute interstitial nephritis) or obstructive kidney injury (obstructive uropathy) and to then distinguish between prerenal azotemia and HRS (the two functional types of AKI in cirrhosis).

7. Renal dysfunction in HRS is functional. The pathophysiology of cirrhosis involves portal hypertension leading to splanchnic arterial vasodilatation. The resultant primary systemic arterial vasodilatation leads to systemic hypotension which in turn causes activation of the neurohumoral axis with stimulation of the renin–angiotensin–aldosterone system (RAAS), sympathetic nervous system (SNS), and arginine vasopressin (AVP). Stimulation of the RAAS, SNS, and AVP contributes to maintenance of blood pressure by increasing systemic vascular resistance along with the secondary increase in cardiac output. While this compensatory neurohumoral activation attenuates any hypotension secondary to arterial vasodilatation, renal vasoconstriction with sodium and water retention also occurs. This resultant diminished renal function is, however, of a functional nature and thus should not be considered ATN in the initial phases. Prolonged and severe HRS can then lead to ATN [4, 5].

8. The **RIFLE** criteria were created by the **Acute Dialysis Quality Initiative (ADQI)** in 2002 to define AKI.

Stage	GFR	Urine output
Risk	1.5–2 × Serum Cr increase or >25% GFR decrease	<0.5 mL/kg/h <6 h
Injury	SCr 2–3 times or GFR >50% decrease	<0.5 mL/kg/h >12 h
Failure	SCr >3 times or >4 mg/dL or GFR 75% decrease	<0.3 mL/kg/h 24 h or anuria for 12 h
Loss of function	Persistent acute renal failure: complete loss of kidney function >4 weeks (requiring dialysis)	
End-stage renal disease	Complete loss of kidney function >3 months (requiring dialysis)	

The limitations include a need for a baseline creatinine level, smaller increases in creatinine (0.3 mg/dL) which can worsen outcome is not included in RIFLE; it is a retrospective tool and does not discriminate between the nature or the site of AKI.

In 2007 the **Acute Kidney Injury Network** changed the RIFLE criteria to stages in AKI [6, 7, 8].

Stage one—Increase in serum creatinine of more than or equal to 0.3 mg/dL or increase to more than or equal to 150% to 200% (1.5- to 2-fold) from baseline. Urine output <0.5 mL per kg per hour for more than 6 h.

Stage two—Increase in serum creatinine to more than 200% to 300% (>2- to 3-fold) from baseline. Urine output <0.5 mL per kg per hour for more than 12 h.

Stage three—Increase in serum creatinine to more than 300% (>3-fold) from baseline (or serum creatinine of more than or equal to 4.0 mg/dL or commencement of acute renal replacement therapy (irrespective of the preceding increase in serum creatinine level or urine output).

More recently, the Kidney Disease: Improving Global Outcomes **(KDIGO)** Acute Kidney Injury Work Group proposed changes to the staging for AKI. KDIGO covers both the AKIN and RIFLE criteria, taking into account changes in creatinine within 48 h or a decline in the glomerular filtration rate (GFR) over 7 days [9, 10].

RIFLE, AKIN, and KDIGO scores were all good predictors of mortality in critically ill patients, and there were no differences among them in terms of predicting death [11, 12].

References

1. Schönermarck U, Kehl K, Samtleben W. Diagnostic performance of fractional excretion of urea and sodium in acute kidney injury. Am J Kidney Dis. 2008;51:870.
2. Vanmassenhove J, Glorieux G, Hoste E, et al. Urinary output and fractional excretion of sodium and urea as indicators of transient versus intrinsic acute kidney injury during early sepsis. Crit Care. 2013;17:R234.
3. Gupta RK, Bang TJ. Prevention of contrast-induced nephropathy (CIN) in interventional radiology practice. Semin Intervent Radiol. 2010;27(4):348–59.
4. Munoz SJ. The hepatorenal syndrome. Med Clin North Am. 2008;92(4):813–37.
5. Low G, Alexander GJM, Lomas DJ. Hepatorenal syndrome: aetiology, diagnosis, and treatment. Gastroenterol Res Pract. 2015;2015:1–11. Web
6. Goren O, Matot I. Perioperative acute kidney injury. Br J Anaesth. 2015;115(Suppl):3–14.
7. Mehta RL, Kellum JA, Shah SV, Molitoris BA, Ronco C, Warnock DG, Levin A. Acute kidney injury network: report of an initiative to improve outcomes in acute kidney injury. Crit Care. 2007;11(2):R31. doi:10.1186/cc5713.
8. Schrier RW. ARF, AKI, or ATN? Nat Rev Nephrol. 2010;6(3):125. doi:10.1038/nrneph.2010.1.
9. Hoste EA, Kellum JA. Acute kidney injury: epidemiology and diagnostic criteria. Curr Opin Crit Care. 2006;12(6):531–7.
10. Roy AK, Mc Gorrian C, Treacy C, Kavanaugh E, Brennan A, Mahon NG, et al. A comparison of traditional and novel definitions (RIFLE, AKIN, and KDIGO) of acute kidney injury for the prediction of outcomes in acute decompensated heart failure. Cardiorenal Med. 2013;3(1):26–37.
11. Shah SR, Tunio SA, Arshad MH, Moazzam Z, Noorani K, et al. Acute kidney injury recognition and management: a review of the literature and current evidence. Glob J Health Sci. 2015;8(5):120–4.
12. Levi TM, de Souza SP, de Magalhaes JG, et al. Comparison of the RIFLE, AKIN and KDIGO criteria to predict mortality in critically ill patients. Rev Bras Ter Intensiva. 2013;25(4):290–6.

Chapter 33
Drug Testing

Alberto J. de Armendi and Gulshan Doulatram

Fig. 33.1 Which drugs?

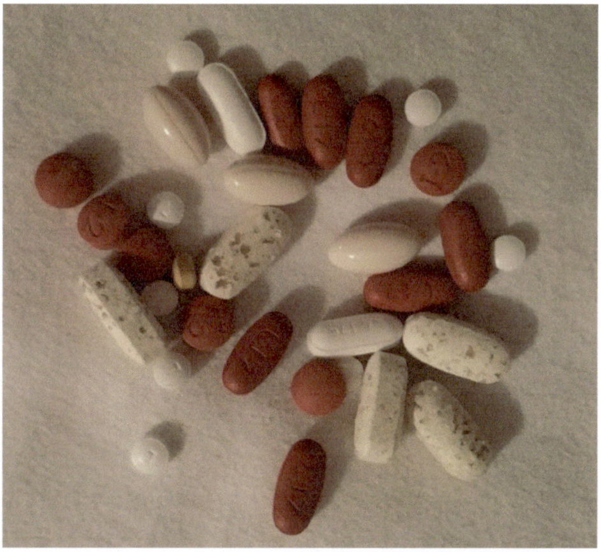

A.J. de Armendi, MD, PhD, MBA (✉)
Department of Anesthesiology, The Children's Hospital, University of Oklahoma Health Sciences Center, 750 NE 13th Street, Suite 200, PO Box 5318, Oklahoma City, OK 73104, USA
e-mail: Alberto-dearmendi@ouhsc.edu

G. Doulatram, MD
Department of Anesthesiology, University of Texas Medical Branch, 301 University Blvd, Galveston, TX, USA
e-mail: gdoulatr@utmb.edu

T.D. Raj (ed.), *Data Interpretation in Anesthesia*,
DOI 10.1007/978-3-319-55862-2_33

Drug Testing Questions

1. How does substance abuse affect anesthesiology as a specialty?
2. What test would you order for suspected fentanyl substance abuse in your patients?
3. What test would you order for suspected cocaine substance abuse in your patients?
4. How do you test for marijuana drug use in your patients?
5. According to the American College of Surgeons certified Level I Trauma Centers, what percentage of patients screened are positive for both alcohol and illicit drug misuse?
6. How do you group illicit drugs and what are their anesthetic implications?

Answers

1. Eighty percent of anesthesia residency programs have at least one resident with substance abuse. One to two percent of anesthesia residents have a problem with substance abuse. The Massachusetts General Hospital has instituted a preplacement (preemployment) and post-employment random urine testing in an attempt to lower the incidence of substance abuse among anesthesia residents [1]. Twenty-nine percent of anesthesia residents relapse after being allowed to return/continue in an anesthesia residency program. For residents that are allowed to return to their residency program, the initial presentation is death (10%). Forty-three percent of program directors feel that residents in recovery should be allowed to attempt reentry, while 30% feel that they should not [2].

2. Fentanyl can be detected by radioimmunoassay or more selective gas chromatographic techniques. Urine and blood screening involving a novel enzyme-linked immunosorbent assay (ELISA) coupled with nanoparticles for fentanyl detection has the advantage of being simple, sensitive, inexpensive, and capable of detecting metabolites [3]. Fentanyl concentrations as low as 5 pg/well can be detected in urine and serum samples.

3. Urine radioimmunoassay test is the initial screening test for cocaine abuse and is positive for up to 72 h after exposure. Benzoylecgonine is the main cocaine urine metabolite tested in cocaine drug screening [4]. Gas chromatography coupled with mass spectrometry (GC-MS) or liquid chromatography coupled with a mass spectrometry (LC/MS) is more sensitive and sophisticated than immunoassay and can be done for confirmation of various drugs and their metabolites including cocaine. The window of testing is 1–3 days for urine testing. Although hair testing is the most sensitive for cocaine and has the widest detection window indicating chronic use, it is not done routinely compared to urine.

4. Urine is the preferred medium to test for marijuana use because of higher concentrations, longer detection time of metabolites, ease of sampling, and higher sensitivity compared to blood [5]. The major metabolite tested in marijuana use is tetrahydrocannabinol (THC) and carboxy tetrahydrocannabinol (THCCOOH). The detection window for urine testing is 10 h for THC and 25 days for THCCOOH. While immunoassay is adequate for preliminary testing, advanced chromatographic techniques are used for quantitation of levels.

5. Eleven percent of the patients screened at Level I Trauma Centers are found to be positive for both legally intoxicated levels of alcohol and illicit drugs [6]. The use of alcohol and illicit drugs is especially concerning due to higher incidence of fatal and nonfatal motor vehicle accidents and higher perioperative morbidity.

6. Illicit drugs may be grouped into opioids, barbiturates, cocaine, benzodiazepines, ephedrine groups, cannabinoids, and hallucinogenic drugs [7].

Opioid drugs (codeine, oxycodone, pentazocine, fentanyl, propoxyphene, methadone, heroin, morphine, meperidine) are used for analgesia. They can cause euphoria, respiratory depression, seizures, stupor, coma, and death. Treatment for opioid withdrawal includes clonidine, diphenhydramine, doxepin, and/or opioids (methadone or buprenorphine).

Barbiturates (secobarbital, pentobarbital, phenobarbital) are central nervous system depressants and can cause sedation, hypotension (central vasomotor depression and cardiac depression), and altered drug metabolism (fluoride, warfarin, digitalis, phenytoin).

Cocaine is a central nervous system stimulant (arterial vasoconstriction) with anesthetic concerns for increased MAC, sympathetic hyperactivity causing hypertension/hypotension, tachycardia, increased myocardial oxygen demand, myocardial infarction, cardiac depression, angina, coronary spasms, thrombus, arrhythmias, and death. Other anesthetic implications include psychosis, nasal septum perforation, restlessness, anxiety, irritability, confusion, pupillary dilatation, seizures, asthma, and pulmonary hemorrhage.

Benzodiazepines (diazepam, midazolam, flunitrazepam) are antianxiety agents and may result in respiratory depression especially with concurrent opioid use.

Ephedrine drugs (pseudoephedrine, methamphetamines) can cause hypertension, cardiac arrhythmias, dilated pupils, hyperthermia, and cardiac arrest in the perioperative setting. The response to treatment of hypotension with vasopressors is unpredictable in amphetamine-abusing patients. Acute intake of amphetamines increases the minimum alveolar concentration (MAC) of potent inhaled anesthetics. In contrast, chronic intake decreases the dose requirement for general anesthetic.

Cannabinoids have some antiemetic and analgesic properties and are the most commonly abused drugs. They can cause hallucinations and severe perioperative complications including cardiac arrhythmias, cardiac depression, hypotension, bradycardia, respiratory depression, bronchospasm, and pulmonary edema.

Hallucinogens [lysergic acid diethylamide (LSD), phencyclidine (PCP, ketamine), psilocybin, mescaline, 3,4-methylenedioxymethamphetamine (MDMA, ectasy), γ-hydroxybutyrate (GHB)] are psychedelic drugs used for recreational purposes. They can cause anxiety, paranoia, delusions, panic attacks, and psychosis. The effects of acute drug intake usually develop over 1 to 2 h and last for approximately 12 h. Ingestion of these drugs activates the sympathetic nervous system causing increased body temperature, tachycardia, hypertension, and dilated pupils. This is treated with fluids, pressors, vasodilators, and sympatholytics. Exaggerated response to sympathomimetic drugs should be expected. These drugs also prolong the analgesic and respiratory depressants effects of opioids. Inhibition of plasma cholinesterase activity can cause prolongation of succinylcholine action in some patients.

References

1. Fitzsimons MG, Baker KH, Lowenstein E, Zapol WM. Random drug testing to reduce the incidence of addiction in anesthesia residents: preliminary results from one program. Anesth Analg. 2008;107(2):630–5. doi:10.1213/ane.0b013e318176fefa.
2. Bryson EO. Should anesthesia residents with a history of substance abuse be allowed to continue training in clinical anesthesia? The results of a survey of anesthesia residency program directors. J Clin Anesth. 2009;21(7):508–13.
3. Mao CL, Zientek KD, Colahan PT, Kuo MY, Liu CH, Lee KM, Chou CC. Development of an enzyme-linked immunosorbent assay for fentanyl and applications of fentanyl antibody-coated nanoparticles for sample preparation. J Pharm Biomed Anal. 2006;41(4):1332–41.
4. Bruns AD, Zieske LA, Jacobs AJ. Analysis of the cocaine metabolite in the urine of patients and physicians during clinical use. Otolaryngol Head Neck Surg. 1994;111(6):722–6.
5. Sharma P, Murthy P, Bharath MM. Chemistry, metabolism, and toxicology of cannabis: clinical implications. Iran J Psychiatry. 2012;7(4):149–56.
6. Langdorf MI, Rudkin SE, Dellota K, Fox JC, Munden S. Decision rule and utility of routine urine toxicology screening of trauma patients. Eur J Emerg Med. 2002;9(2):115–21.
7. Kuczkowski KM. Anesthetic implications of drug abuse in pregnancy. J Clin Anesth. 2003;15(5):382–94.

Chapter 34
Chest Pain Profiles

John David Srinivasan

A 78-year-old male underwent an open AAA repair for an 8 cm infrarenal aneurysm. His preoperative echo showed normal EF and no wall motion abnormality. During the surgery he had an episode of surgical bleeding and hypotension with transient ST depression which resolved with hypotension treatment and PRBC transfusion. On postoperative day 1, the patient developed chest pain with ST depression and elevated cardiac troponin I (cTnI) which was 15 ng/mL. An echocardiography showed severe anteroseptal hypokinesia.

Questions

1. Has this patient suffered an acute myocardial infarction (MI)?
2. What are troponins?
3. What is the 2012 universal classification of myocardial infarction?
4. What conditions can raise troponin levels other than MI?
5. How would you classify this patient's perioperative MI?
6. What should be done next?

J.D. Srinivasan, MD, FRCA
Assistant Professor, Department of Anesthesiology and Critical Care,
Saint Louis University, School of Medicine, 3635 Vista Ave., PO Box 15250, St. Louis, MO 63110-0250, USA
e-mail: srinivjd@slu.edu

T.D. Raj (ed.), *Data Interpretation in Anesthesia*,
DOI 10.1007/978-3-319-55862-2_34

Answers

1. Yes, this patient has elevated cardiac biomarkers along with symptoms of cardiac ischemia (chest pain) with imaging evidence of regional wall motion abnormality in the anterioseptal wall. The term acute MI is used when there is evidence of myocardial necrosis in a clinical setting consistent with acute myocardial ischemia, detection of a rise and/or fall of cardiac biomarker values (preferably cardiac troponin) above the 99th percentile upper reference limit with at least one of the following:

   (a) Symptoms of cardiac ischemia
   (b) EKG changes: new significant ST-segment–T wave changes, new left bundle branch block, or development of pathological Q waves
   (c) Imaging evidence of new regional wall motion abnormality
   (d) Identification of an intracoronary thrombus by angiography or autopsy

2. Troponins are protein molecules that are part of cardiac and skeletal muscle. Smooth muscle cells do not contain troponins. Three types of troponins exist—troponin I, troponin T, and troponin C. Each subunit has a unique function: Troponin T binds the troponin components to tropomyosin, troponin I inhibits the interaction of myosin with actin, and troponin C contains the binding sites for Ca^{2+} that help initiate contraction. Raised troponin levels indicate cardiac muscle cell injury and/or death as the molecule is released into the blood upon injury to the heart. Troponins will begin to increase within 3 h following an MI. The recommended cutoff value for an elevated cardiac troponin is the 99th percentile of a control reference group. As the troponin test kits are made by many manufacturers, the cutoff values suggested by the laboratory should be used as reference [1].

3. Universal Classification of Myocardial Infarction [2]

   Type 1 (spontaneous myocardial infarction): Spontaneous myocardial infarction related to atherosclerotic plaque rupture, ulceration, erosion, or dissection with resulting intraluminal thrombus in one or more of the coronary arteries leading to decreased myocardial blood flow or distal platelet emboli with ensuing myocyte necrosis. The patient may have underlying severe CAD but on occasion non-obstructive or no CAD.

   Type 2 (myocardial infarction secondary to an ischemic imbalance): In instances of myocardial injury with necrosis where a condition other than CAD contributes to an imbalance between myocardial oxygen supply and/or demand, e.g., coronary endothelial dysfunction, coronary artery spasm, coronary embolism, tachy-/brady-arrhythmias, anemia, respiratory failure, hypotension, and hypertension with or without LVH.

   Type 3: Myocardial infarction results in death when biomarker values are unavailable.

   Type 4a: Myocardial infarction related to percutaneous coronary intervention (PCI).

   Type 4b: Myocardial infarction related to stent thrombosis.

   Type 5: Myocardial infarction related to coronary artery bypass grafting (CABG)

4. Causes of troponin elevation other than MI include the following:
   (a) Myocarditis
   (b) Pericarditis
   (c) Cardiac contusion/trauma
   (d) Aortic dissection
   (e) Endocarditis
   (f) Cardiac surgery
   (g) Pulmonary embolism
   (h) Stroke (ischemic or hemorrhagic)
   (i) Cardiopulmonary resuscitation (CPR)
   (j) Defibrillation
   (k) Chronic severe heart failure
   (l) Cardiac arrhythmias (tachyarrhythmias, brady-arrhythmias, heart blocks)
   (m) Sepsis
   (n) Renal failure
   (o) Hypertrophic obstructive cardiomyopathy (HOCM)
   (p) Takotsubo cardiomyopathy
   (q) Burns
   (r) Extreme exertion
   (s) Infiltrative diseases such as amyloidosis
   (t) Medications and toxins such as doxorubicin, trastuzumab, and snake venom
   (u) Transplant vasculopathy
   (v) Critical illness

5. This patient has suffered a perioperative MI, either Type 1 or type 2.

   Acute Coronary Syndrome (Type 1 PMI)

   Acute coronary syndrome occurs when an unstable or vulnerable plaque undergoes spontaneous rupture, fissuring, or erosion, leading to acute coronary thrombosis, ischemia, and infarction. Although it is currently widely accepted that intraplaque inflammation plays a pivotal role in plaque instability and spontaneous acute coronary syndrome, external stressors such as those occurring postoperatively are believed to contribute.
   (a) Physiological and emotional stresses are known to predispose to MI, likely because of the sympathetic induced hemodynamic, coronary vasoconstrictive, and prothrombotic forces thought to promote plaque disruption. These conditions are common perioperatively. Catecholamines and cortisol increase after surgery and may remain elevated for days. Stress hormones increase with pain, surgical trauma, anemia, and hypothermia.
   (b) Tachycardia and hypertension, common in the perioperative period, may exert shear stress, leading to rupture of plaques with outward (positive) remodeling, thin fibrous caps, and high circumferential tensile stress or to endothelial stripping/erosion caused by high blood velocities around plaques with inward (negative) remodeling and severe coronary stenosis.

Myocardial Oxygen Supply-Demand Imbalance (Type 2 PMI) [3]

Numerous studies using perioperative Holter monitoring in high-cardiac-risk patients undergoing major surgery showed that silent, heart rate-related ST-segment depression is common postoperatively and is associated with in-hospital and long-term morbidity and mortality. Postoperative cardiac complications, including sudden death, occurred after prolonged silent ST-segment depression. These findings were further corroborated by studies that correlated continuous, online 12-lead ST-segment analysis with serial cardiac troponin measurements after major vascular surgery. Cardiac troponin elevations occurred after prolonged transient, postoperative ST-segment depression, and peak troponin elevations correlated with the duration of ST depression. ST elevation occurred in <2% of postoperative ischemic events and was a rare cause of PMI. Hence, prolonged, ST-depression-type ischemia is the most common cause of PMI.

6. There are no clear algorithms or guidelines to navigate treatment in perioperative MIs. This is also addressed in Chap. 15. The cardiology team is consulted and involved early. Steps should be taken to ensure adequate oxygen supply to the myocardium by addressing issues with oxygen saturation and anemia. Myocardial oxygen demand should be reduced by controlling tachycardia and hypertension. There are no randomized controlled trials to clarify if PCI or systemic anticoagulation is beneficial in the perioperative setting. Retrospective analysis of over 1000 cases of perioperative MI showed that the 30-day mortality of patients who received diagnostic catheterization was 5.2%. Those who received PCI had a 30-day mortality of 11.3%. Part of this mortality is attributed to the large postoperative hemorrhage risk of anticoagulation. Clinical decision making should be made on a case by case risk benefit analysis [4, 5].

References

1. Priebe HJ. Perioperative myocardial infarction—aetiology and prevention. Br J Anaesth. 2005;95(1):3–19.
2. Thygesen K, Alpert JS, Jaffe AS, Simoons ML, Chaitman BR, White HD, Writing Group on behalf of the Joint ESC/ACCF/AHA/WHF Task Force for the Universal Definition of Myocardial Infarction. Third universal definition of myocardial infarction. J Am Coll Cardiol. 2012;60(16):1581–98.
3. Landesberg G, Mosseri M, Zahger D, Wolf Y, Perouansky M, Anner H, Drenger B, Hasin Y, Berlatzky Y, Weissman C. Myocardial infarction after vascular surgery: the role of prolonged stress-induced, ST depression-type ischemia. J Am Coll Cardiol. 2001;37(7):1839–45.
4. Adesanya AO, Lemos JA, Greilich NB, Whitten CW. Management of perioperative myocardial infarction in noncardiac surgical patients. Chest. 2006;130(2):584–96.
5. Dauerman HL. The expanding universe of perioperative myocardial infarction. J Am Coll Cardiol. 2016;68(4):339–42. doi:10.1016/j.jacc.2016.03.601.

Chapter 35
BNP

Teodora Nicolescu and Tilak D. Raj

A 67-year-old man presented to the ER with increasing shortness of breath, tiredness, and weight gain. Immunoassay for BNP showed a value of 800 pg/mL.

Questions

1. What is BNP and NT-proBNP?
2. What are the normal levels and conditions that cause elevated levels?
3. How do these markers aid in the diagnosis of heart failure?
4. What are the other uses outside diagnosing heart failure?
5. Are there limitations?
6. What is heart failure and why is it important to diagnose it?

T. Nicolescu, MD (✉)
Department of Anesthesiology, Oklahoma University Health Sciences Center,
750 NE 13th Street, Suite 200, Oklahoma City, OK, USA
e-mail: teodora-nicolescu@ouhsc.edu

T.D. Raj, MD, MRCP, FRCA
Department of Anesthesiology, Alliance Health Midwest, Midwest City, OK, USA
e-mail: tilakdraj@gmail.com

T.D. Raj (ed.), *Data Interpretation in Anesthesia*,
DOI 10.1007/978-3-319-55862-2_35

Answers

1. B-type natriuretic peptide is also called brain-type natriuretic peptide (BNP) as it was first described in 1988 after isolation from porcine brain. However, it was soon found to originate mainly from the heart. B-type natriuretic peptide (BNP) and N-terminal proBNP (NT-proBNP) are released by the ventricular myocardium in response to myocardial wall stress initially as a 108 amino acid prohormone. It is cleaved by enzymes corin/furin to BNP the 32 amino-acid, biologically active part of the prohormone and NT-proBNP which is the 76 amino acid, biologically inactive compound. BNP produces a variety of biological effects by interaction with the natriuretic peptide receptor type A (NPR-A) causing intracellular cGMP production. These include natriuresis/diuresis, peripheral vasodilatation, and inhibition of the renin–angiotensin–aldosterone system (RAAS) and the sympathetic nervous system (SNS).

   All effects ultimately lead to decreased afterload.

   BNP has a half-life of 20 min and is cleared by binding to the natriuretic peptide receptor type C (NPR-C) and through proteolysis by endopeptidases. NT-proBNP has a half-life of 120 min and is cleared by renal excretion [1, 2].

2. BNP levels are normally less than 100 pg/mL and the NT-proBNP is less than 300 pg/mL [2]. The levels are higher in:

   (a) females due to differences in metabolism
   (b) advancing age
   (c) worsening renal function (NT-proBNP affected more due to renal clearance)
   (d) LV hypertrophy
   (e) Systolic and diastolic dysfunction
   (f) Fluid overload

3. BNP and NT pro BNP serve as good markers of heart failure. The levels for both markers are different to exclude or confirm the diagnosis of heart failure [3].

   BNP—level < 100 pg/mL heart failure (HF) unlikely; level > 500 pg/mL HF very likely.

   Levels 100–500 use clinical judgment.

   NT-proBNP—level < 300 pg/mL HF unlikely

   Age < 50 years, level > 450 pg/mL—HF likely
   Age 50–75 years, level > 900 pg/mL—HF likely
   Age > 75 years, level > 1800 pg/mL—HF likely

   A good correlation has been made between increasing levels of BNP and functional class of NYHA classification as depicted in the Fig. 35.1.

4. BNP and NT-proBNP provide strong **prognostic information**, and elevated levels are associated with an unfavorable outcome (death, sudden cardiac death, readmission, or cardiac events) in patients with heart failure or asymptomatic left ventricular dysfunction [3, 4].

   They are also useful for choosing optimal treatment and monitoring its effects in heart failure.

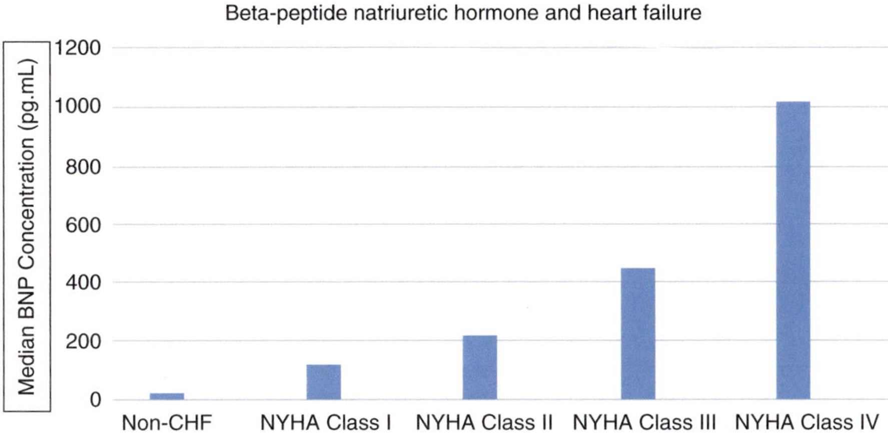

Fig. 35.1 BNP and heart failure

The current American College of Cardiology/American Heart Association (ACC/AHA) guidelines for managing heart failure have incorporated using natriuretic peptide levels in establishing the prognosis and disease severity of chronic heart failure.

In patients with severe heart failure BNP and NT-proBNP assays can be used in **resynchronization therapy**.

Both are also used as markers and to aid in prognosis in acute and stable **coronary heart disease**. Higher values are associated with worse outcomes [5].

In **aortic stenosis**, the levels indicate disease severity, progression, functional status, and also the optimum time for valve replacement after which the levels decline.

In **atrial fibrillation**, the levels are elevated and predict the success of cardioversion.

5. Limitations include **false low levels** in:

   (a) Obesity
   (b) Early acute heart failure
   (c) Heart failure due to causes upstream from the left ventricle, e.g., mitral valve or pericardial disease

False high levels as already mentioned in:

   (a) Females
   (b) Advancing age
   (c) Renal failure

6. Heart failure affects approximately 5.7 million Americans, and about 670,000 new cases are diagnosed annually in the United States. It is a leading cause of

hospital admissions and readmissions in people over 65 years. The estimated total health-care cost of HF in the United States in 2010 was $39.2 billion or 1–2% of all health-care expenditures. The risk of death is about 35% in the year after diagnosis after which it decreases to below 10% each year.

HF is either diastolic, decreased left ventricular filling, or systolic, decreased pump function. It is a diagnosis that is made clinically by history (breathlessness and fatigue) and physical exam (elevated jugular venous pressure and lung crackles). These features are not sensitive or specific, and there is no gold standard investigation to make the diagnosis. The severity is classified based on symptoms and functional limitations into four grades according to the New York Heart Association. Patients with heart failure suffer a decreased quality of life with significantly reduced physical and mental health. So, early diagnosis of heart failure, identification of the cause to determine reversibility, and institution of appropriate management strategies which include lifestyle changes, medications, and/or surgery can potentially make a big impact on the quality and duration of life.

References

1. Klabunde R. Cardiovascular physiology concepts. 2nd ed. Philadelphia, PA: Lippincott Williams & Wilkins; 2011.
2. Weber M, Hamm C. Role of B-type natriuretic peptide (BNP) and NT-proBNP in clinical routine. Heart. 2006;92:843–9.
3. Van Kimmenade R, Pinto YM, Bayes-Genis A. Usefulness of intermediate amino-terminal pro-brain natriuretic peptide concentrations for diagnosis and prognosis of acute heart failure. Am J Cardiol. 2006;98:386–90.
4. Oremus M, McKelvie R, Don-Wauchope A. A systematic review of BNP and NT-proBNP in the management of heart failure: overview and methods. Heart Fail Rev. 2014;19:413–9.
5. Berry C. Predictive value of plasms brain natriuretic peptide receptors for cardiac outcome after vascular surgery. Heart. 2005;92(3):401–23.

Chapter 36
Blood Gas I

Tanmay Shah

A 36-year-old woman presents to the emergency room with severe abdominal pain, nausea, vomiting, anorexia, and somnolence.

ABG: pH 7.20, PCO_2 35 mmHg, pO_2 68 mmHg on room air

Laboratory values: Na 130 mEq/L, Cl 80 mEq/L, HCO_3 10 mEq/L

1. How do you diagnose a simple acid–base disorder?
2. What blood gas abnormality does this patient have?
3. How do you calculate anion gap and corrected anion gap?
4. How do you diagnose a mixed acid–base disorder and does this patient have mixed acid–base disorder?
5. What is Winter's formula?
6. Is there any compensation in this blood gas value?
7. What are the possible causes of metabolic acidosis?
8. What are the possible causes of respiratory acidosis?

T. Shah, MD, MBBS
Department of Anesthesiology, University of Oklahoma Health Sciences Center, 750 NE 13th Street, Suite 200, Oklahoma City, OK 73104, USA
e-mail: Tanmay-Shah@ouhsc.edu

T.D. Raj (ed.), *Data Interpretation in Anesthesia*,
DOI 10.1007/978-3-319-55862-2_36

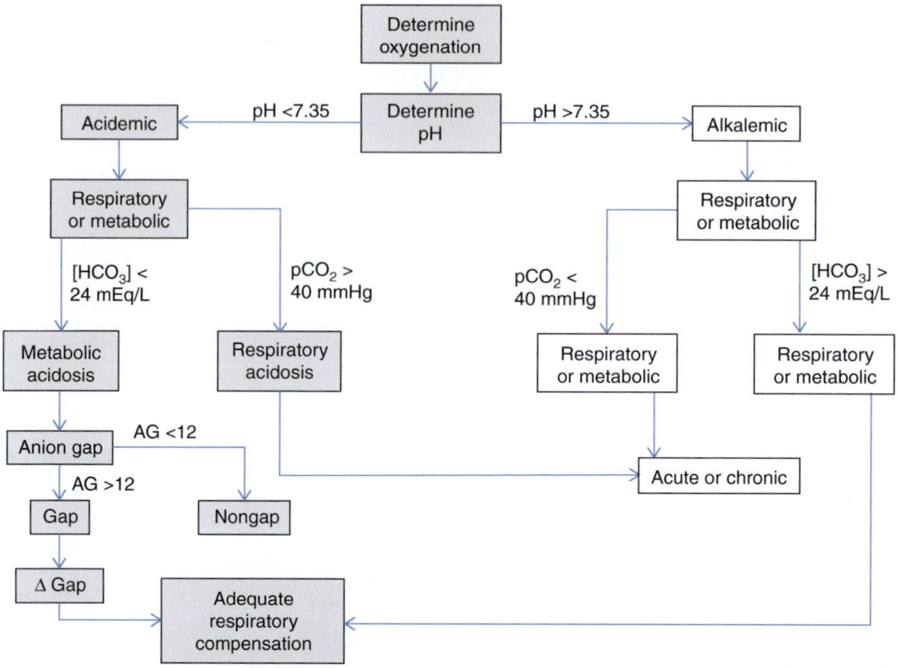

Fig. 36.1 Diagnosis of acid–base disorders (This figure was published in Miller textbook, Chap. 21 in 2011. Permission obtained from Elsevier to reproduce the image.)

Answers

1. Initially the pH is used to determine acidosis or alkalosis, and then the value of $PaCO_2/HCO_3$ is used to determine if the derangement is metabolic or respiratory. If it is of respiratory origin, then we will have to determine whether the process is acute or chronic. If it is due to a metabolic component, then respiratory compensation should be calculated using the appropriate formula.

2. Our patient has a pH less than 7.4, which signifies acidosis. The HCO_3 is less than 24 mEq/L; therefore the primary abnormality in this patient is metabolic acidosis. This chart (Fig. 36.1) shows the steps to follow in order to diagnose an acid–base disorder [1].

3. Anion gap (AG) = Na − (Cl + HCO_3)

   (a) AG is the difference in the 'routinely measured' **cations** (Na) and 'routinely measured' **anions** (Cl and HCO_3) in the blood and depends on serum phosphate and albumin concentrations [2]. Determination of AG is useful in determining the cause of acidosis [3, 4]. The normal value for serum AG is usually 8–12 mEq/L. In our patient, AG = 130 − (80 + 10) = 40 mEq/L. So, this patient has a high AG, most likely due to starvation or diabetic ketoacidosis.

(b) In a normal healthy patient, negatively charged albumin is the single largest contributor to the AG [5]. Hypoalbuminemia causes a decrease in AG; hence AG is corrected to albumin level using the equation of Figge as follows: corrected AG = AG + [0.25 × (44 – Albumin)] [6].

- If corrected AG >16, there is high AG acidosis.
- If corrected AG <16, non-AG acidosis.

4. Delta gap formula can be used to assess mixed acid–base disorder.

(a) Δ gap = AG − 12 + HCO_3 (12 is normal serum AG value)

- If Δ gap <22 mEq/L, then concurrent non-gap metabolic acidosis exists.
- If Δ gap >26 mEq/L, then concurrent metabolic alkalosis exists.

(b) In our patient, Δ gap = 40 − 12 + 10 = 38 mEq/L. So, there is a concurrent metabolic alkalosis probably from vomiting in addition to high AG metabolic acidosis in this patient.
So, there is a concurrent metabolic alkalosis probably from vomiting in addition to high AG metabolic acidosis in this patient.

5. Winter's formula is used to determine whether there is an appropriate respiratory compensation during metabolic acidosis [1].

(a) Winter's formula: $PCO_2 = (1.5 \times HCO_3) + 8$

- If measured PCO_2 > calculated PCO_2, then concurrent respiratory acidosis is present.
- If measured PCO_2 < calculated PCO_2, then concurrent respiratory alkalosis is present.

6. In our patient, calculated $PCO_2 = (1.5 \times 10) + 8 = 23$ mmHg according to Winter's formula.
Our measured PCO_2 of 35 mmHg is higher than the calculated PCO_2 of 23 mmHg, so our patient also has concurrent respiratory acidosis. Usually, metabolic acidosis is compensated by respiratory alkalosis, but due to somnolence in this patient, concurrent respiratory acidosis exists.

7. Causes of anion gap metabolic acidosis are easily remembered by pneumonic MUDPILES [1].

M: methanol
U: uremia
D: diabetic ketoacidosis
P: paraldehyde
I: infection, INH therapy
L: lactic acidosis
E: ethanol, ethylene glycol
S: salicylates (aspirin)

Causes of non-gap metabolic acidosis:

- Excessive administration of 0.9% normal saline
- GI losses: diarrhea, ileostomy, neobladder, pancreatic fistula
- Renal losses: renal tubular acidosis
- Drugs: acetazolamide

8. Respiratory acidosis which is from increased CO_2 is due either to increased production or decreased elimination [2].

   (a) Increased production of CO_2:

   - Malignant hyperthermia
   - Hyperthyroidism
   - Sepsis
   - Overfeeding

   (b) Decreased elimination of CO_2:

   - Intrinsic pulmonary disease (pneumonia, ARDS, fibrosis, edema)
   - Upper airway obstruction (laryngospasm, foreign body, OSA)
   - Lower airway obstruction (asthma, COPD)
   - Chest wall restriction (obesity, scoliosis, burns)
   - CNS depression (anesthetics, opioids, CNS lesions)
   - Decreased skeletal muscle strength (myopathy, neuropathy, residual effects of neuromuscular blocking drugs)
   - Rarely, an exhausted soda–lime or incompetent one-way valve in an anesthesia delivery system can contribute to respiratory acidosis.

References

1. Miller RD, Pardo MC Jr. Basics of anesthesia. 6th ed. Philadelphia: Elsevier Saunders; 2011.
2. Morgan GE, Mikhail MS, Murray MJ. Clinical anesthesiology. 4th ed. New York: McGraw-Hill; 2006.
3. Emmett M, Narins RG. Clinical use of the anion gap. Medicine (Baltimore). 1977;56(1):38–54.
4. Barash PG, et al. Clinical anesthesia. 6th ed. Philadelphia: Lippincott Williams & Wilkins; 2009.
5. Feldman M, Soni N, Dickson B. Influence of hypoalbuminemia or hyperalbuminemia on the serum anion gap. J Lab Clin Med. 2005;146(6):317–20.
6. Hatherill M, Waggie Z, Purves L, et al. Correction of the anion gap for albumin in order to detect occult tissue anions in shock. Arch Dis Child. 2002;87(6):526–9.

Chapter 37
Blood Gas II

Daniel A. Biggs

A patient is unresponsive and taking shallow breaths in the recovery room. Arterial blood gas shows:

pH—7.26, CO_2—69, O_2—54, HCO_3^-—25

Questions

1. What does the blood gas show?
2. What is the difference between hypoxia and hypoxemia?
3. What is the most common cause of hypoxia seen in the perioperative period?
4. What are some other possible causes of hypoxia?
5. What are some of the physiologic effects, signs, and symptoms?
6. How would you treat hypoxia?
7. What is the alveolar gas equation and how might it help in identifying the cause of hypoxia?

D.A. Biggs, MD, MSc
Department of Anesthesiology, Oklahoma University Medical Center,
750 NE 13th Street, Suite 200, Oklahoma City, OK 73104, USA
e-mail: Daniel-biggs@ouhsc.edu

T.D. Raj (ed.), *Data Interpretation in Anesthesia*,
DOI 10.1007/978-3-319-55862-2_37

Answers

1. The blood gas shows hypoxia (pO_2 less than 60) along with respiratory acidosis with little metabolic compensation [1].

2. Hypoxia is a failure of the delivery of adequate amounts of oxygen to tissue. This can be local, regional, or global. Hypoxemia is a low blood oxygen content. SaO_2 <90%, PaO_2 <60 mmHg.

3. Hypoventilation is a common problem noted in the postoperative period. There are a number of possible causes [1]. Some of the more common etiologies that might be seen in the PACU:
   (a) Poor respiratory drive—may be caused by narcotics, sedatives, and inhalational anesthetic agents.
   (b) Muscle weakness—most commonly related to residual neuromuscular blockade. It could also be seen in patients with neuromuscular disease.
   (c) Airway obstruction—could be secondary to residual muscle weakness, airway surgery, or laryngospasm. The patient could have a history of obstructive sleep apnea.

4. Hypoxia can be divided [2]:
   (a) Hypoxic hypoxia—an inadequate amount of oxygen getting to the lungs [1]
      - Low inspired oxygen concentration, e.g., high altitude
      - Airway obstruction
      - Hypoventilation [3]
      - Neuromuscular disease
      - Shunting and V/Q mismatch [1, 3]
      - Interstitial lung disease
   (b) Anemic hypoxia
      - Low hemoglobin level
      - Abnormal hemoglobin, e.g., methemoglobin or carbon monoxide poisoning [1]
   (c) Stagnant or circulatory hypoxia—inadequate blood flow to the tissues
      - Generalized—causes
         – Low cardiac output—heart failure, MI [3]
         – Poor cardiac venous return
         – Shock
      - Localized—causes
         – Anything which limits flow to the local tissue
   (d) Histotoxic hypoxia
      - Cells are unable to utilize oxygen, e.g., cyanide toxicity

5. Effects will vary based on the cause and what tissues are hypoxic.
   (a) Generalized hypoxia—signs and symptoms [1]
      - Tachypnea
      - Tachycardia
      - Shortness of breath
      - Sweating

- Cyanosis (cherry red skin color in cyanide toxicity)
- Headache
- Confusion
- Restlessness
- Seizure
- Coma

6. Initial treatment is oxygen administration. Further therapy may be required depending on the cause. Examples:
   (a) Acute asthma exacerbation—bronchodilators
   (b) Embolus or thrombus—removal
7. Alveolar gas equation [3]
   (a) $P_AO_2 = F_iO_2\left(P_{atm} - P_{H_2O}\right) - P_aCO_2 / R$

   P_AO_2—partial pressure of alveolar O_2
   F_iO_2—fraction of inspired O_2
   P_{atm}—atmospheric pressure
   P_{H_2O}—partial pressure of water vapor
   P_aCO_2—partial pressure CO_2 in arterial blood
   R—respiratory exchange ratio, usually 0.8

   Alveolar–arterial gradient [3]
   (b) A–a gradient = $P_AO_2 - P_aO_2$
   P_aO_2—partial pressure of arterial O_2

   A–a gradient may be used to help determine the cause of hypoxia. The gradient increases with age. Normal gradient is less than 10 mmHg plus 1 mmHg per decade of life.

   Hypoxia with normal A–a gradient

   - Hypoventilation
   - Low partial pressure of inspired O_2 such as at high altitudes

   Hypoxia with high A–a gradient

   - Diffusion impairment in alveolus
   - V/Q mismatch
   - Right to left shunt

References

1. Barash PG, Cullen BF, Stoelting RK, Cahalan MK, Stock MC, Ortega R, editors. Clinical Anesthesia. 7th ed. Philadelphia: Lippincott Williams & Wilkins; 2013.
2. Federal Aviation Administration [Internet]. Beware of Hypoxia [2015 Jul 21, cited 2016 Jul 24]; [3 screens]. Available from: https://www.faa.gov/pilots/training/airman_education/topics_of_interest/hypoxia/
3. Miller RD. Miller's Anesthesia. 8th ed. Philadelphia: Elsevier Saunders; 2015.

Chapter 38
Blood Gas III

Pramod Chetty

A patient with closed fracture of the lower extremity is scheduled for an ORIF. The patient is an unaccompanied, slender, 26-year-old male who cannot give a good history due to confusion and has deep, rapid breathing with a distinctive odor. His vital signs show mild hypotension, tachycardia, and low-grade fever. Investigations demonstrate Na^+ 132, K^+ 4.8, Cl^- 92, HCO_3^- 12, BUN 24 mg, creatinine 1.6 mg, Ca^{++} 7.8 mg, and blood sugar of 318 mg/dl. Arterial blood gas shows a pH of 7.24, PCO_2 28, PO_2 76, HCO_3 12, BE of 14, and O_2 sat of 93%. His CBC is normal with mild leukocytosis and evidence of hemoconcentration. The chest X-ray is unremarkable and EKG shows sinus tachycardia.

1. What is the likely initial diagnosis of this patient and how can you confirm the diagnosis?
2. What are abnormal laboratory values in the BMP and ABGs that are seen in this condition?
3. What is the major differential diagnosis in this clinical condition?
4. What are the principles in the treatment of this condition?
5. How do the results of the BMP and ABG trend during the treatment of this condition?
6. How will you continue management of this patient with the planned surgery?

P. Chetty, MD
Department of Anesthesiology, OU Health Sciences Center,
750 NE 13th Street, Suite 200, PO Box 53168, Oklahoma City, OK 73104, USA
e-mail: Pramod-chetty@ouhsc.edu

T.D. Raj (ed.), *Data Interpretation in Anesthesia*,
DOI 10.1007/978-3-319-55862-2_38

Answers

1. The presentation of this young patient with altered sensorium, "Kussmaul" breathing, hyperglycemia, and metabolic acidosis strongly suggests diabetic ketoacidosis (DKA). The diagnosis can be *confirmed by the presence of ketone bodies* in the urine and serum [1]. Concomitant lactic acidosis must also be investigated [2, 3]. As with any patient with a traumatic injury and altered sensorium, radiological testing for cervical spine and cranial pathology must be done.

2. The laboratory values in DKA will show evidence of metabolic acidosis, electrolyte derangements, and evidence of severe dehydration [4].

   (a) BMP

   - Na^+—there is a total body loss of Na^+; the levels can be low normal. Correction must be made for undermeasurement of Na^+ due to hyperglycemia (add 1.6 meq/L to the measured Na^+ for every 100 mg of glucose above 100 mg/dl level).
   - K^+—there can be a significant total body loss of 3–10 meq/kg of K^+. The initial serum K^+ level may be paradoxically high due to both volume contraction and decreased movement into the intracellular compartment [1].
   - Cl^-—will be decreased.
   - HCO_3^-—will be decreased.
   - Anion gap—will be increased above normal 10–14 meq/L [5]. This gap is calculated by the formula:

   $$AG = Na^+ - (Cl^- + HCO_3^-)$$

   - BUN—will be increased.
   - Creatinine—may be mildly increased.
   - Ca^{++}—may be decreased. Additionally magnesium and phosphate depletion can also occur.
   - Glucose—increases to levels greater than 250–600 mg/dl [4] but *rarely* may be normal, when called euglycemic DKA [6].

   (b) ABG

   - pH—usually less than 7.3
   - $PaCO_2$—usually lower due to respiratory compensation for metabolic acidosis
   - PaO_2—usually low normal unless a pneumonic process causes it to be low
   - HCO_3—will be lower due to metabolic acidosis
   - BE—will be lower to indicate significant metabolic acidosis
   - O_2 saturation—will be in the low 90 s with O_2 supplementation unless a pneumonic process causes it to be lower

3. The major differential diagnosis in this scenario would be non-ketotic hyperosmolar hyperglycemia (NHH) [1]. In this condition the patient is generally a type 2 diabetic and as such would likely be an older and often overweight patient. The patient can

present with altered mentation or in a coma. The blood sugar levels are frequently higher (>600 mg/dl) and there is no ketone body formation [4]. Therefore metabolic acidosis if present would likely be due to the precipitant cause such as infection with lactic acidosis. The reason for the absence of ketone bodies is due to the presence of some circulating insulin. This insulin can prevent the alteration in fatty acid metabolism leading to ketosis but due to peripheral insulin resistance still leads to very high serum glucose levels [6]. The presence of increased insulin counter regulatory hormones (esp. glucagon) exacerbates the hyperglycemia due to increased hepatic gluconeogenesis [7, 8]. The resultant osmotic diuresis leads to the severe dehydration (~12 L loss), azotemia, and hyperosmolarity (>330 mOsm/L) [4].

Serum osmolarity is calculated by the formula $2(Na^+ + K^+) + Glucose/18 + BUN/2.8$.

The precipitating causes can be infection, stoppage of medication, newly diagnosed diabetes, stroke, MI, subdural hematoma, and GI diseases. The treatment of this condition is hydration, correction of electrolyte aberrations, and treatment of the causative process. Insulin use will be needed to gradually bring down the blood sugar.

4. The principles for treatment of DKA are

   (a) Insulin therapy to decrease hyperglycemia and stop production of ketone bodies.
   (b) Hydration with isotonic solutions. Deficit may be up to 9 L in the average adult.

       Start with saline and convert to isotonic fluids with K^+ when K^+ levels start to decrease, and urine output is maintained [9]. Change to hypotonic solution if Na^+ level >150 meq/L [6].

       Bicarb therapy is only reserved for severe acidosis ($pH < 7.1$).
   (c) Replacement of other specific electrolytes Ca^{++}, Mg^{++}, PO_4.
   (d) Treatment of precipitating cause—infections, interruption of insulin, MI, trauma, stress.
   (e) Mental status changes—may need to have airway protected and ventilator assistance.
   (f) Ileus and other GI presentations, e.g., acute cholecystitis, either due to systemic ketosis or incidental, must be clinically managed.

5. The trending changes for electrolytes and the ABG with treatment will be:

   (a) BMP

   - Na^+—should be in the upper normal range.
   - K^+—after initial fluid resuscitation with use of NS (first 4 h), the K^+ levels will drop associated with the intracellular migration due now to the presence of insulin. K^+ can be added to IV fluids once the level goes below 4 meq/L, and a steady urine output is maintained.
   - Cl^-—will increase with use of normal saline (NS). Excessive use of NS can lead to hyperchloremic acidosis.
   - HCO_3—use of replacement $NaHCO_3$ is not required unless acidosis is severe (<pH7.1).

- Anion gap—will move toward normal gap of <11 meq/L.
- BUN—azotemia, if present, will normalize with hydration and increased urine production.
- Creatinine—as volume status and GFR improves, it should normalize unless kidneys are affected.
- Ca^{++}—can be low due to loss from osmotic diuresis—careful augmentation along with associated Mg^{++} and phosphate supplementation for their measured deficiencies.
- Glucose—the target is to gradually bring the blood sugar (BS) level down ~75–100 mg/h using regular insulin as an IV bolus (0.1 u/kg) followed by continuous infusion IV (0.1 u/kg/h) [4]. Rates of insulin infusion can be progressively ramped up with use of any standard protocol. Once BS levels reach the lower 200 s/dl, then 5% glucose should be added to the IV fluids to prevent hypoglycemia [10]. Target blood sugar is in the range 120–150 mg/dl.

(b) ABG

- pH—with hydration alone, the acidosis should start to correct. Insulin is needed to prevent further ketone production and bring down glucose levels.
- $PaCO_2$—as metabolic acidosis is corrected, the respiratory alkalosis should normalize.
- PaO_2—with normalization of vascular volume, the oxygenation should improve.
- HCO_3—if there is severe metabolic acidosis, then correction with exogenous bicarb will be required. Level should normalize with decreased ketone body formation and elimination of the same by the normal buffer systems.
- BE—abnormality will normalize with therapy.
- O_2 saturation—with fluid resuscitation the maintenance of normal O_2 saturation will be easier.

6. Once the patient has had definitive treatment for DKA and has shown metabolic stabilization, surgery can proceed. The principles for perioperative management would include:

(a) Continuing the use of appropriate fluids and electrolyte and IV insulin administration by infusion.
(b) Precautions for a full stomach before induction if not already intubated.
(c) Type 1 diabetics can have a difficult airway due to stiffening of tissues of the upper airway and rigidity of the cervical spine [7].
(d) Arterial line and good venous access for this particular case would be appropriate. Central venous access for volume estimation in major surgery or in patients with comorbidity would be appropriate.

(e) Glucose checks at least hourly under anesthesia with BMP and ABG at regular intervals.
(f) At the end of the procedure, extubation would depend on preinduction status, intraoperative course, and emergence profile. The postoperative care should continue in an ICU setting with treatment for both initiating and coexisting clinical issues.
(g) Once stable, the diet and treatment plan must be made with type, amount, and route of administration of insulin determined.

References

1. Magee MF, Bhatt BA. Management of decompensated diabetes. Diabetic ketoacidosis and hyperglycemic hyperosmolar syndrome. Crit Care Clin. 2001;17(1):75–106.
2. Lu J, Zello GA, Randell E, Adeli K, Krahn J, Meng QH. Closing the anion gap: contribution of D-lactate to diabetic ketoacidosis. Clin Chim Acta. 2011;412(3–4):286–91.
3. Cox K, Cocchi MN, Salciccioli JD, Carney E, Howell M, Donnino MW. Prevalence and significance of lactic acidosis in diabetic ketoacidosis. J Crit Care. 2012;27(2):132–7.
4. Kasper DL, Jameson JL, Hauser S, Loscalzo J, Fauci AS, Longo D, editors. Harrison's principles of internal medicine. 19th ed. New York: McGraw-Hill Medical; 2015. Chap. 418.
5. Roizen MF, Fleisher LA. Anesthetic implications of concurrent disease. In: Miller RD, editor. Miller's anesthesia. 8th ed. Philadelphia: Churchill Livingstone/Elsevier; 2015.
6. Delaney MF, Zisman A, Kettyle WM. Diabetic ketoacidosis and hyperglycemic hyperosmolar nonketotic syndrome. Endocrinol Metab Clin N Am. 2000;29(4):683–705.
7. McAnulty GR, Robertshaw HJ, Hall GM. Anaesthetic management of patients with diabetes mellitus. Br J Anaesth. 2000;85(1):80–90.
8. Nattrass M. Diabetic ketoacidosis. Medicine. 2010;38(12):667–70.
9. Chua HR, Venkatesh B, Stachowski E, Schneider AG, Perkins K, Ladanyi S, et al. Plasma-Lyte 148 vs 0.9% saline for fluid resuscitation in diabetic ketoacidosis. J Crit Care. 2012;27(2):138–45.
10. Nyenwe EA, Kitabchi AE. Evidence-based management of hyperglycemic emergencies in diabetes mellitus. Diabetes Res Clin Pract. 2011;94(3):340–51.

Chapter 39
Blood Gas IV

Ranganathan Govindaraj

Below are the values obtained on arterial blood gas measurement of a patient on cardiopulmonary bypass (CPB).

pH	7.44
pCO_2	30.8 mmHg
pO_2	354 mmHg
BE	3 mmol/L
HCO_3	27 mmol/L
SpO_2	100%

Sample type: arterial

F_iO_2: 35
Temp: 30°C

1. What type of clinical test is this and what does it measure?
2. What is the importance of temperature in the reported result?
3. What is the pH-stat approach?
4. What is the α-stat approach?
5. Which is better?

R. Govindaraj, MD, FRCA
Associate Professor for Anesthesia and Pain, Department of Anesthesiology, UTMB, Galveston, TX, USA

Director for Ultrasound Guided Regional Anesthesia, Galveston, TX 77555, USA
e-mail: gorangan@utmb.edu

T.D. Raj (ed.), *Data Interpretation in Anesthesia*,
DOI 10.1007/978-3-319-55862-2_39

Answers

1. This is an arterial blood gas (ABG) analysis; it gives information about the adequacy of a patient's gas exchange and acid–base status. It is used perioperatively, during CPB and also in severe lung disease (severe asthma in the ER), cardiac and kidney failure, uncontrolled diabetes, severe infections, drug overdose, and also in the ICU. An abnormal pH value as in acidosis or alkalosis can occur in disease states. ABG helps us to determine if the acid–base derangement is respiratory or metabolic in origin. The result is always reported taking into consideration the temperature of the patient at the time of collection.

2. The arterial blood sample is preheated to 37°C prior to measurement. If the actual patient temperature is keyed in, modern blood gas machines will report the pH value for that temperature as well. This is calculated mathematically from the pH measured at 37°C. For clinical use, the Rosenthal correction factor is recommended and is done as follows:

   Change in pH = 0.015 pH units per degree Celsius change in temperature.

   According to Henry's law, the solubility of a gas increases with decrease in temperature. PO_2 is 5 mmHg lower and PCO_2 is 2 mmHg lower for each degree below 37°. Hypothermia causes a decrease in the PCO_2 (hypocarbia) and a concomitant increase in the pH (alkalemia), yet the total body CO_2 content remains the same. There are two blood gas management strategies in hypothermia—temperature correction (pH stat) or not (α stat). These have different effects on cerebral blood flow, oxygen dissociation curve, and intracellular enzyme and protein activity.

3. In the pH-stat strategy (in hypothermic CPB or deep hypothermic circulatory arrest [DHCA]), blood gases are corrected to patient's temperature by decreasing the CPB gas sweep rate (which *decreases* the removal of CO_2) or adding CO_2 to the oxygenator to maintain a constant pH of 7.4 and PCO_2 of 40 mmHg at varying patient temperature. pH stat requires an increased total body CO_2 content to maintain neutrality during hypothermia thereby producing an acidotic state.

   The increased PCO_2 exerts a cerebral vasodilatory effect (loss of autoregulation). Proposed benefits of pH stat include rightward shift of the oxyhemoglobin dissociation curve increasing oxygen delivery, increased cerebral blood flow (CBF) decreasing the risk of cerebral ischemia during CPB, more complete and faster cooling, and greater suppression of cerebral metabolic rate [1–3].

4. In the α-stat approach, there is no temperature correction; blood gases are always interpreted at the same normal (37°C) temperature irrespective of the actual patient temperature. Neutrality is maintained only at 37°C permitting the hypothermic alkaline drift. No CO_2 is added and cerebral autoregulation is maintained.

   Alpha is the ratio of protonated to total imidazole of histidine (degree of dissociation) residues among protein molecules at 37°C. At the normal intracellular pH of 6.8, it is 0.55. The alpha value remains constant despite changes in temperature as the pK (dissociation constant) changes with temperature. This is optimal for intracellular enzyme structure and function which is the reason cited by its proponents who also argue that the increased CBF with the pH stat strategy may put the brain at risk from microemboli or cerebral edema. They also argue that the alkaline pH in the α-stat approach is beneficial before the ischemic insult of circulatory arrest [4, 5].

5. The debate over the optimal blood gas management is not over. This may not be important in moderate hypothermia but may be critical in deep hypothermia. In adults α-stat strategy is preferred to maintain cerebral autoregulation and limit cerebral embolic load, and in neonates and children, the pH-stat strategy demonstrated better outcomes. The reason for the difference may be related to the differences in the mechanism of brain injury on CPB. In children, due to the aortopulmonary collaterals causing hypoperfusion, the pH-stat strategy with its increased CBF seemed to provide benefit [6].

Easy way to remember: In pH stat you pour CO_2 into the circulation. In Alpha stat you don't.

References

1. Abdul Aziz KA, Meduoye A. Is pH-stat or alpha-stat the best technique to follow in patients undergoing deep hypothermic circulatory arrest? Interact Cardiovasc Thorac Surg. 2010;10(2):271–82. doi:10.1510/icvts. 2009.214130.
2. Sakamoto T, Kurosawa H, Shin'oka T, Aoki M, Isomatsu Y. The influence of pH strategy on cerebral and collateral circulation during hypothermic cardiopulmonary bypass in cyanotic patients with heart disease: results of a randomized trial and real-time monitoring. J Thorac Cardiovasc Surg. 2004;127(1):12–9. doi:10.1016/j.jtcvs. 2003.08.033.
3. Murkin JM, Martzke JS, Buchan AM, et al. A randomized study of the influence of perfusion technique and pH management strategy in 316 patients undergoing coronary artery bypass surgery: neurological and cognitive outcomes. J Thorac Cardiovasc Surg. 1995;110:349–62.
4. Reeves R. An imidazole alphastat hypothesis for vertebrate acid-base regulation: tissue carbon dioxide content and body temperature in bullfrogs. Respir Physiol. 1972;14(1–2):219–36.
5. Rahn H. Body temperature and acid-base regulation. Pneumologie. 1974;151(2):87–94.
6. Hensley FA, Martin DE, Gravlee GP. A practical approach to cardiac anesthesia. 5th ed. Philadelphia: Lippincott Williams & Wilkins; 2013.

Chapter 40
CBC/Chemistries I

Daniel A. Biggs

You are asked to see a healthy female at 38-weeks gestation. She has the following lab results:

Complete blood count (CBC)

- White blood count (WBC)—12,800 × 10^3/mm^3
- Hemoglobin (Hgb)—9.5 g/dL
- Hematocrit (Hct)—28.5%
- Platelets—148 × 10^9/L

Chemistries

- Sodium (Na)—136 meq/L
- Potassium (K)—3.9 meq/L
- Chloride (Cl)—108 meq/L
- Bicarbonate (HCO_3)—21 mmol/L
- Anion gap (AG)—7 mmol/L
- Blood urea nitrogen (BUN)—6 mg/dL
- Creatinine (Cr)—0.6 mg/dL
- Glucose—91 mg/dL
- Total protein—5.8 g/dL
- Albumin—3.2 g/dL
- Calcium (Ca)—8.7 mg/dL
- Total bilirubin—0.4 mg/dL
- Aspartate transaminase (AST/SGOT)—20 U/L
- Alanine transaminase (ALT/SGPT)—12 U/L
- Alkaline phosphatase (AP)—165 U/L

D.A. Biggs, MD, MSc
Department of Anesthesiology, Oklahoma University Medical Center,
750 NE 13th Street, Suite 200, Oklahoma City, OK 73104, USA
e-mail: Daniel-biggs@ouhsc.edu

T.D. Raj (ed.), *Data Interpretation in Anesthesia*,
DOI 10.1007/978-3-319-55862-2_40

Questions

1. What is the upper limit of normal for a WBC count in a term patient?
2. In a term patient what is the normal hemoglobin range? What level is considered to be anemia?
3. What is the normal lower limit of a platelet count?
4. How does pregnancy affect the serum bicarbonate level?
5. How do the renal function tests change BUN and creatinine?
6. Are the plasma proteins affected by pregnancy?
7. Which liver function test is frequently affected?

Answers

1. The upper limit for WBC increases through pregnancy. In the third trimester, this reaches 16,900/mm^3. This is primarily from an increase in neutrophils [1]. There is frequently a spike in labor.

2. The normal hemoglobin range during the third trimester is 9.5–15 gm/dL [1]. Anemia in pregnancy is defined as a Hgb below 11 gm/dL (compared to a threshold of below 12 gm/dL for the non-parturient) by the American College of Obstetrics and Gynecology and the World Health Organization [2]. The most common cause of anemia in pregnancy is iron deficiency. Other causes include micronutrient deficiencies, chronic inflammation, and inherited disorders such as sickle cell and the thalassemias. The increase in blood volume in pregnancy results in a relatively lower Hct when compared with nonpregnant females. This is because the plasma volume increases at a higher percentage than does the red cell mass [3].

3. Platelet count normal range changes very little in pregnancy. This range is 146–429 × 10^9/L near term [1]. Approximately 8% of pregnant patients at term will have platelet counts <150,000 and in about 1% it will be <100,000 [3].

4. Bicarbonate levels are decreased throughout pregnancy [1]. Tidal volume increases by about 1/3, and the respiratory rate increases slightly resulting in a 30–50% increase in minute ventilation. The CO_2 decreases to approximately 30 mmHg. Metabolic compensation results in a bicarbonate level of about 20 meq/L [3].

5. Both levels are decreased because of an increase by 50% in the glomerular filtration rate (GFR) and the increase in creatinine clearance from 120 ml/min to greater that 150 ml/min [3].

Test	Nonpregnant adult normal range	Third trimester pregnancy normal range
Blood urea nitrogen	7–20 mg/dL	3–11 mg/dL
Creatinine	0.5–0.9 mg/dL	0.4–0.9 mg/dL (commonly 0.5–0.6 mg/dL)

6. Total plasma proteins and albumin are both decreased.

Test	Nonpregnant adult normal range	Third trimester pregnancy normal range
Total plasma proteins	6.7–8.6 g/gL	5.6–6.7 g/dL
Albumin	4.1–5.3 g/dL	2.3–4.2 g/dL

7. Alkaline phosphatase (AP) is commonly increased 2–4 times above nonpregnant values because of production by the placenta [3].

References

1. Abbassi-Ghanavati M, Greer LG, Cunningham FG. Pregnancy and Laboratory Studies: a Reference Table for Clinicians. Obstet Gynecol. 2009;114:1326–31.
2. ACOG Practice Bulletin #95, Anemia in Pregnancy. Obstet Gynecol. 2008;112:201–7.
3. Chestnut DH, et al. Chestnut's Obstetric Anesthesia: Principles and Practice. 5th ed. Philadelphia: Elsevier Saunders; 2014.

Chapter 41
CBC/Chemistries II

Tanmay Shah

A 27-year-old G4P3 presented to antepartum clinic with high blood pressure and epigastric pain. On physical examination the patient had mild epigastric tenderness and 2+ edema over both lower extremities.

Vital signs: BP 170/120 mmHg, HR 90 bpm, RR 20 bpminute, SpO_2 95% on room air

Hb 11 mg/dL
Hct 33
Platelets 90 K
Creatinine >1.2 mg/dL
Billirubin >1.2 mg/mL
Uric acid >6 mg/mL
LDH >600 IU/L
Elevated AST/ALT
Proteinuria >0.3 g in a 24 h urine specimen

1. What laboratory work-up is needed to confirm your diagnosis?
2. How will you differentiate mild vs severe forms of the condition based on proteinuria?
3. What is important to look for in the complete blood count (CBC)?
4. How are blood urea nitrogen (BUN), creatinine, and uric acid levels affected in this condition?
5. Is the epigastric pain significant in this patient?
6. What is HELLP syndrome and what are some of the diagnostic criteria?
7. What will you look for in the DIC panel?

T. Shah, MD, MBBS
Department of Anesthesiology, University of Oklahoma Health Sciences Center,
750 NE 13th Street, Suite 200, Oklahoma City, OK 73104, USA
e-mail: Tanmay-Shah@ouhsc.edu

T.D. Raj (ed.), *Data Interpretation in Anesthesia*,
DOI 10.1007/978-3-319-55862-2_41

Answers

1. Complete blood cell count (CBC), serum electrolytes, blood urea nitrogen, creatinine, liver function test, serum uric acid, urine analysis—microscopic and 24 h specimen for protein and creatinine clearance. According to the American Congress of Obstetricians and Gynecologists (ACOG) practice bulletin in 2002, preeclampsia is defined as the new onset of hypertension and proteinuria after 20 weeks' gestation [1]. Proteinuria is a key factor in order to differentiate preeclampsia vs gestational hypertension and chronic hypertension in pregnancy. However in 2013 ACOG guidelines, proteinuria was removed from the diagnostic criteria of preeclampsia as it is nonspecific and doesn't always correlate with maternal and fetal outcomes. ACOG has suggested that any parturient with new-onset hypertension at 20 weeks of pregnancy or beyond, along with either of the following conditions, should be diagnosed with preeclampsia even in the absence of proteinuria.
   (a) Reduced platelet counts
   (b) Renal insufficiency
   (c) Severe headache
   (d) Cardiopulmonary compromise
   (e) Impaired liver function

2. Mild preeclampsia: BP ≥140/90 mmHg after 20 weeks of gestation
   (a) Proteinuria 300 mg/24 h or 1+ result on urine dipstick
   Severe preeclampsia: BP ≥160/110 mmHg
   (b) Proteinuria >5 g/24 h

3. Thrombocytopenia is present in 15–30% of women with preeclampsia, and it is the most common hematologic abnormality [2]. Platelet counts of less than 100,000/mm^3 occur mostly in severe preeclampsia or HELLP syndrome. Platelet counts also correlate with the severity of the disease process and the incidence of placental abruption [3]. Therefore, serial CBC (6 h apart) should be drawn in a patient with severe preeclampsia to follow the progression of the disease.

   Women with preeclampsia are usually intravascular volume depleted which causes hemoconcentration with false elevation of Hb and Hct [4]. It is also an indicator of severity, although measurements are decreased if hemolysis is present with HELLP syndrome.

4. Glomerular filtration rate (GFR) increases by 40–60% during the first trimester of pregnancy which causes a decrease in levels of BUN, creatinine, and uric acid [5]. These are the serum markers of renal clearance. In preeclampsia, GFR is 34% lower than in normal pregnancy. Decrease in GFR contributes to higher BUN and creatinine levels in women with preeclampsia. Abnormal or rising creatinine level suggests severe preeclampsia, especially in the presence of oliguria.

   Urate clearance decreases in women with preeclampsia with resulting increase in serum uric acid concentration which is possibly an early indicator of preeclampsia. Serum urate greater than 5.5 mg/dL is diagnostic of preeclampsia.

5. Epigastric or subcostal pain is an ominous symptom and is usually caused by the distension of the liver capsule by edema or subcapsular hemorrhage [6]. Hepatic dysfunction is frequently seen manifested as an increase in serum transaminase levels in patients with preeclampsia which should be followed serially to assess the disease progression to HELLP syndrome, if it occurs.

6. HELLP syndrome is a variant of severe preeclampsia characterized by *hemolysis*, *elevated liver enzymes*, and *low platelet counts*. It is associated with rapid clinical deterioration.
   (a) Diagnostic criteria:
      - Hemolysis:
        - Bilirubin >1.2 mg/dL
        - Lactic dehydrogenase >600 IU/L
        - Abnormal peripheral blood smear
   (b) Elevated liver enzymes:
      - Serum glutamic oxaloacetic transaminase (SGOT) ≥70 IU/L
   (c) Low platelet counts:
      - <100,000/mm^3

   Hemolysis is usually reflected as microangiopathic hemolytic anemia on peripheral blood smear which demonstrates schistocytes, burr cells, and echinocytes.

7. Patients with severe preeclampsia and HELLP syndrome can develop disseminated intravascular coagulation, and its presence should be confirmed by laboratory work-up. Blood work will show a decrease in fibrinogen level and severe thrombocytopenia as these procoagulants are decreased in DIC along with an increase in D-dimer level and fibrinogen degradation product (FDP) [1–3].

References

1. ACOG practice bulletin. Diagnosis and management of preeclampsia and eclampsia. Number 33, January 2002. American College of Obstetricians and Gynecologists. Int J Gynaecol Obstet. 2002 Apr;77(1):67–75.
2. Chestnut DH, et al. Chestnut's obstetric anesthesia: principles and practice. 4th ed. Philadelphia: Mosby; 2009.
3. Barash PG, et al. Clinical anesthesia. 6th ed. Philadelphia: Lippincott Williams & Wilkins; 2009.
4. Yao FSF. Yao & Artusio's anesthesiology: problem-oriented patient management. 7th ed. Philadelphia: Lippincott Williams & Wilkins; 2012.
5. Moran P, Lindheimer MD, Davison JM. The renal response to preeclampsia. Semin Nephrol. 2004;24:588–95.
6. Walters BN. Preeclamptic angina—a pathognomonic symptom of preeclampsia. Hypertens Pregnancy. 2011;30:117–24.

Chapter 42
Blood Gas: Fetal

Tanmay Shah

A 27-year-old woman, G1P0, had an emergent cesarean section with an epidural anesthesia for severe fetal heart rate deceleration. A nuchal cord was found at the time of delivery by the obstetrician and an umbilical blood gas was ordered.

Umbilical artery blood gas values were as follows:

pH 7.27, PCO_2 50 mmHg, pO_2 20 mmHg, HCO_3 23 mEq/L, Base excess −3.6 mEq/L

1. How will you interpret this blood gas value and what are the different types of acidosis?
2. What are the different methods to assess fetal acid–base balance?
3. In the newborn, is blood sampling for blood gas analysis performed from the umbilical artery or vein?
4. Is fetal blood gas estimation more reliable than Apgar scores in assessing a newborn's condition?
5. Is umbilical blood gas analysis done for every newborn?
6. What is the implication of fetal blood gas acidosis?
7. Does fetal acidosis have long-term sequelae on neonatal outcome?
8. What should you do as an anesthesiologist during routine/urgent cesarean section to improve fetal outcome?

T. Shah, MD, MBBS
Department of Anesthesiology, University of Oklahoma Health Sciences Center,
750 NE 13th Street, Suite 200, Oklahoma City, OK 73104, USA
e-mail: Tanmay-Shah@ouhsc.edu

T.D. Raj (ed.), *Data Interpretation in Anesthesia*,
DOI 10.1007/978-3-319-55862-2_42

Answers

1. The given values are representative of a normal blood gas for a newborn. The table below lists normal findings for a fetal blood gas at term gestation [1].

	Umbilical artery	Umbilical vein
pH	7.27	7.34
PCO_2 (mmHg)	50	40
pO_2 (mmHg)	20	30
Bicarbonate (mEq/L)	23	21
Base excess (mEq/L)	−3.6	−2.6

During oxidative metabolism, carbonic acid is produced, which is usually cleared by the placenta as carbon dioxide [2]. If placental blood flow is not adequate, then CO_2 elimination can be affected leading to **respiratory acidosis**. Lactic and beta-hydroxybutyric acids are produced as a result of anaerobic metabolism [3], which requires hours of metabolic clearance and contributes to **metabolic** and **mixed acidosis**.

2. Fetal acid–base balance can be accessed via a number of ways:
   (a) Antepartum: by percutaneous umbilical cord blood sampling
   (b) Intrapartum: by fetal scalp blood sampling (after membranes have ruptured)
   (c) Postpartum: by umbilical cord blood sampling

3. Usually, blood samples from both umbilical artery and vein are collected, which represent the fetal and maternal condition, respectively. In addition to maternal condition, umbilical vein blood samples also represent the utero-placental gas exchange.

   In order for blood samples to be accurate, the umbilical cord should be double clamped at least 10–20 cm apart immediately after delivery, and the blood samples should be drawn via heparinized syringe within 15 min of delivery [3]. For accuracy, the samples should be analyzed within 30–60 min. Air bubbles should also be removed from the syringe to get accurate pO_2 measurement.

   In low birth weight infant, it can be difficult to obtain blood sample from the umbilical artery, especially if it is small. In such situations, the newborn should be carefully evaluated for arterial academia, since isolated venous blood gas pH can be normal.

4. Umbilical cord blood gas analysis is routinely ordered by obstetricians if there is suspicion of neonatal depression. It reflects the fetal condition immediately before delivery and is a more objective indication of a newborn's condition than Apgar score, as Apgar score is usually done after the delivery at 1 min, 5 min,

and 10 min interval. However, there is usually a time lag between blood gas sampling and analysis. In the meantime neonatal condition should be assessed by the Apgar score.

Another factor that can affect umbilical arterial blood pH is the mode of delivery. A fetus that is delivered via spontaneous vaginal delivery will have a lower pH than the one delivered by elective cesarean section as the former has to go through the stress of labor. Duration of labor can also affect pH measurement, as prolonged labor in nulliparous women will lower the fetal pH.

5. In 2006, the American Congress of Obstetricians and Gynecologists (ACOG) recommended cord blood gas for:
   (a) Cesarean delivery for fetal compromise
   (b) Low 5-min Apgar score
   (c) Severe growth restriction
   (d) Abnormal FHR tracing
   (e) Maternal thyroid disease
   (f) Intrapartum fever
   (g) Multiple gestation

6. The type of acidosis, if present, should be ascertained, as metabolic and mixed acidosis are associated with an increased incidence of neonatal complications and death [4]. One study found a higher incidence of neonatal death when the pH of umbilical arterial blood was less than 7.00. Seizures were also reported in infants with pH of less than 7.05.

7. According to the ACOG Task Force in 2006, an umbilical artery pH of less than 7.0 and a base deficit of greater than or equal to 12 mmol/L at delivery pointed toward an acute intrapartum hypoxic event which could eventually cause cerebral palsy [5, 6].

   Whenever pH is less than 7.00, the base deficit and bicarbonate values are the predictors for neonatal morbidity [7]. Moderate to severe complications occur in 10% of infants when base deficit is 12–16 mmol/L, which increases to 40% when base deficit is more than 16 mmol/L.

8. There are certain things that can be done by an anesthesiologist to improve the fetal outcome during routine/urgent c-section to maintain adequate placental perfusion.
   (a) Provide left uterine displacement to avoid aorto–caval compression by gravid uterus
   (b) Support the hemodynamics by intravenous administration of fluids and vasopressors if needed to maintain utero-placental circulation (as it is MAP dependent)
   (c) If general anesthesia is chosen, then maintain proper oxygenation by providing at least 50% oxygen when mixed with 50% N_2O to avoid hypoxia

References

1. Miller RD, Pardo MC Jr. Basics of anesthesia. 6th ed. Philadelphia: Elsevier Saunders; 2011.
2. Morgan GE, Mikhail MS, Murray MJ. Clinical anesthesiology. 4th ed. New York: McGraw-Hill; 2006.
3. Chestnut DH, et al. Chestnut's obstetric anesthesia: principles and practice. 4th ed. Philadelphia: Mosby; 2009.
4. Victory R, Penava D, Da Silva O, et al. Umbilical cord pH and base excess values in relation to adverse outcome events for infants delivering at term. Am J Obstet Gynecol. 2004;191:2021.
5. American College of Obstetricians and Gynecologists (ACOG) and American Academy of Pediatrics (AAP). Neonatal encephalopathy and neurologic outcome. 2nd ed. Washington, DC: ACOG; 2014.
6. Low JA, Lindsay BG, Derrick EJ. Threshold of metabolic acidosis associated with newborn complications. Am J Obstet Gynecol. 1997;177:1391.
7. Wiberg N, Källén K, Olofsson P. Base deficit estimation in umbilical cord blood is influenced by gestational age, choice of fetal fluid compartment, and algorithm for calculation. Am J Obstet Gynecol. 2006;195:1651.

Part III
Imaging

Chapter 43
Ultrasound: Abnormal Placenta

Madhumani Rupasinghe

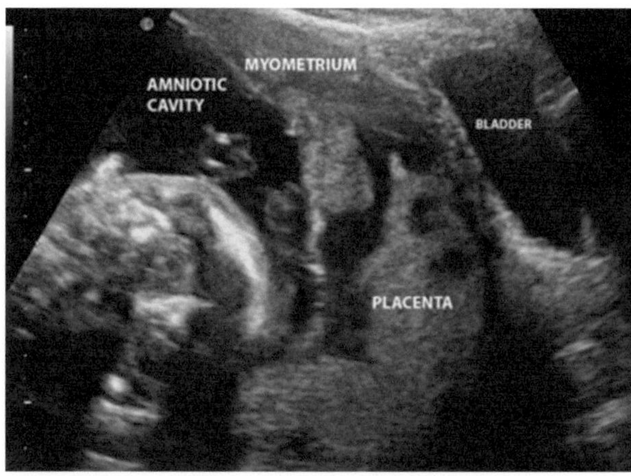

Fig. 43.1 Abnormal placental implantation (Reproduced with permissions from Elsevier [1])

1. What is concerning regarding the ultrasound image in Figs. 43.1 and 43.2?
2. What risk factors are implicated in this presentation?
3. What is the classification/grading and common sonographic findings?
4. What is the frequency of this presentation?
5. How does coagulation change during pregnancy?
6. What is your choice of anesthesia?

M. Rupasinghe, MBBS, FRCA
Department of Anesthesiology, University of Texas Health Science Center at Houston, 6431 Fannin Street, MSB 5.020, Houston, TX 77030, USA
e-mail: Madhumani.Rupasinghe@uth.tmc.edu

T.D. Raj (ed.), *Data Interpretation in Anesthesia*,
DOI 10.1007/978-3-319-55862-2_43

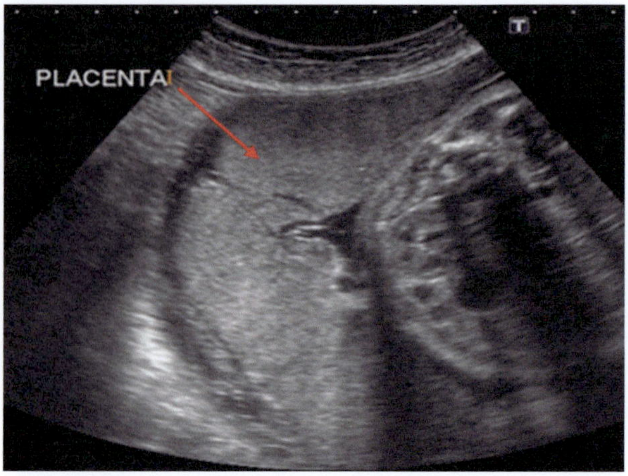

Fig. 43.2 Normal pregnancy ultrasound image

Answers

1. The ultrasound image depicts abnormal placental attachment to the uterine wall, which is characterized by invasion of trophoblast into the uterine myometrium.

2. The incidence of placenta accreta has been increasing and seems to parallel the increasing cesarean section rate. A low-lying placenta (placenta previa) and any condition or surgeries resulting in myometrial tissue damage, along with advanced maternal age and multiparity have been implicated as risk factors.

3. Diagnosis of placenta accreta is usually established by transabdominal and transvaginal ultrasonography and may be supplemented by magnetic resonance imaging (MRI). Abnormal placental attachment is defined according to the depth of myometrial invasion as:

    (a) Accreta: Chorionic villi attach to the myometrium
    (b) Increta: Chorionic villi invade into the myometrium
    (c) Percreta: Chorionic villi invade through the myometrium

    The common sonographic findings being:

    (a) Loss of normal hypoechoic retro placental zone
    (b) Multiple vascular lacunae within placenta, giving "Swiss cheese" appearance
    (c) Blood vessels or placental tissue bridging uterine-placental margin
    (d) Retro placental myometrial thickness of <1 mm

4. Frequency of placenta accreta according to number of cesarean deliveries and presence or absence of placenta previa [2]:

Cesarean delivery	Placenta previa	No placenta previa
First (primary)	3.3	0.03
Second	11	0.2
Third	40	0.1
Fourth	61	0.8
Fifth	67	0.8
≥Sixth	67	4.7

5. Pregnancy is a relatively hypercoagulable state characterized by an increased activity of clotting factors (I, VII, VIII, IX, X, XII), increased levels of fibrinogen, and decreased activity of physiologic anticoagulants (significant reduction in protein S activity and acquired activated protein C resistance).

    Procoagulant changes are balanced by significant activation of fibrinolytic system and deactivation of natural antifibrinolytics via decrease in activity of factors XI and XIII.

    Platelet count can be low or normal. There is a dramatic short-term increase in coagulability immediately after delivery due to increase in factor V and VIII activity.

6. There is no single optimal anesthetic plan for all patients; both general anesthesia and neuraxial techniques have been used successfully. Involvement of a multidisciplinary team which consists of MFM, anesthesiology, urology, general surgery, and interventional radiology improves outcome. One of the primary anesthetic considerations is the potential for significant blood loss necessitating preparation for volume resuscitation which may require multiple large bore venous access and invasive arterial monitoring. Appropriate preparations may include arterial occlusion techniques, arterial embolization, skilled surgical personnel, cell salvage, as well as availability of blood products. In addition, use of point of care monitoring (TEG) and adjuncts to transfusion such as recombinant Factor VIIa and antifibrinolytics should be considered in cases of massive hemorrhage [3].

References

1. Jauniaux E, Jurkovic D. Placenta accreta: pathogenesis of a 20th century iatrogenic uterine disease. Placenta. 2012;33(4):244–51. doi:10.1016/j.placenta.2011.11.010.
2. Belfort MA, et al. Placenta accreta. Am J Obstet Gynecol. 2010;203(5):430–9. doi:10.1016/j.ajog.2010.09.013.
3. Snegovskikh D, Clebone A, Norwitz E. Anesthetic management of patients with placenta accreta and resuscitation strategies for associated massive hemorrhage. Curr Opin Anesthesiol. 2011;24(3):274–81. doi:10.1097/ACO.0b013e328345d8b7.

Chapter 44
CXR I

Raghuvender Ganta

Fig. 44.1

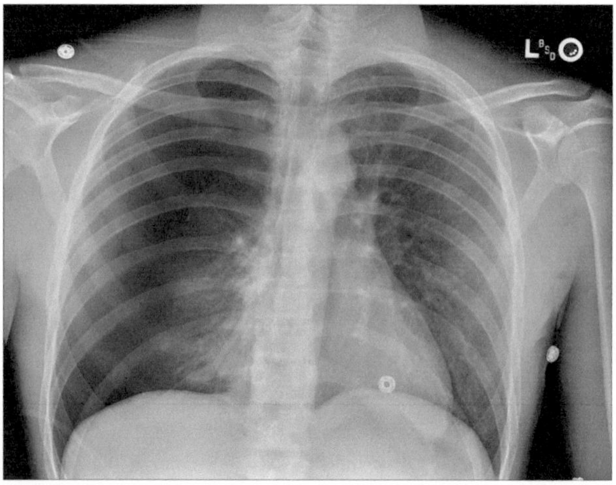

1. What does above image Fig. 44.1 show?
2. Is there a way to classify this condition?
3. What are the causes and the clinical presentation of this condition?
4. What are the indications for surgical intervention?
5. How do you treat tension pneumothorax?

R. Ganta, MD, FRCA
Department of Anesthesiology, VA Hospital, OUMC,
921 NE 13th Street, Oklahoma City, OK 73104, USA
e-mail: raghuvender-Ganta@ouhsc.edu

T.D. Raj (ed.), *Data Interpretation in Anesthesia*,
DOI 10.1007/978-3-319-55862-2_44

Answers

1. The image shows a large right-sided pneumothorax with visible margins of the collapsed lung. Pneumothorax is the presence of gas within the pleural space owing to disruption of the parietal or visceral pleura.

2. Classification
   Neonatal, spontaneous, traumatic

   - Pediatric pneumothorax – neonates with respiratory distress syndrome, especially if they are mechanically ventilated with positive and expiratory pressure and are prone to pneumothorax.
   - Congenital diaphragmatic hernia results in underdeveloped lung ipsilateral to the defect in diaphragm. The more compliant contralateral lung is prone to barotrauma and pneumothorax.

   Spontaneous pneumothorax occurs without trauma and most often in males between 20 and 35 years of age. These patients are often tall and slender, and most of the patients are smokers. Recurrent spontaneous pneumothorax is common during the first year after the initial event.

   Primary spontaneous pneumothorax occurs in tall, thin males aged 20–40 and who are smokers. Secondary spontaneous pneumothorax occurs in patients with underlying pulmonary disease, and the presentation may be more serious with symptoms and sequelae due to comorbid conditions.

   Traumatic pneumothorax

   Blunt or penetrating trauma to the chest wall can cause a pneumothorax; the most common cause is iatrogenic and is caused by subclavian line placement.

   Tension pneumothorax

   This occurs when air enters the pleural cavity on inspiration but, because of a ball-valve mechanism, is unable to exit. This progressively enlarges the pleural space, shifting the mediastinum and trachea to the contralateral side and also decreasing venous return. Tension pneumothorax is a medical emergency and without prompt intervention leads to rapid deterioration in the patient's condition leading to death [1].

3. Some causes of pneumothorax were mentioned under the classification. Other causes may include laparoscopic intra-abdominal surgical procedures such as cholecystectomy, nephrectomy, adrenalectomy, hiatal hernia repair, or positive end expiratory pressure (PEEP) [2].

   The clinical presentation of pneumothorax can vary depending on the type and severity and can range from no symptoms to acute distress which can be life-threatening. Symptoms may include sudden and severe pleuritic chest pain accompanied by dyspnea and cough.

   The hemithorax is hyperresonant to percussion, with tracheal shift away from the affected side. Neck veins may become distended. Breath sounds may be diminished or absent. There may be increased airway pressure, decreased pulmonary compliance, cyanosis, and hypotension during the intraoperative period. Blood gases show hypoxia and hypercarbia in severe cases. Radiographic examination is the best diagnostic tool. Other modalities for diagnosis include chest ultrasonography and computed tomography.

Treatment of pneumothorax is with a chest tube, when large amounts of lung are collapsed. The spontaneous pneumothorax usually gets absorbed when the collapsed lung is estimated to be less than 20%. Spontaneous resorption may be accelerated by the administration of supplemental oxygen.

4. An air leak from the lung that persists for more than 10 days may be an indication for surgical intervention. Recurrent pneumothorax can be treated by chemical pleurodesis without a thoracotomy by instilling tetracycline into the pleural space [3].

5. Tension pneumothorax (Fig. 44.2) is a surgical emergency, and if suspected on clinical grounds, time should not be spent seeking radiological evidence. A large-bore needle should be placed in the second intercostal space in the midclavicular line, allowing air to drain freely (Fig. 44.3). The needle should be left in place until a tube thoracotomy is performed.

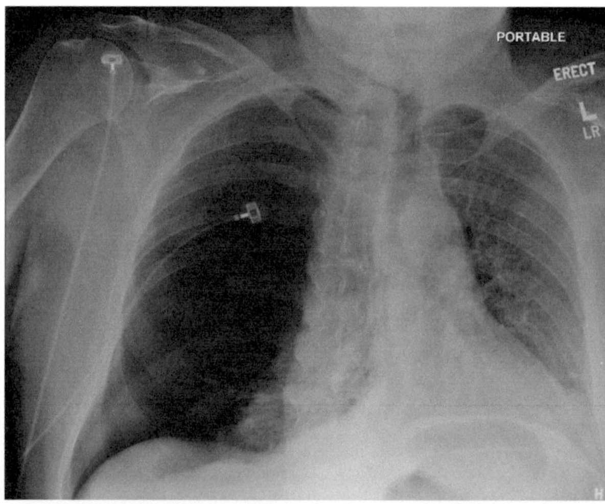

Fig. 44.2 Tension pneumothorax

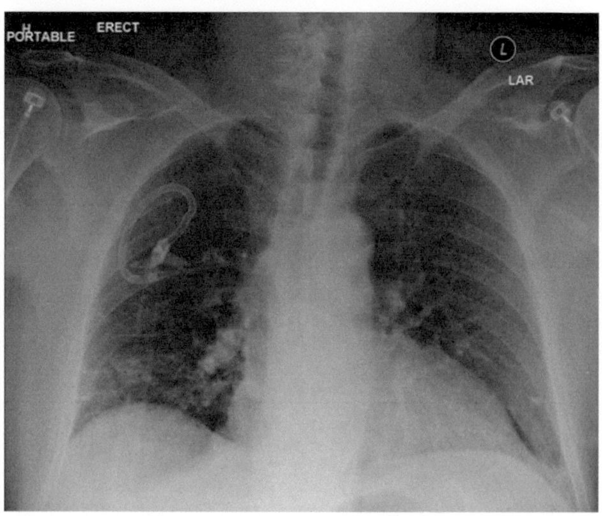

Fig. 44.3 After treatment with a chest tube

References

1. Krasnik M, Christensen B, Halkier E, et al. Pleurodesis in spontaneous pneumothorax by means of tetracycline: follow-up evaluation of a method. Scand J Thorac Cardiovasc Surg. 1987;21:181–8.
2. Marshall BE, Longnecker NE, Fairley HB. Anesthesia for thoracic procedures. Boston: Blackwell Scientific; 1988.
3. Roberts DJ, Leigh-Smith S, Faris PD, et al. Clinical manifestations of tension pneumothorax: protocol for a systematic review and meta-analysis. Syst Rev. 2014;3:3.

Chapter 45
CXR II

Marcos E. Gomes

Below is an image of a chest x-ray of an ICU patient on a ventilator.

1. Name some causes for the changes seen in the image?
2. What's the most valuable x-ray finding used to help differentiate the etiology of this finding?
3. What is the differential diagnosis of this finding when there is no tracheal deviation or mediastinal shift on chest x-ray?
4. What is the differential diagnosis when there is mediastinal shift away from the opacity?
5. What is the differential diagnosis when there is mediastinal shift toward the opacity?

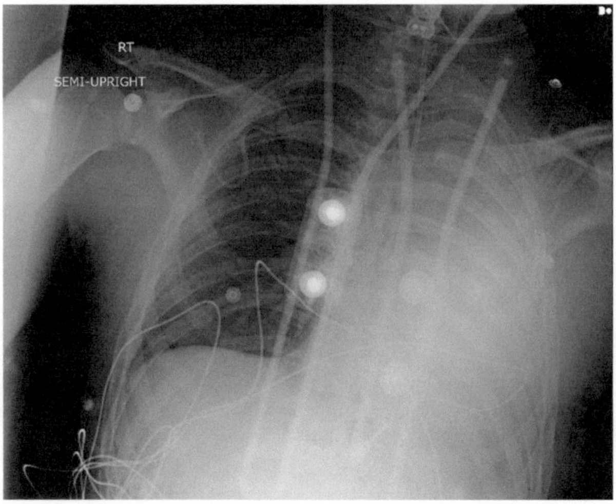

Fig. 45.1 Chest x-ray (AP view)

M.E. Gomes, MD
Department of Anesthesiology, University of Oklahoma Health Sciences Center, 750 NE 13th Street, Suite 200, Oklahoma City, OK 73104, USA
e-mail: mewgomes@gmail.com

T.D. Raj (ed.), *Data Interpretation in Anesthesia*,
DOI 10.1007/978-3-319-55862-2_45

Answers

1. The most common causes of unilateral lung whiteout on chest radiograph (Fig. 45.1) are pneumonia, pleural effusion (including hemothorax), and collapse/atelectasis. The ability to differentiate between collapse and pleural effusion is essential because they require distinct treatments, which, if applied erroneously, could harm the patient [1].
2. The most important finding that may help differentiate the etiology of unilateral whiteout is tracheal deviation or mediastinal shift.
3. With a finding of *central* mediastinum, diagnostic considerations include consolidation/pneumonia, pulmonary edema/ARDS, small to moderate pleural effusions (most likely would cause a partial rather than a complete whiteout), and mesothelioma. Small and moderate pleural effusions tend to gravitate posteriorly without producing mediastinal shift. Encasement of the lung in a mesothelioma patient limits mediastinal shift [2, 3].
4. With tracheal displacement *away* from the diffuse opacity, diagnostic considerations include a moderate to large pleural effusion, large pulmonary mass, and a diaphragmatic hernia. Diaphragmatic hernias on the right side usually consist of liver herniation, while on the left, from herniated bowel [2, 3].
5. Mediastinal shift *toward* the side of the opacity is seen in lung collapse (endobronchial intubation, mucus plugging), post-pneumonectomy, and pulmonary agenesis/hypoplasia. The figure above (Fig. 45.1) illustrates a case of mucus plugging in the ICU in a young patient with high-level spinal cord injury compromising the strength of his cough and therefore his ability to clear secretions. This scenario can be encountered by the anesthesiologist quite often. Endotracheal tube repositioning with or without bronchoscopy is a simple fix to main stem intubation, whereas endotracheal suctioning or bronchoscopy are easily performed to clear secretions and/or mucus plugs [1, 2, 3].

References

1. Fazili T, Dehadrai G. Unilateral white out on chest radiograph. Hosp Physician. 2009;45(5):27.
2. Drury N, et al. A unilateral whiteout: when not to insert a chest drain. J R Soc Med. 2010;103(1):31–3.
3. Khan AN, et al. Reading chest radiographs in the critically ill (Part II): radiography of lung pathologies common in the ICU patient. Ann Thorac Med. 2009;4(3):149–57.

Chapter 46
CXR III

German Barbosa-Hernandez

Abbreviations

AV block	Atrioventricular block
BiV ICD	Biventricular implantable cardio-defibrillator
CHF	Congestive heart failure
CXR	Chest x-ray
EF	Ejection fraction
EKG	Electrocardiogram
EP	Electrophysiology dept
ICD	Implantable cardio-defibrillator
PEA	Pulseless electrical activity
VT/VF	Ventricular tachycardia/ventricular fibrillation

A 65-year-old female after a motor vehicle collision requires emergency surgery for an open lower extremity fracture; the patient tells you she has a "bad heart," she has no history in your institution, and no signs of heart failure. An EKG shows wide QRS with dual-chamber pacing. A CXR on admission show (See Fig. 46.1).

1. What type of device is shown in the image?
2. What are the indications for cardiac implantable electronic device placement?
3. What is the effect of placing a magnet over the device (pacemaker and/or ICD)?
4. In the OR, you place a magnet over the device. The patient goes pulseless after prolonged use of electrocautery. What is your diagnosis?

G. Barbosa-Hernandez, MD
Department of Anesthesia, Oklahoma University Health and Science Center,
800 NE 10th Street, Oklahoma City, OK 73102, USA
e-mail: German-BarbosaHernandez@ouhsc.edu

T.D. Raj (ed.), *Data Interpretation in Anesthesia*,
DOI 10.1007/978-3-319-55862-2_46

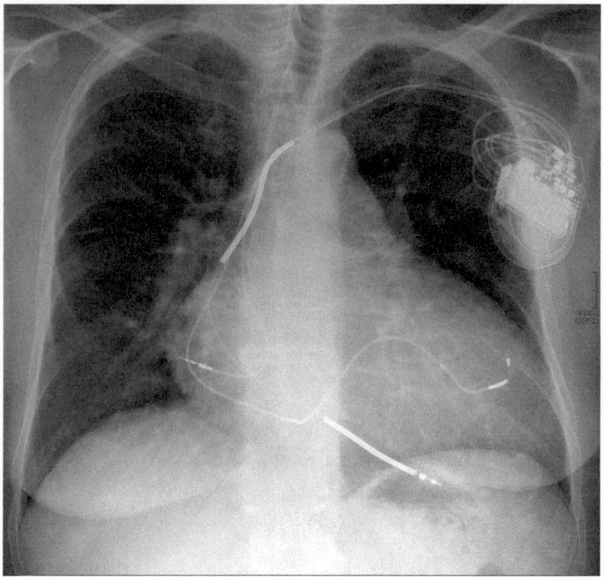

Fig. 46.1 Anterior posterior chest x-ray showing a cardiac device

5. What are the effects of electrocautery, radiation therapy, and radiofrequency on a pacemaker and an ICD?
6. What measures can you take to ensure proper intraoperative device functioning?

Answers

1. This patient has an implantable biventricular cardio-defibrillator (BiV ICD) [1].

   (a) The radiographic image of a pacemaker would show (See Fig. 46.2):

   - Smaller generator
   - Discreet right ventricular lead (stable diameter)
   - With or without right atrial lead or coronary sinus lead

   (b) The radiographic image of an ICD would show (See Fig. 46.3):

   - Larger generator.
   - Prominent right ventricular lead, otherwise known as shock coils. They appear as two metallic segments along the length of the ICD lead.

   (c) The radiographic image of a BiV ICD would show (See Fig. 46.4):

   - Larger generator
   - Prominent right ventricular lead (shock coils)
   - Right atrium lead
   - Coronary sinus lead

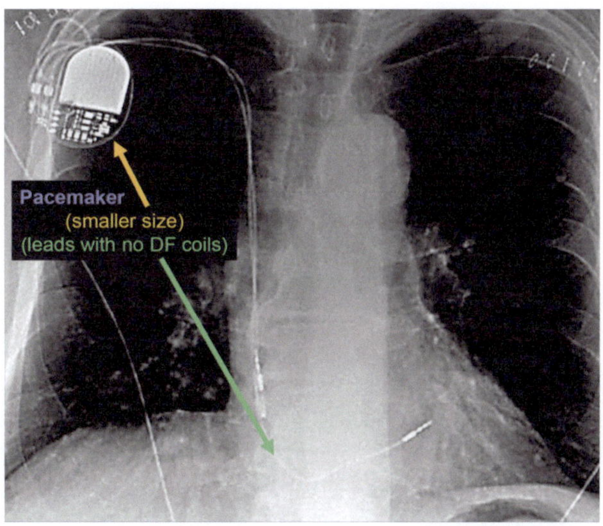

Fig. 46.2 Anterior posterior chest x-ray showing a pacemaker

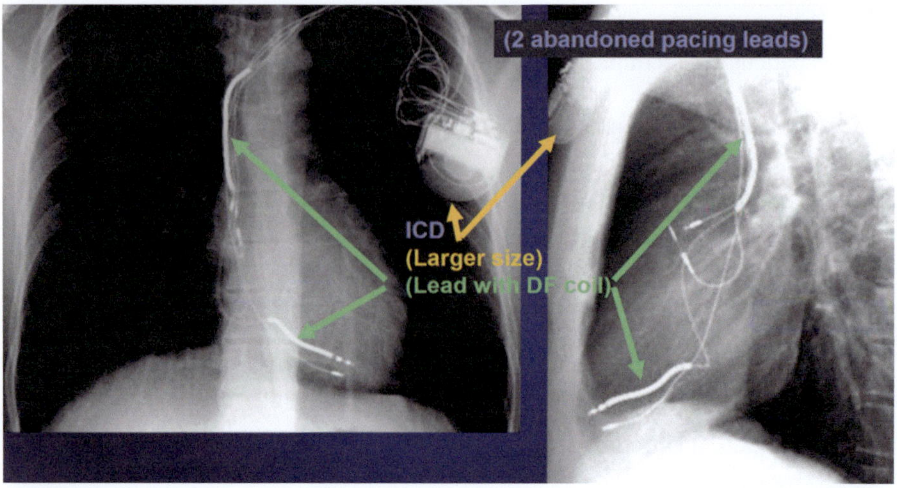

Fig. 46.3 Anterior posterior and lateral chest x-ray showing an ICD

Manufacturer ID can be seen in the CXR as well (See Fig. 46.5).

2. Indications for cardiac implantable electronic device placement [2]:

   (a) Pacemaker:

   - Patients with symptomatic sinus node dysfunction and bradycardia
   - Patients with complete AV block (symptoms less relevant)
   - Hypersensitive carotid sinus syndrome and neurocardiogenic syncope

   (b) ICD:

   - Patients at risk of sudden cardiac death: Prior ventricular tachycardia or fibrillation, low ejection fraction [3]
   - Long QT syndrome
   - Hypertrophic cardiomyopathy
   - Arrhythmogenic right ventricular dysplasia
   - Cardiac transplantation
   - Primary electrical disease: idiopathic ventricular fibrillation, short QT syndrome, Brugada syndrome, and catecholaminergic polymorphic ventricular tachycardia

   (c) BiV ICD:

   - Treatment of left ventricular dysfunction and heart failure, with prolonged ventricular conduction and heart failure symptoms.
   - Required ventricular pacing and low EF:
     - RV pacing in patients with low EF increases CHF admissions and mortality.
   - Cardiac resynchronization therapy [4]:
     - Improved exercise tolerance and mortality.
     - Continuous pacing provides better hemodynamic stability.

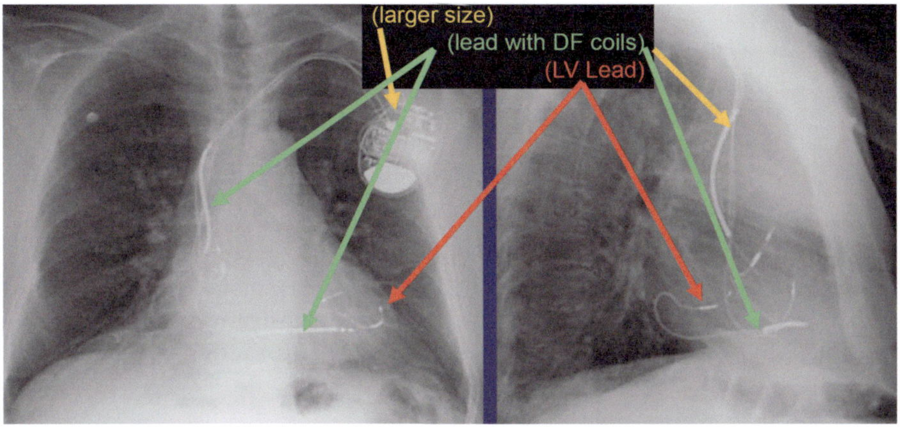

Fig. 46.4 Anterior posterior and lateral chest x-ray showing a BiV ICD

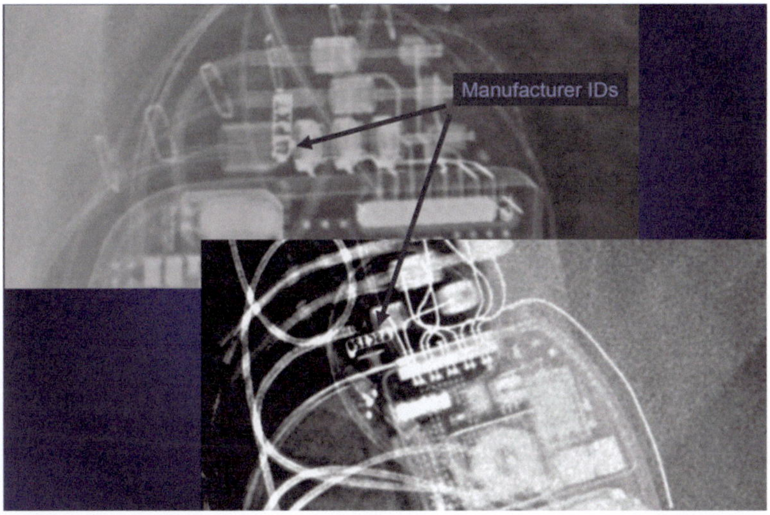

Fig. 46.5 Magnified view of a chest x-ray showing manufacturer ID of a cardiac implantable electronic device

3. Effect of a magnet on a device [5]:

   (a) Pacemaker:

   - Suspend sensing of intrinsic rhythm.
   - Pacing in an asynchronous mode: the rate depends on the manufacturer and the battery life; if the battery life is low, the rate may not be adequate for surgery.
   - Turns off "rate response."

   (b) ICD:

   - Varies depending on device, manufacturer, and programming of the device.

- In general it turns off detection of tachycardia and tachycardia therapy (discharge and pacing).
- In general, it has no effect on the pacemaker (pacing will not become asynchronous). In patients that are pacemaker dependent due to the risk of electrical interference and pacemaker malfunction, it is best to reprogram the device to address both the tachycardia and bradycardia therapy.

4. Most probably this patient has a BiV ICD and low ejection fraction and is pacemaker dependent. The device functioned appropriately with the magnet, which suspended the tachyarrhythmia detection. Pacing was inhibited by the prolonged use of electrocautery. Pacing returns to an unresponsive myocardium, after a prolonged period of asystole that might have led to PEA arrest.

5. Pacemaker [1, 6]:

   (a) Electrocautery:

   - Faulty sensing of intrinsic activity causing inappropriate inhibition of pacemaker activity
     – More prominent with monopolar cautery
     – More likely with above the waist surgery
   - Possible device reset or damage to the generator, or the leads, but unlikely

   (b) Radiation therapy:

   - Possible device reset when performed near the device

   (c) Radiofrequency:

   - Electrocautery-like electromagnetic interference that could cause inappropriate inhibition of pacemaker activity which is more likely with procedures above the waist
   - Possible device reset or damage to the generator, or the leads, but unlikely

ICD:

   (a) Electrocautery:

   - Faulty sensing of intrinsic activity causing inappropriate sensing of arrhythmias
     – More prominent with monopolar cautery
   - Possible device reset or damage to the generator, or the leads, but unlikely

   (b) Radiation therapy:

   - Possible device reset when performed near the device

   (c) Radiofrequency:

   - Electrocautery-like electromagnetic interference that could cause inappropriate arrhythmia sensing inhibition
   - Possible device reset or damage to the generator, or the leads, but unlikely

6. When facing a patient with a device one must ascertain [1, 5]:

   (a) Device type (see answer to question 1) and obtain as much information as possible

   - Is there a history of cardiac arrest, arrhythmias, or VT/VF?
   - Evaluate medical record, registration card.
   - Contact the manufacturer.

   (b) Procedure type: Location and presence of electromagnetic interference
   (c) Patients characteristics:

   - Pacemaker dependence:
     – Usually can tell just from the monitor or EKG. If pacing spikes are not visible, then usually they are not dependent.
     – If there are spikes in front of all or most P waves and/or QRS complexes, then assume pacemaker dependency.
   - Chambers being paced
   - Presence of low EF?

   (d) Urgency of the case

   - Elective cases:
     – Contact patient's provider, pacemakers should be seen every year, and ICDs every 6 months.
     – Follow recommendations.
   - Emergency cases:
     (1) General recommendations:

       a. Have magnet immediately available.
          i. If magnet impossible to place, must call EP; the device might require reprograming before the procedure.
       b. Monitor patient with plethysmography or arterial line.
          i. All other forms of monitoring are unreliable due to noise with electromagnetic interference.
       c. Transcutaneous pacing and defibrillation pads should be placed (anterior/posterior).
       d. Evaluate the pacemaker or ICD before leaving a cardiac-monitored environment.
       e. ICD patients should be on monitor at all times while ICD is deactivated.
       f. If any device is programmed specifically for surgery, patient cannot be taken off the monitor until the device is reprogrammed.

     (2) Recommendations for patients—not pacemaker dependent

       a. No ICD present:
          i. If the surgery is not within 6 inches (15 cm) of the device, then no other actions are necessary.

    ii. If the surgery is within 6 inches of the device, then a magnet can be placed or the device reprogramed by a device specialist to asynchronous mode (AOO, VOO, DOO).
  b. ICD or BiV ICD present:
    i. Place magnet to stop tachyarrhythmia detection.
    ii. If magnet is impossible to place, or surgery is within 6 inches of the device, or is a cardiac/thoracic procedure, then you must call the device specialist to turn off the tachyarrhythmia detection to avoid unwarranted discharges during the procedure if electrical interference is present.

(3) Recommendations for patients—pacemaker dependent

  a. No ICD present:
    i. Use short electrosurgical bursts.
    ii. Place magnet over device for procedures not within 6 inches (15 cm) of the device.
    iii. If magnet is impossible to place or surgery is within 6 inches of the device, then the device specialists must be called to reprogram to an asynchronous mode.

  b. ICD or BiV ICD present:
    i. Use short electrosurgical bursts.
    ii. If the surgery is not within 6 inches of the device, then place magnet over device to suspend tachyarrhythmia detection and contact the device specialist to reprogram the device to an asynchronous mode.
    iii. If magnet is impossible to place or surgery within 6 inches of the device, then contact in-hospital device specialist to reprogram the device to an asynchronous mode to avoid electrical interference and to turn off tachyarrhythmia detection to avoid unwarranted discharges during the procedure.

References

1. Aguilera AL, Volokhina YV, Fisher KL. Radiography of cardiac conduction devices: a comprehensive review. Radiographics. 2011;31(6):1669–82. doi:10.1148/rg.316115529.
2. Epstein AE, DiMarco JP, Ellenbogen KA, Estes NA 3rd, Freedman RA, Gettes LS, et al. 2012 ACCF/AHA/HRS focused update incorporated into the ACCF/AHA/HRS 2008 guidelines for device-based therapy of cardiac rhythm abnormalities: a report of the American College of Cardiology Foundation/American Heart Association Task Force on Practice Guidelines and the Heart Rhythm Society. J Am Coll Cardiol. 2013;61(3):e6–75. doi:10.1016/j.jacc.2012.11.007.
3. Moss AJ, Zareba W, Hall WJ, Klein H, Wilber DJ, Cannom DS, et al. Prophylactic implantation of a defibrillator in patients with myocardial infarction and reduced ejection fraction. N Engl J Med. 2002;346(12):877–83. doi:10.1056/NEJMoa013474.

4. Cleland JG, Daubert JC, Erdmann E, Freemantle N, Gras D, Kappenberger L, et al. The effect of cardiac resynchronization on morbidity and mortality in heart failure. N Engl J Med. 2005;352(15):1539–49. doi:10.1056/NEJMoa050496.
5. Crossley GH, Poole JE, Rozner MA, Asirvatham SJ, Cheng A, Chung MK, et al. The Heart Rhythm Society (HRS)/American Society of Anesthesiologists (ASA) Expert Consensus Statement on the perioperative management of patients with implantable defibrillators, pacemakers and arrhythmia monitors: facilities and patient management this document was developed as a joint project with the American Society of Anesthesiologists (ASA), and in collaboration with the American Heart Association (AHA), and the Society of Thoracic Surgeons (STS). Heart Rhythm. 2011;8(7):1114–54. doi:10.1016/j.hrthm.2010.12.023.
6. Costa A, Richman DC. Implantable devices: assessment and perioperative management. Anesthesiol Clin. 2016;34(1):185–99. doi:10.1016/j.anclin.2015.10.014.

Chapter 47
CXR/CT IV

Marcos E. Gomes

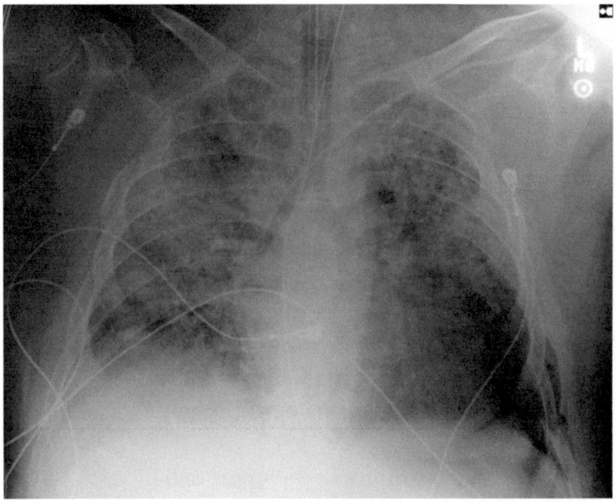

Fig. 47.1 Chest X-ray

M.E. Gomes, MD
Department of Anesthesiology, University of Oklahoma Health Sciences Center,
750 NE 13th Street, Suite 200, Oklahoma City, OK 73104, USA
e-mail: mewgomes@gmail.com

T.D. Raj (ed.), *Data Interpretation in Anesthesia*,
DOI 10.1007/978-3-319-55862-2_47

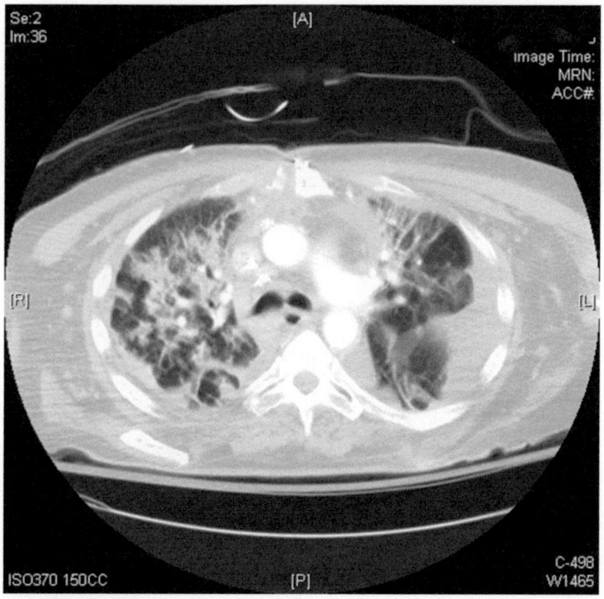

Fig. 47.2 Chest computed tomography

1. What do the images above show and what is the differential diagnosis based on the appearance seen in the images above?
2. What is the current definition of acute respiratory distress syndrome?
3. Name some common triggers for the development of ARDS.
4. What is the approach for mechanical ventilation on patients with the above diagnosis?
5. Is there an indication for steroids, statins, or neuromuscular blockade (NMB) in ARDS?
6. Which nonconventional therapies can be used to enhance oxygenation in severe ARDS?
7. What is the role of nitric oxide and prostaglandins in ARDS?

Answers

1. The chest X-ray (Fig. 47.1) shows diffuse bilateral coalescent opacities, whereas the CT chest (Fig. 47.2) shows ground-glass opacification, reflecting an overall reduction in the air content of the affected lung. It is also possible to visualize bronchial dilatation within areas of ground-glass opacification. Differential diagnosis include (a) ARDS, (b) congestive heart failure, (c) pulmonary hemorrhage, (d) pneumonia, (e) transfusion-related acute lung injury, and (f) non-cardiogenic pulmonary edema.

2. The Berlin definition, dated 2012, states that acute respiratory distress syndrome is an entity characterized by hypoxemia and stiff lungs that occurs within a week of a known clinical insult or new/worsening respiratory symptoms. It presents with bilateral opacities on the chest X-ray involving at least three quadrants that are not fully explained by effusions, atelectasis, or nodules. Chest computed tomography (CT) findings are opacification that is denser in the most dependent regions as compared to more normal and hyper-expanded lung in the nondependent ones. In addition, CT chest shows widespread ground-glass attenuation, which is a nonspecific sign that reflects an overall reduction in the air content of the affected lung. Respiratory failure in ARDS must not be fully explained by cardiac failure, and an objective assessment for exclusion of such cause may be necessary by echocardiography. Finally, ARDS is classified as mild, moderate, or severe based on PaO_2/FiO_2 ratio and PEEP. If PaO_2/FiO_2 ratio is between 200 and 300 mmHg with PEEP ≥ 5, it is classified as mild. If PaO_2/FiO_2 ratio between 100 and 200 mmHg with PEEP ≥ 5, it is moderate. PaO_2/FiO_2 ratio less than 100 mmHg with PEEP ≥ 5 is classified as severe. Note that the term acute lung injury has been removed, as well as the requirement of pulmonary capillary wedge pressure ≤ 18 mmHg [1].

3. Common risk factors for ARDS are divided into two categories: direct and indirect.
   (a) Direct causes are pneumonia, aspiration of gastric contents, inhalational injury, pulmonary contusion, pulmonary vasculitis, and drowning.
   (b) Indirect causes are non-pulmonary sepsis, major trauma, pancreatitis, severe burns, non-cardiogenic shock, drug overdose, and multiple transfusions or transfusion-associated acute lung injury (TRALI).

4. Protective lung strategy (also known as open lung approach or lung protective ventilation) is the standard of care for the management of patients with ARDS. The ARDS Network was a randomized controlled trial designed based on the concept that the limitation of end inspiratory lung stretch may reduce mortality in this patient population. Patients that received lower tidal volume (Vt 4–6 ml/kg ideal body weight) and maintenance of plateau pressure between 25 and 30 mmHg had a survival benefit, with a decrease in mortality from 40% to 31% [2]. Drawbacks from this mode of ventilation were hypoventilation leading to permissive hypercapnia and shear injury due to repetitive opening and closing of alveoli with each cycle. For that reason, PEEP should be set at above lower

inflection point to prevent cyclic atelectasis. It is difficult to describe an efficient method of applying optimal PEEP in any given patient. Applying the highest PEEP that allows for maintenance of goal plateau pressure could be a reasonable approach. In that study, the survival benefit was also associated with a reduction of plasma IL-6, supporting the hypothesis that a lung protective strategy limits the spill of inflammatory mediators into the systemic circulation, which may induce multiple system organ failure. In refractory hypoxemia, prolonging the inspiratory time by increasing the I:E ratio may improve oxygenation; however, close attention must be directed to avoid air trapping, auto-PEEP, barotrauma, and hemodynamic compromise.

5. The use of glucocorticoid treatment for ARDS remains contradictory. The ARDS Network LaSRS study showed no benefit in mortality from the routine use of steroids in patients with ARDS. In addition, it was associated with increased risk of neuromuscular complications, as well as risk of death if started 2 weeks after onset of ARDS. The potential adverse effects of steroids also include immunosuppression, superadded infection, and higher blood glucose levels. The mineralocorticoid component contributes to fluid/sodium retention; both of which could result in positive fluid balance, a known factor associated with poor outcomes in lung injury. At the moment, there is insufficient evidence to justify the routine use of steroids in patients with ARDS [3]. The SAILS trial published in 2014 compared statin with placebo in patients with ARDS in the setting of sepsis. Statin therapy did not reduce mortality or increase ventilator-free days; therefore there is no evidence to support its use in ARDS [4]. Neuromuscular blockade therapy for hypoxia has a few potential benefits. Avoidance of large tidal volumes that predispose to volutrauma decreased oxygen consumption from lack of muscle activity and improved patient–ventilator synchrony. Literature shows that the use of NMB in early (first 48 h) ARDS is associated with improved mortality rate. Having said that, judicious use is warranted since paralysis interferes with neurological exam and has been linked to ICU-acquired weakness and posttraumatic stress disorder.

6. Airway pressure release ventilation (APRV) is a combination of pressure-controlled ventilation and inverted ratio ventilation on a time-triggered, pressure-targeted, and time-cycled mode (Fig. 47.3). A higher and a lower PEEP are set, and 80–95% of the respiratory cycle is spent during inspiration at the higher PEEP. The patient is allowed to breathe spontaneously during both high and low PEEP. The mean airway pressure increases without much increase in the peak pressure, favoring lung protection. This mode has been found to be associated with shorter ICU stay and duration of ventilation in patients with ARDS, but contradictory literature still exists, mostly in regard to the lack of evidence of mortality benefit.

   High-frequency oscillatory ventilation (HFOV) has been evaluated recently by two randomized controlled trials (OSCAR, and OSCILLATE) as well as by a meta-analysis. HFOV has failed to show any mortality benefit. The HFOV group in the OSCILLATE trial had higher mortality, higher

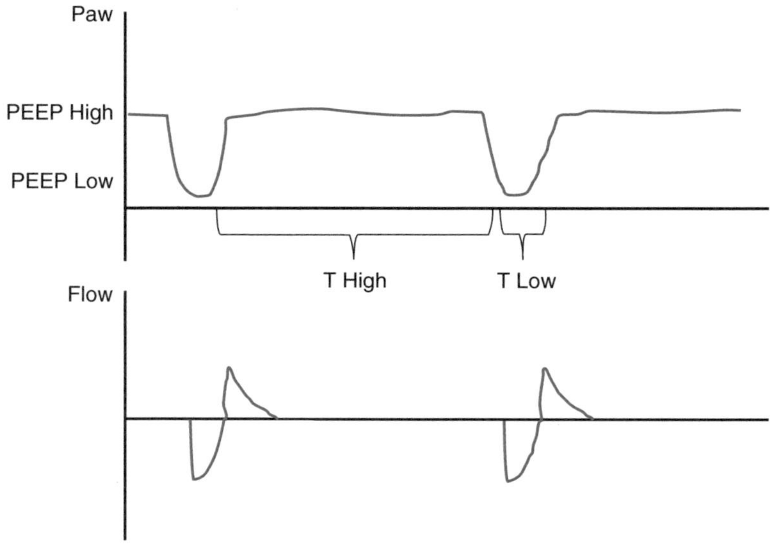

Fig. 47.3 Airway pressure release ventilation (APRV)

requirement for sedatives, paralytics, and vasopressors, and therefore no evidence to support its use.

Prone positioning takes advantage of gravity and repositioning of the heart in the thorax to recruit lung regions and improve ventilation–perfusion matching. The mechanisms for the proposed benefit are change in diaphragm movements, increased functional and residual capacity, better secretion clearance, and reduced ventilator-induced lung injury. The PROSEVA trial, published in 2013, brought attention back to this rescue mode after showing association with major decrease in 28-day and 90-day mortality, increase in ventilation-free days, and reduced time to extubation. An increase in PaO_2 by 10 mmHg over the first 30 min of prone ventilation usually predicts a sustained increase in PaO_2 and deems the patient as a "responder."

Finally, extracorporeal membrane oxygenation (ECMO) remains an important tool for managing refractory hypoxemia that is life-threatening but often considered as a last resort. Literature on its benefit is scarce and controversial. Guidelines suggest it should be used in scenarios that have a potential reversible cause, less than 7 days on mechanical ventilation, age <65 years, no significant comorbidities, no contraindication to anticoagulation, and no significant neurological dysfunction. In case of isolated respiratory failure, a veno-venous approach is advised, whereas in case of hemodynamic instability, a venoarterial approach should be used. More evidence is needed to support its use as standard of care [5].

7. Inhaled vasodilators reduce pulmonary arterial pressure and redistribute blood flow to well-ventilated lung regions with little to no systemic side effects, improving the ventilation–perfusion matching. Inhaled nitric oxide has been shown to improve oxygenation as measured by PaO_2/FiO_2 ratio and

oxygenation index. It is expensive, gets rapidly inactivated by hemoglobin, can result in methemoglobinemia, and carries an increased risk of renal failure. No beneficial effect on mortality or ventilator-free days has been shown with the use of nitric oxide. Inhaled prostaglandins demonstrate similar vasodilator effects when compared to nitric oxide, including improved oxygenation and reduction in pulmonary hypertension; however evidence with large randomized clinical trials is lacking. Patients on these vasodilators are considered "responders" if an improvement on oxygenation is observed within the first 1 h of administration. Based on current evidence, inhaled vasodilators must be considered only as a rescue and temporary therapy for patients with refractory hypoxemia (with or without pulmonary hypertension) when other methods have failed.

References

1. Fanelli V, et al. Acute respiratory distress syndrome: new definition, current and future therapeutic options. J Thorac Dis. 2013;5(3):326–34.
2. Donahoe M. Acute respiratory distress syndrome: a clinical review. Pulm Circ. 2011;1(2):192–211.
3. Bihari S, et al. Steroids in ARDS: to be or not to be. Intensive Care Med. 2016;42(5):931–3.
4. Truwit J, et al. SAILS: statins for acutely injured lungs (ARDS) from sepsis. Am J Respir Crit Care Med. 2014;189:A5088.
5. Mehta C, et al. Management of refractory hypoxemia. Ann Card Anesth. 2016;19(1):89–96.

Chapter 48
CT I

Pramod Chetty

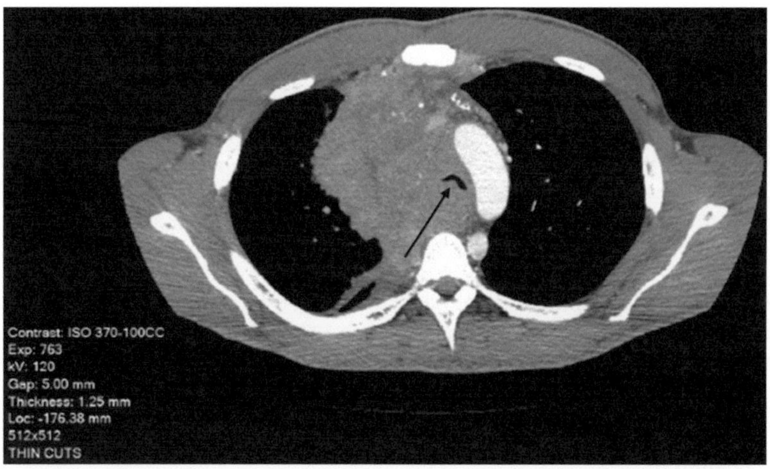

Fig. 48.1 CT showing mediastinal mass causing deviation and crescentic compression of the trachea

P. Chetty, MD
Department of Anesthesiology, OU Health Sciences Center,
750 NE 13th Street, Suite 200, PO Box 53168, Oklahoma City, OK 73104, USA
e-mail: Pramod-chetty@ouhsc.edu

T.D. Raj (ed.), *Data Interpretation in Anesthesia*,
DOI 10.1007/978-3-319-55862-2_48

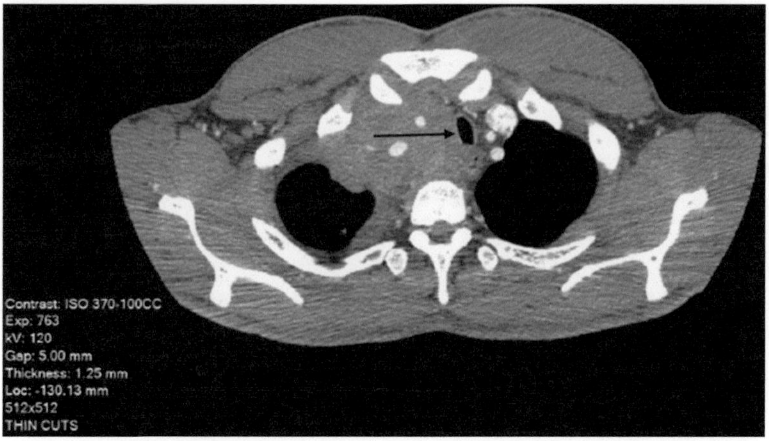

Fig. 48.2 CT showing mediastinal mass posttreatment with less deviation and loss of crescentic compression

A 58-year-old man with a diagnosis of Hodgkin's disease presents to the anesthesia preoperative clinic prior to placement of a port. He complains of mild difficulty in sleeping totally supine and clinically shows fullness of the veins of the neck. CT scan (Fig. 48.1) shows that he has a mediastinal mass with both tracheal deviation and crescentic compression.

1. What are the symptoms of a mediastinal mass?
2. What are the physical ramifications of a significant mediastinal mass on the airway?
3. What are the anesthesia considerations for a significant mediastinal mass?
4. What are techniques for the safe administration of an anesthetic for a significant mediastinal mass?

Answers

1. Symptoms of a mediastinal mass:
   (a) A mediastinal mass may be asymptomatic even when it reaches a significant size. It may be discovered during routine radiological testing for the disease causing the mass or just incidentally [1].
   (b) When the mass reaches a critical size within the restricted mediastinal space, it can cause signs and symptoms related primarily to the cardiac or pulmonary system. This can include diminished venous return via the superior vena cava (SVC) leading to fullness of the neck veins and in extreme cases cardiac dysfunction from direct compression. Respiratory symptoms could range from dyspnea, progressive orthopnea, voice changes (nerve palsy), and in late stages stridor.

2. Physical ramifications of the mediastinal mass on the intrathoracic airway:
   (a) Deviation of the trachea. This could include:
      - "C"-shaped bowing of the trachea
      - "S"-shaped trachea
   (b) Narrowing and invasion of the lumen of the trachea and/or major bronchus:
      - The trachea when externally compressed becomes crescentic as the membranous posterior wall is the first to collapse.
      - Narrowing can be a short segment or a long segment of the trachea.
      - Encroachment can be around the entire carinal trifurcation of the trachea.

3. Anesthesia considerations for a significant mediastinal mass:
   (a) Lack of symptoms should not be considered as reassuring. This is especially true with superior or anterior mediastinal masses. With spontaneous ventilation, the mechanics of thoracic cage cause a distracting force on the larger airways by maintaining the intrapleural pressure gradient, helping to maintain the patency of the lumen. The loss of bronchial tone due to general anesthesia can also decrease lumen size. Thirdly, the distension of the major airways will be diminished with smaller ventilatory volumes [2]. The loss of normal spontaneous ventilation during general anesthesia can thus precipitate intrathoracic airway obstruction in such cases with catastrophic results [3].
   (b) Once the airway has been secured, the anesthetic plan is determined by the surgery and patient's other comorbidities.
   (c) Placement of a regular endotracheal tube (ETT) in a trachea with "S"-shaped deviation can lead to the distal bevel end pushing up against the wall of the trachea leading to obstruction.
   (d) A smaller ETT size must be chosen against the measured diameter of the lumen by CT scan.
   (e) Securing the "lost" airway can possibly be done only by rigid bronchoscopy (RB).

(f) Long-segment tracheal narrowing is a cause for concern for ETT placement or for the performance of rescue rigid bronchoscopy.
(g) Extracorporeal oxygenation (ECO) which takes time with significant prior organization and access placement is the only rescue for loss of the intrathoracic airway with failed rigid bronchoscopy [4, 5].
(h) Significant and chronic tracheal compression can lead to tracheomalacia [6]. This weakness of tracheal wall and airway swelling due to the ETT in a narrowed lumen must be considered before extubation.
(i) Occlusion beyond the carina in one of the major bronchi is significant but less concerning than total tracheal obstruction.
(j) Intravenous lines should be placed in the lower extremities if the SVC is compromised.

4. Techniques for safe administration of anesthesia in a patient with a significant mediastinal mass:
   (a) Ascertain the significance of the mass and its encroachment of the airway preoperatively—this consultation should include the surgeon (and CVT surgeon), radiologist, and anesthesiologist [7]. The factors in risk assessment include symptoms, type of tumor, and airway compromise.
   (b) Many tumor masses will show amazing resolution with chemotherapy or radiation prior to surgery. The CT scan in the above patient was repeated after short definitive therapy and showed near-total resolution of tracheal deviation and compression (Fig. 48.2). This should be done if appropriate.
   (c) When feasible, consider avoidance of general anesthesia. In the case presented, if venous access for treatment was critically needed, this should be done under monitored anesthesia care (MAC). If SVC drainage is compromised, venous access should be secured in the lower extremity.
   (d) Even if MAC or regional anesthesia is considered, every precaution to prevent loss of spontaneous ventilation must be employed. Rigid bronchoscopy must be available in the OR.
   (e) If MAC or regional anesthesia is not feasible, the choices are maintenance of spontaneous ventilation with either an inhalational induction or perform awake fiber-optic intubation followed by general anesthesia with appropriate ETT placement. This should include proper selection of the appropriate ETT for size and made with reinforced material.
   (f) In cases of significant compromise or long-segment stenosis, awake fiber-optic intubation after placement of access catheters for extracorporeal oxygenation in the groin is warranted [5, 8]. In extreme cases of carinal encroachment, the patient can be placed on ECO and rigid bronchoscopy performed under TIVA for airway securement (personal experience).

   After the anesthetic, due caution must be given to the airway, as described above (3H), before removing the ETT which must preferably be done in the fully awake and recovered patient.

References

1. Cooper JC, et al. The use of computed tomography in the evaluation of large multinodular goiters. Ann R Coll Surg Engl. 1991;73:32–5.
2. Miller's anesthesia, 8th ed. – Chapter anesthesia for thoracic surgery – Mediastinal masses.
3. Keon TP. Death on induction of anesthesia for cervical node biopsy. Anesthesiology. 1981;55:471–2.
4. Bouaggad A, et al. Prediction of difficult tracheal intubation in thyroid surgery. Anesth Analg. 2004;99:603–6.
5. Shoa Y, et al. Extracorporeal membrane oxygenation-assisted resection of goiter causing severe extrinsic airway compression. Ann Thorac Surg. 2009;88:659–61.
6. Lee C, Cooper RM, Goldstein D. Management of a patient with tracheomalacia and supraglottic obstruction after thyroid surgery. Can J Anesth. 2011;58:1029–33.
7. Seong Tan PC, Esa N. Anesthesia for massive retrosternal goiter with severe intrathoracic tracheal narrowing: the challenges imposed. Korean J Anesthesiol. 2012;62(5):474–8.
8. Wang G, et al. Surgical management of tracheal compression caused by mediastinal goiter: is extra-corporeal circulation requisite? J Thorac Dis. 2009;1:48–50.

Chapter 49
CT II

Ankur Garg

Case presentation: A 44-year-old man was brought into the hospital after being hit by a truck while riding a bicycle. Glasgow Coma Scale (GCS) was 5 on presentation. CT images of his head on arrival are shown below (Fig. 49.1A–C).

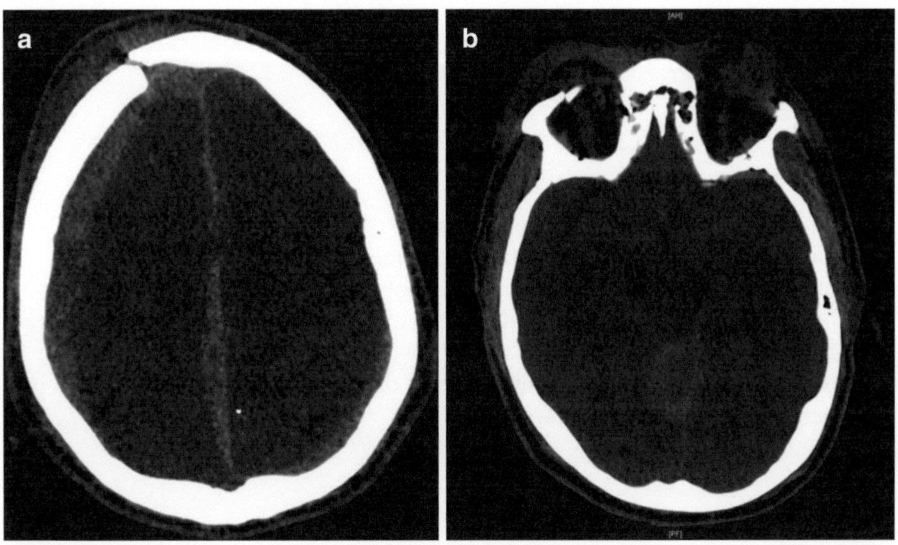

Fig. 49.1 CT head images of a patient following motor vehicle collision

A. Garg, MD
Orlando Neurosurgery, 1605 W. Fairbanks Ave,
Orlando, FL, USA
e-mail: dr.garg@orlandoneurosurgery.com

T.D. Raj (ed.), *Data Interpretation in Anesthesia*,
DOI 10.1007/978-3-319-55862-2_49

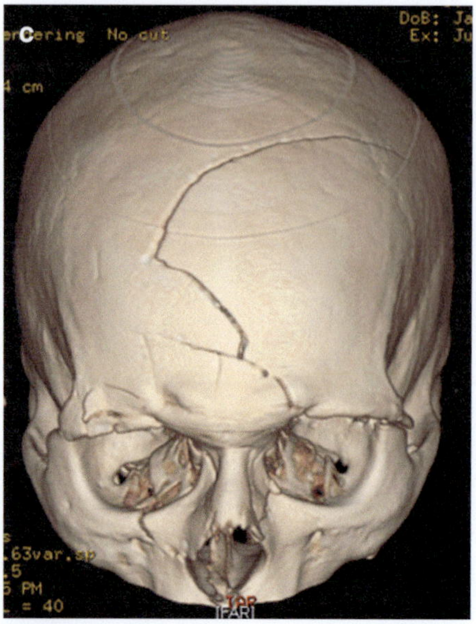

Fig. 49.1 (continued)

Questions

1. Define Glasgow Coma Scale.
2. How do you grade traumatic brain injury?
3. What are the common types of traumatic brain injuries?
4. What are the abnormal findings in the images shown above?
5. What are the usual aspects of medical care of a patient with acute traumatic brain injury?
6. Describe some of the important elements of perioperative anesthetic care in a patient with acute traumatic brain injury.

Answers

1. Teasdale and Jennett [3] first described the Glasgow Coma Scale (GCS) in 1974 as a neurological tool to assess the level of consciousness following head injury. The scale is since widely used by medical professionals worldwide as a reliable and objective way of recording the conscious state of a person for initial as well as subsequent assessments. The scale ranges from a minimum score of 3 (*not* zero) to a maximum score of 15. As described in Fig. 49.2, GCS has three elements: eye response, verbal response, and motor response.

Glasgow coma scale		
Response	**Scale**	**Score**
I. Eye opening response	Spontaneously	4
	Opens to voice	3
	Opens to pain	2
	No eye opening	1
II. Best verbal response	Oriented	5
	Confused, but able to answer	4
	Inappropriate words	3
	Incomprehensible sounds	2
	No verbal output	1
III. Best motor response	Follows commands	6
	Localizes to noxious stimuli	5
	Withdraws to noxious stimuli	4
	Flexor posturing (decorticate)	3
	Extensor posturing (decerebrate)	2
	No motor response	1
Total GCS score = eye opening score + verbal score + motor score		

Fig. 49.2 Glasgow Coma Scale

2. Traumatic brain injury (TBI) can be classified as mild, moderate, or severe, based on patient's Glasgow Coma Scale (GCS) on presentation. A TBI with a GCS of 13 or above is classified as mild, 9–12 as moderate, and 8 or below as severe [4]. The patient described above, therefore, has suffered a severe traumatic brain injury. Other classification systems exist secondary to the limited ability of GCS alone in predicting the outcome. The model developed by the US Department of Defense and Department of Veterans Affairs uses three criteria: GCS after resuscitation, duration of post-traumatic amnesia (PTA), and loss of consciousness (LOC) [5]. It has also been proposed that changes visible on neuroimaging, such as swelling, focal lesions, or diffuse injury, should also be taken into consideration.

3. Some of the common types of traumatic brain injury include epidural hematoma, subdural hematoma, subarachnoid hemorrhage, intraparenchymal hemorrhage, contusion, intraventricular hemorrhage, and diffuse axonal injury. An epidural hematoma is the bleeding from an artery leading to collection of blood between the skull and dura. It can present with the characteristic feature of a lucid interval following which the patient decompensates acutely. It is often a neurosurgical emergency requiring emergent craniotomy and hematoma evacuation. Subdural hematoma is secondary to bleeding from ruptured bridging veins leading to collection of blood between the dura and arachnoid layers of meninges. In elderly, subdural hematomas can occur even from minor trauma and present with symptoms such as new onset headache, seizures, and focal neurological deficits. Subarachnoid hemorrhage is the bleeding into the space between arachnoid membrane and pia mater. Trauma is the leading cause of subarachnoid hemorrhage. Intraparenchymal or intracerebral hemorrhage is the bleeding into the brain tissue itself. A contusion is a small intracerebral hemorrhage commonly noted in orbitofrontal and anterior temporal cortices. Intraventricular hemorrhage is the bleeding into the ventricles of the brain. This is often accompanied by intraparenchymal hemorrhage. An external ventricular drain is usually placed to drain the intraventricular hemorrhage. Diffuse axonal injury (DAI) happens when there is widespread damage to the white matter tracts of the brain secondary to shearing forces. It is one of the most devastating types of traumatic brain injury and can result in persistent vegetative state.

4. The CT images (Fig. 49.3A–C) show some of the common CT findings that can be present in cases of traumatic brain injury following high-velocity motor vehicle collisions. Figure 49.3A shows subdural hematomas (blue arrows) in the midline and bilaterally (right larger than left), skull fracture (red circle), and soft tissue swelling on the right (yellow arrow). Figure 49.3B shows significant subarachnoid hemorrhage in the basal cisterns (blue margins). Figure 49.3C shows a nondepressed skull fracture running obliquely through the bifrontal and left parietal calvarium (blue arrows) and comminuted depressed fractures of the bilateral nasal bones and the nasal septum (green circle).

5. Guidelines for the management of severe traumatic brain injury have been published [6, 7]. Broadly, the acute management of a patient with traumatic brain injury revolves around ensuring hemodynamic stability; airway protection; control of elevated intracranial pressure by emergent medical and surgical measures such as intravenous mannitol/hypertonic infusion, hyperventilation, and place-

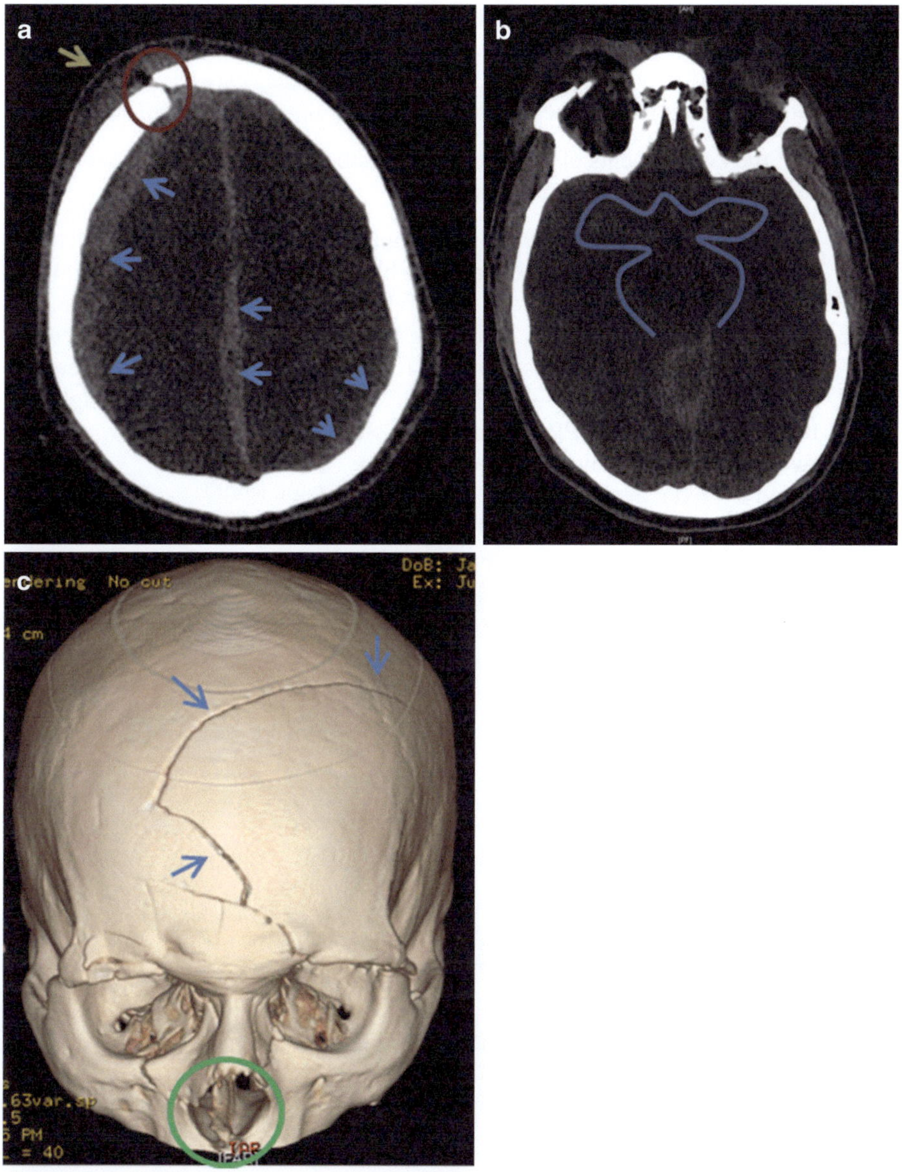

Fig. 49.3 CT findings illustrating the subdural hematomas (*blue arrows* in **A**), subarachnoid hemorrhage (*blue margins* in **B**), scalp swelling (*yellow arrow* in **A**), and fractures (*red circle* in **A** and *green circle* in **C**)

ment of external ventricular drain and/or emergent craniotomy and surgical intervention; rapid identification and management of other injuries; and multimodal monitoring. The initial approach to a trauma patient involves the primary and secondary surveys with rapid assessment of the airway, breathing, circulation, neurologic status (GCS), and associated injuries. Signs and symptoms of severe traumatic brain injury and elevated intracranial pressure (such as low GCS, pupillary dysfunction, Cushing's triad) usually indicate the need for emergent surgical interventions. Airway management in such circumstances may be complicated by the status of the cervical spine, laryngopharyngeal integrity, and full stomach.

6. Some of the key elements of perioperative anesthetic care in a patient with acute severe traumatic brain injury include:
   (a) Treat hypotension first and then intracranial pressure (ICP). The cerebral blood flow is more affected by the decrease in blood pressure than by elevated ICP.
   (b) Intracranial pressure (ICP) and cerebral perfusion pressure (CPP) management: treat if ICP is above 20 mmHg but avoid prophylactic hyperventilation. Define target MAP based on ICP to maintain a normal CPP and cerebral blood flow: CPP = MAP − ICP or CPP = MAP − CVP (take the higher of ICP or CVP). Avoid CPP <50 mmHg or >70 mmHg.
   (c) Avoid hypotension: avoid SBP <90 mmHg.
   (d) Avoid hypoxia: avoid PaO_2 <60 mmHg or O_2 SaO_2 <90%.
   (e) Maintain normovolemia. Avoid using hypotonic solutions such as lactated ringer, free water, or glucose containing intravenous fluids. These can increase ICP by increasing cerebral edema. The first choice for IV fluids in patients with brain injury is normal saline and plasmalyte.
   (f) The objective is to avoid secondary injuries from hypoxemia, hypercapnia, hypotension, elevated ICP, and metabolic derangements.

References

1. Maas AI, Stocchetti N, Bullock R. Moderate and severe traumatic brain injury in adults. Lancet Neurol. 2008;7(8):728–41.
2. Centers for Disease Control and Prevention, National Center for Health Statistics. Mortality in the United States, 2014. NCHS Data Brief No 229; December 2015.
3. Teasdale G, Jennett B. Assessment of coma and impaired consciousness. A practical scale. Lancet. 1974;2(7872):81–4.
4. Parikh S, Koch M, Narayan RK. Traumatic brain injury. Int Anesthesiol Clin. 2007;45(3):119–35.
5. Department of Defense and Department of Veterans Affairs. Traumatic brain injury task force. 2008. www.cdc.gov/nchs/data/icd9/Sep08TBI.pdf.
6. Brain Trauma Foundation, American Association of Neurological Surgeons AANS, Congress of Neurological Surgeons CNS, AANS, CNS Joint Section on Neurotrauma and Critical Care. Guidelines for the management of severe traumatic brain injury. J Neurotrauma. 2007;24(1):S1–S106.
7. Kochanek PM, Carney N, Adelson PD, Ashwal S, Bell MJ, et al. Guidelines for the acute medical management of severe traumatic brain injury in infants, children, and adolescents, 2nd edition. Pediatr Crit Care Med. 2012;13(Suppl 1):S1–82.

Chapter 50
CT/MRI III

Ankur Garg

Case presentation: A 51-year-old woman initially presented to the hospital with 1-month history of confusion. Figure 50.1A, B illustrates the initial CT and MRI findings. She underwent awake craniotomy with maximal resection of the mass followed by outpatient chemotherapy and radiation. She was reoperated 6 months later for recurrence of the lesion noted on surveillance imaging (Fig. 50.1C, D). Eight months after that, she presented with progressive weakness, confusion, aphasia, and gaze preference and was found to have further progression of the disease (Fig. 50.1E, F).

A. Garg, MD
Orlando Neurosurgery, 1605 W. Fairbanks Ave, Orlando, FL, USA
e-mail: dr.garg@orlandoneurosurgery.com

T.D. Raj (ed.), *Data Interpretation in Anesthesia*,
DOI 10.1007/978-3-319-55862-2_50

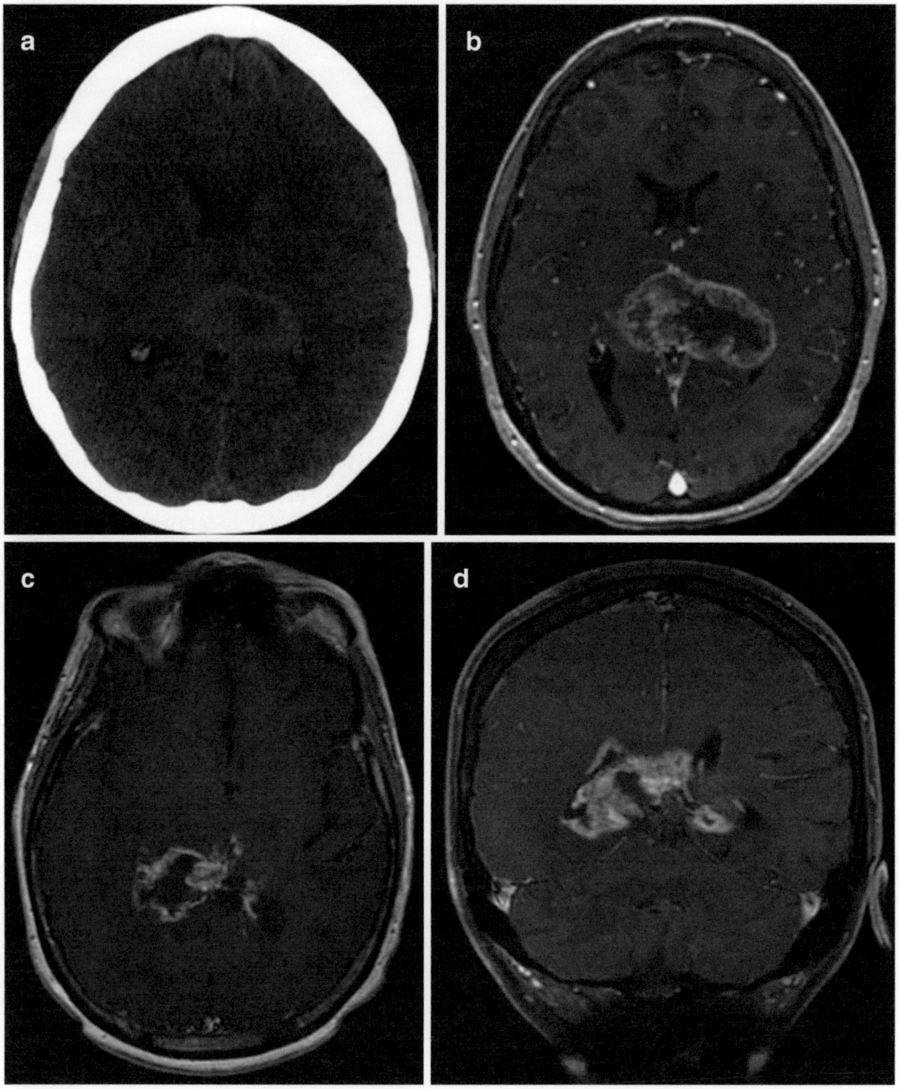

Fig. 50.1 (**a**) and (**b**) are the initial CT and MRI images of the patient presenting with an intracranial mass lesion manifesting as 1 month of confusion. (**c**) and (**d**) are MRI images 8 months later showing local recurrence. (**e**) and (**f**) are MRI images from 6 months later

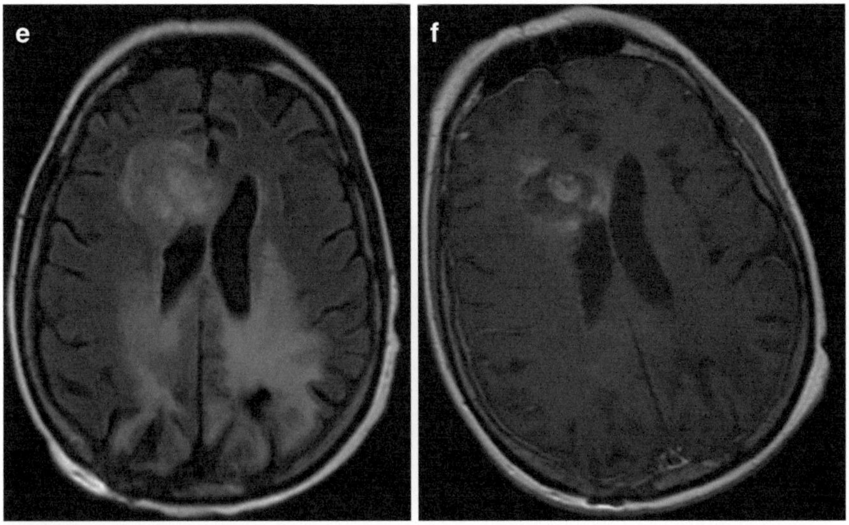

Fig. 50.1 (continued)

Questions

1. Identify and describe the abnormal findings in the images shown above.
2. How are brain tumors classified?
3. List some of the common brain tumors.
4. What is the role of steroids in the acute management of brain tumors?
5. Describe important elements of anesthesia in a patient undergoing awake craniotomy for an intracranial mass lesion.

Answers

1. The CT and MRI images of the brain depicted in Figs. 50.1A, B and 50.2A, B show an irregular heterogeneously enhancing mass lesion centered in the region of the splenium of the corpus callosum, slightly to the left of the midline. This mass extends to involve the left lateral ventricle and bilateral thal-

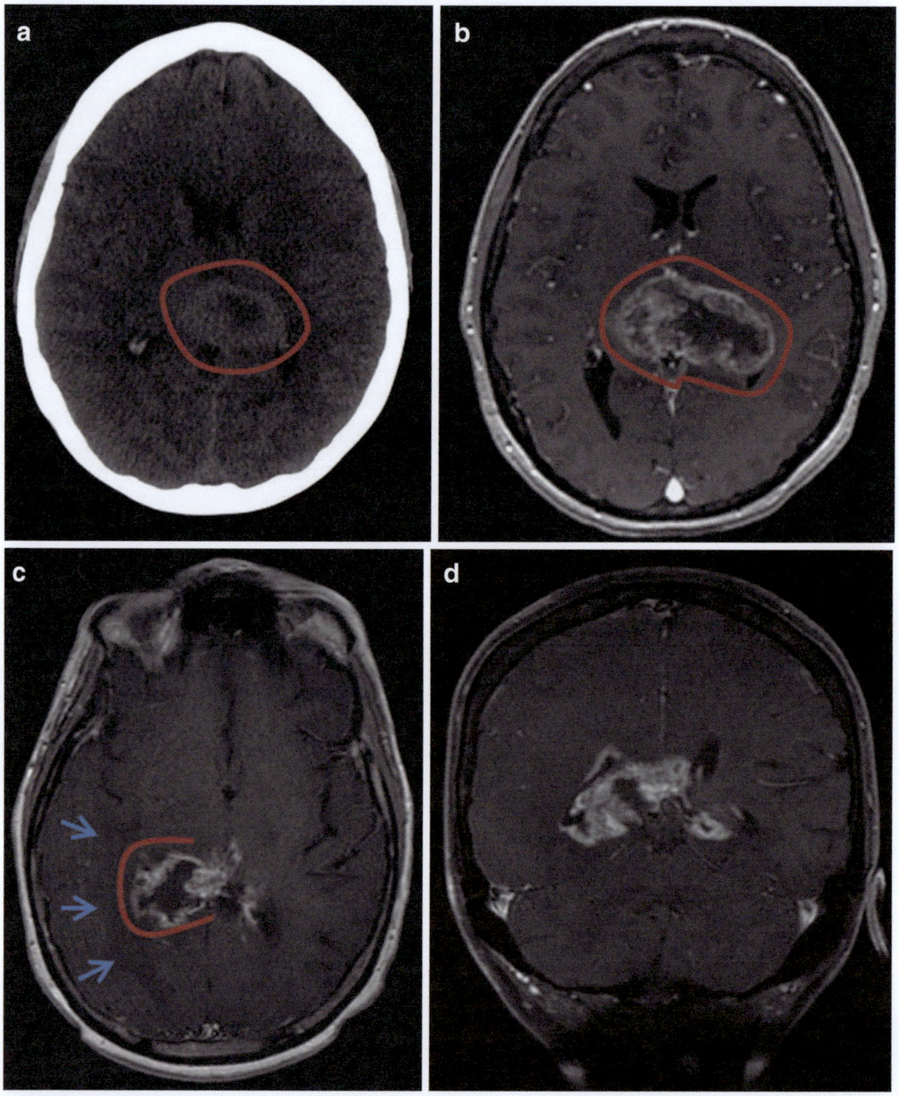

Fig. 50.2 *Encircled region* in (**a**) and (**b**) shows the mass lesion in the region of the splenium of the corpus callosum. *Open circles* in (**c**) and (**d**) illustrate local recurrence, more toward the *right side* and the blue arrows illustrate vasogenic edema. *Circled* regions in (**e**) and (**f**) illustrate the recurrence in the right frontal region, while the *arrows* illustrate radiation-induced changes

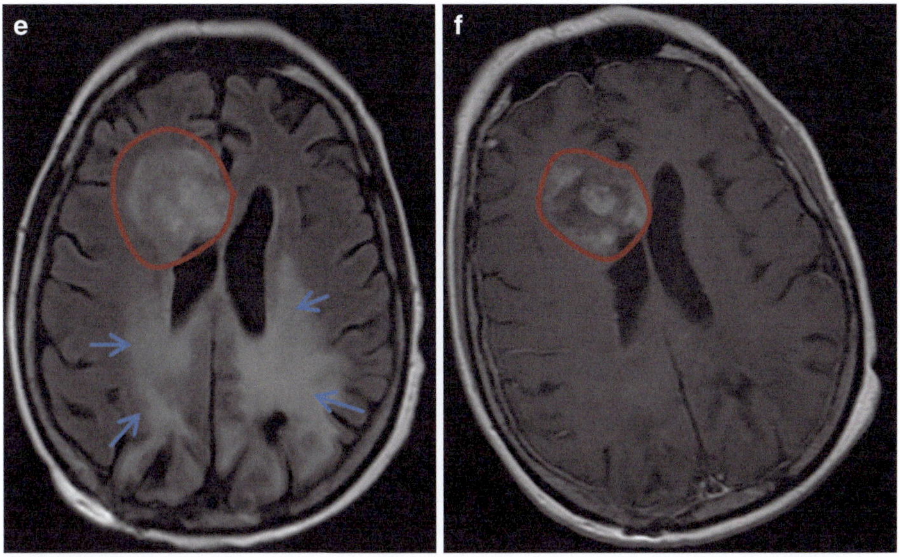

Fig. 50.2 (continued)

ami. These findings are concerning for a high-grade glioma, likely glioblastoma multiforme. This patient underwent awake craniotomy and resection of the mass followed by outpatient chemotherapy and radiation. The pathology confirmed the diagnosis of glioblastoma. Figures 50.1C, D and 50.2C, D depict the local recurrence of the tumor six months later. Following this, the patient underwent repeat craniotomy and tumor resection. Figures 50.1E, F and 50.2E, F depict the pre- and post-contrast MRI images which reveal recurrence in the right frontal region eight months later (encircled region). Radiation-induced changes are also noted (blue arrows). The decision was made to pursue hospice care at this point.

2. Brain tumors can be classified in a number of ways. A primary brain tumor is a tumor that starts in the brain, as opposed to metastatic brain disease. Primary brain tumors can be classified as benign tumors that tend to have slower growth and distinct borders vs. malignant tumors that grow rapidly, invade the surrounding tissues and structures, and have grave prognosis. Brain tumors are also commonly graded using the WHO grading system. Grade I tumors such as craniopharyngiomas and pilocytic astrocytomas grow slowly and are associated with good long-term prognosis. Grade II brain tumors are also slow growing but can spread into adjacent tissue. Grade III and IV tumors are malignant. Glioblastoma is the most common example of a grade IV primary brain tumor. A very extensive WHO classification of brain tumors was recently published and serves as the guideline for neurosurgeons and neuropathologists [1].

3. The most common brain tumors include meningiomas, gliomas, and metastatic brain disease. *Meningiomas* are the most common primary brain tumors. A meningioma is a tumor that arises from the meninges, which are the linings of the brain. They occur most frequently in middle-aged women. They are benign, WHO grade I tumors, and surgery is the usual first-line treatment. Small asymptomatic meningiomas can also just be observed. Approximately 5% of meningiomas are malignant in nature. *Gliomas* are tumors arising from glial cells which form the supportive tissue of the brain. They are the second most common primary brain tumors but comprise the most common malignant brain tumor. An astrocytoma is a glioma arising from the glial cells called astrocytes. A grade IV astrocytoma is also called *Glioblastoma multiforme or GBM*. GBM can present with a variety of neurological signs and symptoms such as headache, seizures, and focal neurologic deficits. Usual treatment is maximal surgical resection followed by radiation and chemotherapy, but recurrence is frequent and prognosis is usually grave. *Craniopharyngioma* is a benign tumor that arises from a nest of cells located near the pituitary stalk. These tumors can present with signs of increased intracranial pressure by causing obstruction of CSF outflow across the foramen of Monro. Surgery is the first-line treatment. *Medulloblastoma* is a high-grade cerebellar tumor usually seen in children. They can extend into the fourth ventricle and cause hydrocephalus by obstructing CSF outflow and metastasize to the spinal cord. Treatment included resection followed by radiation and chemotherapy. *Metastatic brain disease* is the spread of a primary tumor elsewhere in the body to the brain. The common cancers that spread to the brain are those arising in the thyroid, lung, breast, kidney, prostate, and colon, as well as melanomas. The prognosis is grave.

4. Steroids are often used acutely to treat the cerebral edema that can sometimes be caused by a brain tumor. There are two broad categories of cerebral edema: cytotoxic edema and vasogenic edema. Cytotoxic edema happens after neuronal death and involves both grey and white matter. This is usually seen after a stroke. Vasogenic edema involves the white matter only and is often associated with tumors, infections, and hypertensive encephalopathy. Steroids are very effective for vasogenic edema from brain tumors and can temporarily relieve some of the neurologic signs and symptoms. They can be utilized before, during, or after surgery or to treat edema caused by radiation therapy. Steroids can also be prescribed to improve quality of life in patients with advanced primary or metastatic neoplastic brain disease. The usual dose in acute setting is dexamethasone 10 mg IV followed by 4 mg every 6 h.

5. Awake craniotomy is utilized when the brain lesion (such as a tumor) is located in close proximity to an eloquent cortical region such as Broca's area or the motor strip. It provides the neurosurgeon the opportunity to preserve neurological function and limit deficits by performing awake functional cortical mapping during the resection. The procedure, however, poses some unique challenges to the anesthesiologist [2]. Patient cooperation during the procedure is critical, and loss of intraoperative cooperation may result in a failed

awake craniotomy. Well-motivated and mature patients are the best candidates. Preoperative evaluation should include a discussion of the expectations and level of cooperation required during the procedure as well as eliciting risk factors for failed awake craniotomies such as history of alcoholism, low tolerance to pain, and anxiety or psychiatric disorders [3]. Intraoperatively, the most critical element of anesthesia management is provision of a rapid and smooth transition of the anesthetic depth tailored to the different surgical stages while maintaining a stable hemodynamic and cardiopulmonary function. Comfortable positioning is mandatory. Several different anesthetic techniques have been described such as conscious sedation, asleep-awake-asleep technique, and asleep-awake technique. The choice of anesthetic agent is highly dependent upon the requirement for functional cortical mapping and intraoperative electrocorticography. Propofol infusion with a supplementary opioid is a common anesthetic choice for awake craniotomies.

References

1. Louis DN, Perry A, Reifenberger G, Deimling AV, Figarella-Branger D, et al. The 2016 world health organization classification of tumors of the central nervous system: a summary. Acta Neuropathol. 2016;131:803–20.
2. Chui J. Anesthesia for awake craniotomy: an update. Rev Colomb Anestesiol. 2015;43(S1):22–8.
3. Erickson KM, Cole DJ. Anesthetic considerations for awake craniotomy for epilepsy and functional neurosurgery. Anesthesiol Clin. 2012;30:241–68.

Chapter 51
MRI Spine

Gulshan Doulatram

A 38-year-old female has undergone an ORIF of the femur with a general anesthetic and epidural anesthesia for postoperative pain. On the second postoperative day, she is complaining of increasing back pain, numbness, and some weakness on the left leg. Her VSS show a blood pressure of 110/60 mmHg, HR 85, RR 14, T-38.8 C. The surgeon would like you to remove the epidural catheter. She is on aspirin and subcutaneous heparin 5000 units three times a day.

G. Doulatram, MD
Department of Anesthesiology, University of Texas Medical Branch, 301 University Blvd, Galveston, TX, USA
e-mail: gdoulatr@utmb.edu

T.D. Raj (ed.), *Data Interpretation in Anesthesia*,
DOI 10.1007/978-3-319-55862-2_51

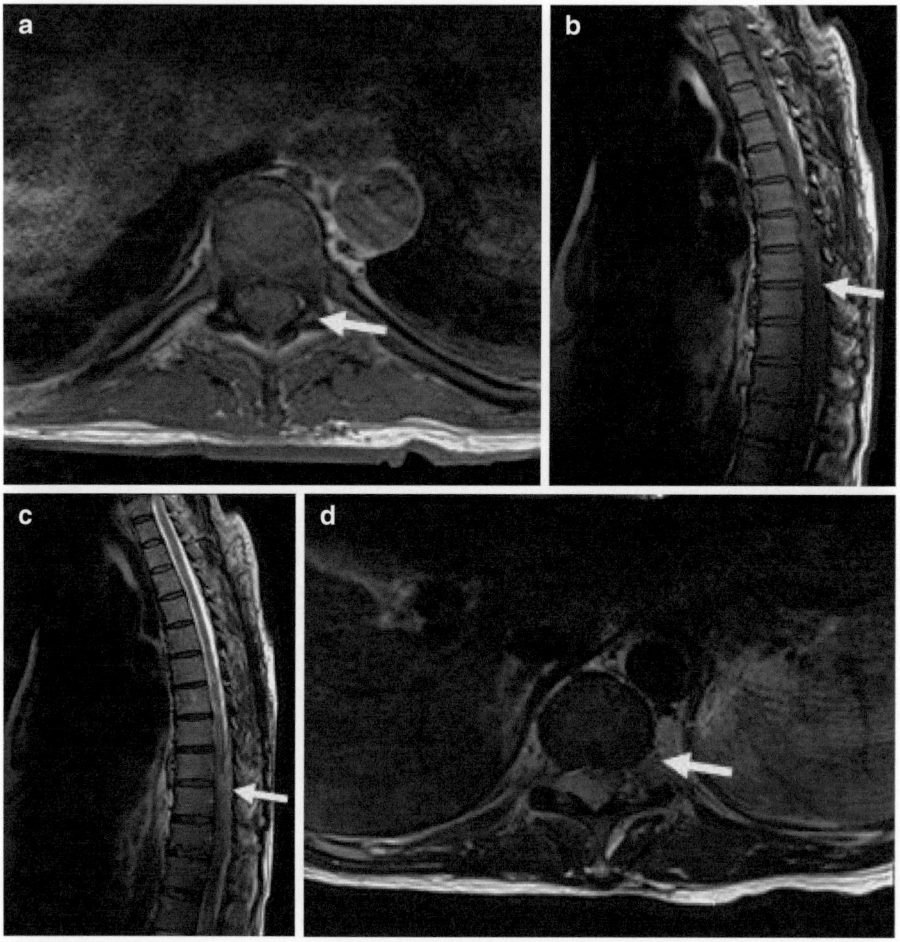

Fig. 51.1 T1 and T2 MR image of the thoracic spine. (**a**) T1-weighted MR image of the thoracic spine in the *axial view*. (**b**) T1-weighted MR image of the thoracic spine in the *sagittal view*. (**c**) T2-weighted MR image of the thoracic spine in the *sagittal view*. (**d**) T2-weighted MR image of the thoracic spine in the *axial view*

1. What does the MRI show you in this picture?
2. What is the incidence of this condition?
3. How does this condition present clinically?
4. What is the differential diagnosis for this patient?
5. What are its risk factors?
6. How could one prevent its occurrence?
7. What treatment options are available?

Answers

1. Figure 51.1A and B shows a fluid collection in the epidural space in the thoracic spine in a T1-weighted image in sagittal and axial views, respectively. Figure 51.1C and D shows a hyperintense mass at the same level in a T2-weighted image. Figure 51.1D shows an intense mass pushing on the anterior aspect of the spinal cord (white arrows). Spinal epidural hematoma can occur spontaneously or may follow spinal or epidural anesthesia [1]. The peridural anterolateral venous plexus usually is most often the primary source, though arterial sources of hemorrhage can occur rarely. This is supported by the fact that hematoma usually develops over hours to days suggesting a slow accumulation of blood from a venous bleed. The hematoma usually extends to the dorsal aspect of thoracic or lumbar region over several vertebral levels. If the patient has any contraindication to obtaining a MRI, then a CT myelography scan may be substituted to make an early diagnosis. MRI is however more specific in detecting the various stages of hematoma compared to CT myelography and is considered the first choice diagnostic step to confirm the presence of an epidural hematoma. An acute hematoma usually presents as low signal intensity signal on T1-weighted image and high signal intensity on T2-weighted image [2].

2. Epidural hematoma after neuraxial anesthesia is fortunately a rare event. The true incidence is unknown but is estimated to occur at an incidence of 1:220,000 after a spinal block and 1:150,000 after an epidural block [3]. The risk is much higher at 1 in 3000 in certain patients with risk factors. The risk is much lower in the obstetric population compared to vascular patients. About 1 in 430 patients with epidural catheters will be suspected to have an epidural hematoma and undergo a workup for it [4].

3. Patients with epidural hematoma present with severe unrelenting, nonpositional, acute onset back pain and varying degrees of lower-limb weakness and sensory deficits. Some patients may have motor weakness as a primary symptom in the absence of back pain [5]. If the compression is extensive, then it could cause bowel and bladder incontinence. Symptoms could be absent or attenuated in the presence of a well-functioning epidural catheter infusing high concentrations of local anesthetics. Symptoms rarely develop in the immediate postoperative period and typically take 2–3 days. Once symptoms begin, they can progress from back pain to a complete or partial paraplegia or even quadriplegia in a few hours [6].

4. The differential diagnosis for this presentation can include epidural abscess, intradural hemorrhage, prolonged and exaggerated neuraxial block, anterior spinal artery syndrome, spinal cord compression due to presence of tumors, disc herniation, worsening of previous spinal stenosis, lumbar radiculopathy, compression fracture of the spine, and spinal cord infarction. There should be a high index of suspicion for an epidural hematoma in an anticoagulated patient who has an epidural catheter and in the presence of back pain with neurological deficits.

Table 51.1 Timeline of use of anticoagulant drugs before and after neuraxial anesthesia

Drug	Time before needle/ catheter placement and manipulation	Epidural catheter maintenance	Time to restart anticoagulant therapy
Antiplatelet drugs			
ASA	No change	Yes	No change
NSAIDs	No change	Yes	No Change
P2Y12 inhibitors			
Clopidogrel (Plavix)	7 d	No	12–24 h
Ticlopidine (Ticlid)	14 d	No	12–24 h
Prasugrel (Effient)	7 d	No	12–24 h
Ticagralor (Brilinta)	7 d	No	12–24 h
Glycoprotein IIB/IIIA inhibitors			
Eptifibatide (Integrilin)	8 h	No	8–12 h
Tirofiban (Aggrastat)	8 h	No	8–12 h
Abciximab	2–5 d	No	8–12 h
Heparin derivatives			
Heparin unfractionated 5000 U SQ Q12 h	8–10 h	Yes	2 h
Heparin unfractionated 5000 U SQ Q8 h	8–10 h	Yes	2 h
Heparin unfractionated 7500 U SQ Q8 h	8–10 h	No	4 h
Heparin IV	4 h	No	4 h
Dalteparin (Fragmin) 5000 U SQ QD Enoxaparin (Lovenox) 40 mg SQ QD	12 h	Must wait 8 h after catheter is placed before giving a dose Must wait 12 h after the last dose before removing the catheter	4 h
Enoxaparin 30 mg SQ Q12	24 h	No	4 h
XA inhibitors			
Fondaparinux (Arixtra) 2.5 mg SQ QD	3 d	No	24 h
Apixaban (Eliquis)	3 d		24 h
Rivaroxaban (Xarelto)	3 d		24 h
Warfarin (Coumadin)	5 d (normal INR)	No (remove the catheter while INR is below 1.5)	Immediately

Table 51.1 (continued)

Drug	Time before needle/ catheter placement and manipulation	Epidural catheter maintenance	Time to restart anticoagulant therapy
Thrombin inhibitors			
Dabigatran (Pradaxa)	3 d 6 d if renal impairment	No	24 h

5. The risk factors for developing an epidural hematoma include "patient-specific" factors or "surgery-related" issues. "Patient-specific factors" include advanced age, needle size, presence of epidural catheter, females, trauma patients, spinal cord and vertebral column abnormalities, preexisting spinal stenosis, organ function compromise, presence of underlying coagulopathy, traumatic or difficult needle placement, as well as indwelling catheter in anticoagulated patient. Spontaneous spinal epidural hematoma can sometimes occur with anticoagulation, thrombolysis, blood dyscrasias, coagulopathies, thrombocytopenia, neoplasms, or vascular malformations. "Surgery-related factors" include prolonged surgery and high intraoperative blood loss.

6. The practice guidelines put forth by the American Society of Regional Anesthesia and Pain Medicine provide several preventive measures to avoid the occurrence of epidural hematoma. The rarity of occurrence mandates that most guidelines come from the collective experience of recognized experts in the field of regional anesthesia and anticoagulation. They are based on case reports, clinical series, pharmacology, hematology, and risk factors for surgical bleeding. The timelines to stopping and restarting anticoagulants after neuraxial anesthesia are summarized in Table 51.1. Multiple anticoagulants always pose an additional risk even in the case of aspirin, selective serotonin reuptake inhibitors, and nonsteroidal anti-inflammatory medications [5, 6]. Several newer anticoagulants in the past few years necessitate a thorough knowledge of these drugs and their impact on neuraxial anesthesia. Optimal coagulation is necessary during needle placement, maintenance, and removal of catheters. Close monitoring of anticoagulation status, frequent and regularly timed neurological checks, and the use of low-concentration local anesthetics are necessary to avoid this dreaded complication.

7. The treatment of epidural hematoma is timely diagnosis, consultation with a neurosurgeon, and an emergency laminectomy to avoid persistent neurological deficits. The prognosis is best when the laminectomy is done within 8 h. Treatment delay greater than 24 h is associated with the worst prognosis [7].

References

1. Matsumura A, Namikawa T, Hashimoto R, Okamoto T, Yanagida I, Hoshi M, Noguchi K, Takami M. Clinical management for spontaneous spinal epidural hematoma: diagnosis and treatment. Spine J. 2008;8(3):534–7.
2. Rothfus WE, Chedid MK, Deeb ZL, Abla AA, Maroon JC, Sherman RL. MR imaging in the diagnosis of spontaneous spinal epidural hematomas. J Comput Assist Tomogr. 1987;11(5):851–4.
3. Bateman BT, Mhyre JM, Ehrenfeld J, Kheterpal S, Abbey KR, Argalious M, Berman MF, Jacques PS, Levy W, Loeb RG, Paganelli W, Smith KW, Wethington KL, Wax D, Pace NL, Tremper K, Sandberg WS. The risk and outcomes of epidural hematomas after perioperative and obstetric epidural catheterization: a report from the Multicenter Perioperative Outcomes Group Research Consortium. Anesth Analg. 2013;116(6):1380–5.
4. Ehrenfeld JM, Agarwal AK, Henneman JP, Sandberg WS. Estimating the incidence of suspected epidural hematoma and the hidden imaging cost of epidural catheterization: a retrospective review of 43,200 cases. Reg Anesth Pain Med. 2013;38(5):409–14.
5. Vandermeulen EP, Van Aken H, Vermylen J. Anticoagulants and spinal-epidural anesthesia. Anesth Analg. 1994;79:1165–77.
6. Horlocker TT, Wedel DJ, Rowlingson JC, Enneking FK, Kopp SL, Benzon HT, Brown DL, Heit JA, Mulroy MF, Rosenquist RW, Tryba M, Yuan CS. Regional anesthesia in the patient receiving antithrombotic or thrombolytic therapy: American Society of Regional Anesthesia and Pain Medicine Evidence-Based Guidelines (Third Edition). Reg Anesth Pain Med. 2010;35(1):64–101.
7. Neal JM, Barrington MJ, Brull R, Hadzic A, Hebl JR, Horlocker TT, Huntoon MA, Kopp SL, Rathmell JP, Watson JC. The second ASRA practice advisory on neurologic complications associated with regional anesthesia and pain medicine: executive summary 2015. Reg Anesth Pain Med. 2015;40(5):401–30.

Chapter 52
TEE I

Kofi B. Vandyck

An 82-year-old man with a history of hypertension, hyperlipidaemia and COPD presented from a nursing home for an emergent laparotomy for a ruptured appendix. A transoesophageal echocardiography (TEE) probe was placed intraoperatively for diagnosis and monitoring after several attempts at managing hypotension proved futile.

Questions

1. What are some of the benefits of using TEE in managing patients for non-cardiac surgery?
2. What physics principles underlie the calculation of valve area, stroke volume and cardiac output using TEE? (See Figs. 52.1, 52.2, 52.3, 52.4 and formula illustration)
3. Intraoperative echo showed a severely calcified aortic valve with a left ventricular outflow tract diameter (LVOT) of 2.59 cm, an LVOT VTI of 17.5, maximum LVOT velocity (Vmax) of 69.2 cm/s, aortic valve VTI of 152 cm and an aortic valve Vmax of 533 cm/s. The heart rate on the monitor was 97 beats/min. How would you calculate the stroke volume and cardiac out?

K.B. Vandyck, MD
Department of Anesthesiology, University of Oklahoma Health Sciences Center, 750 NE 13th Street, Suite 200, Oklahoma City, OK 73104, USA
e-mail: Kofi-Vandyck@ouhsc.edu

T.D. Raj (ed.), *Data Interpretation in Anesthesia*,
DOI 10.1007/978-3-319-55862-2_52

Answers

1. TEE can provide immediate and accurate haemodynamic measurement of cardiac function including cardiac output and left ventricular filling pressure, chamber preload, atrial interaction and pulmonary arterial pressures. Doppler ultrasound principles are used to derive intracardiac flow across orifices and valves in order to calculate orifice area, stroke volume and cardiac output. Intraoperative cardiac output measurement provides a tool for assessing global cardiac function. The information obtained from the cardiac output measurement can be used in guiding therapeutic decision during cardiac and non-cardiac surgery. The use of TEE for cardiac output measurement thus provides a simple and reliable minimally invasive method of assessing cardiac function. Intraoperatively, TEE can be used to diagnose or redefine the cause of haemodynamic instability and detect new or unsuspected pathology like valvular (stenosis or regurgitation) and other lesions.

2. Blood flow across valves and orifices of the heart can be obtained using the Doppler capabilities of echocardiography and applying the basic principle of physics and fluid dynamics.

According to the principles of physics and fluid dynamics,

$$\text{Volume in a cylinder} = \text{cross-sectional area of the cylinder or vessel} \times \text{length of cylinder or vessel} = \pi r^2 \times L,$$

where r is the radius of the cylinder or vessel and L is the distance between the two point (or the length of the cylinder or vessels).

Also, flow rate (Q) is calculated as

$$\text{Flow rate}\left(Q\right) = \frac{\text{volume}}{t} = \frac{\text{Area} \times L}{t} = \frac{\pi r^2 \times L}{t}$$

where t is time for fluid to traverse from point A to B.

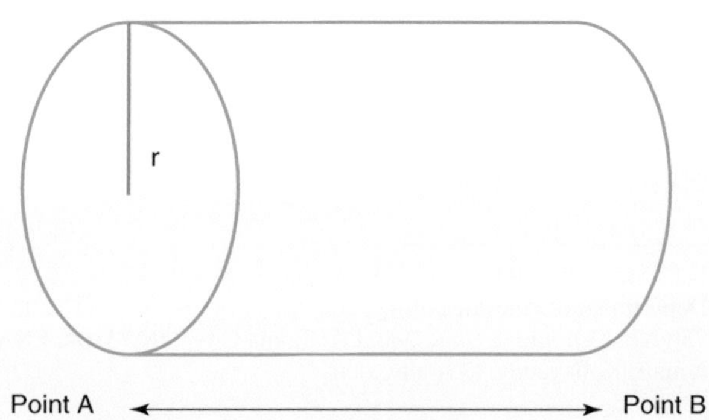

Fig. 52.1 Illustration of a cylinder with parameters used in calculating area and flow across two points in the cylinder where r is cross-sectional radius of cylinder and L is distance between point A and point B [1–3]

Using the law of conservation of mass (continuity equation) and assuming laminar flow,

$$Q_A = Q_B$$

$$\frac{\left(\pi r^2 \times L\right)_A}{t} = \frac{\left(\pi r^2 \times L\right)_B}{t}$$

$$\text{velocity} = L / t$$

Therefore, the formula can be simplified to read;

$$\left(\pi r^2 \times v\right)_A = \left(\pi r^2 \times v\right)_B$$

The velocity (and distance L) that blood travels in a blood vessel can be measured by TEE using continuous or pulse wave Doppler. Continuous wave uses two crystals; one crystal continuously transmits ultrasound wave and the other crystal continuously receives ultrasound waves thus allowing for measurement of high-frequency Doppler velocities along the entire length of the ultrasound beam [1]. In contrast to continuous wave measurement, pulse wave measurements use one ultrasound crystal for both transmitting and receiving ultrasound waves. This allows for measurement of low-frequency Doppler velocity (v) from a specific region of blood flow.

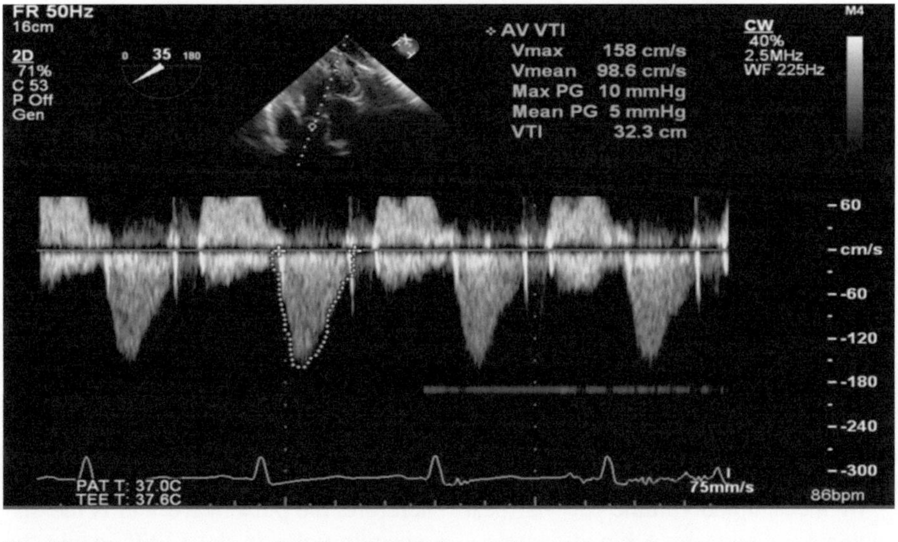

Fig. 52.2 Continuous wave Doppler through the annulus of the aortic valve. V_{max} = maximum velocity through aortic valve; V_{mean} = mean velocity at aortic valve; max PG = maximum pressure gradient at aortic valve; mean PG = mean pressure gradient at aortic valve; VTI = volume time integral at aortic valve

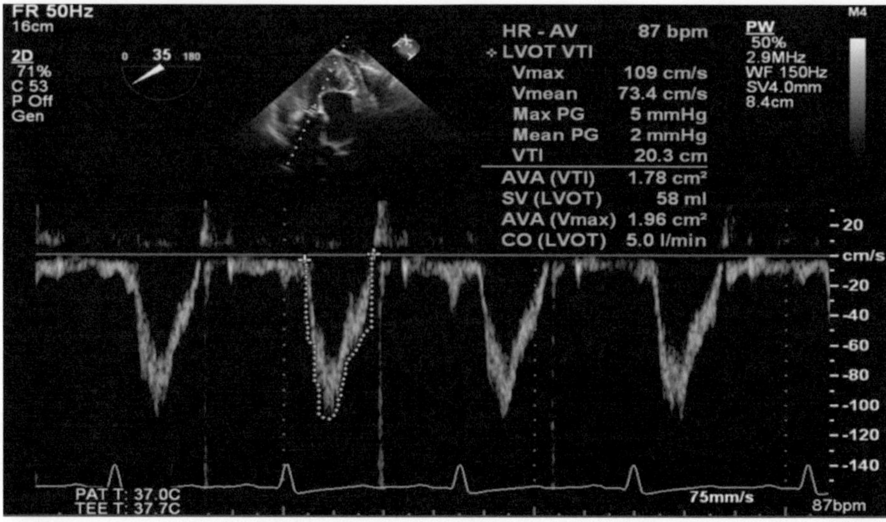

Fig. 52.3 Pulse wave Doppler through the left ventricular outflow tract (LVOT). V_{max} = maximum velocity in LVOT; V_{mean} = mean velocity in LVOT; max PG = maximum pressure gradient in LVOT; mean PG = mean pressure gradient; VTI = volume time integral; AVA = aortic valve area; SV = stroke volume; CO = cardiac output

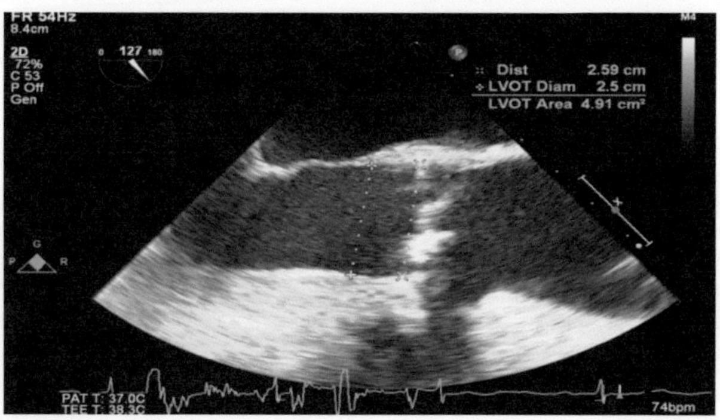

Fig. 52.4 Mid-esophageal aortic valve long (ME AVLAX) axis view of the left ventricular outflow tract (LVOT) with measurement of the LVOT diameter and area

Using either continuous or pulse wave Doppler allows for the measurement of velocity (v) and distance (measured by the echo machine as velocity time integral (VTI)). The VTI and v are obtained by tracing the area under the Doppler signal obtained. The VTI is also called the stroke distance that is the distance travelled by the sampled volume per heartbeat. Therefore, the pulse wave VTI is the distance travelled by a blood sample at a specific point in the LVOT, while the continuous wave VTI (usually measured across the aortic valve) is the longest distance travelled by blood across the aortic valve [1–3].

Blood volume at a point in a vessel can be measured using the formula;

$$\text{Volume} = \pi r^2 \times VTI\left(\text{stroke distance}\right)$$

The stroke volume (SV) across the left ventricular outflow tract (LVOT) is therefore;

$$SV_{\text{LVOT}} = \pi r_{\text{LVOT}^2} \times VTI_{\text{LVOT}}$$

where r_{LVOT} is the diameter of the left ventricular outflow tract proximal to the aortic annulus

$$\text{Cardiac output}\left(CO\right) = \text{Stroke volume}\left(SV\right) \times \text{Heart Rate}\left(HR\right)$$

Therefore, the cardiac output (CO) at the LVOT is;

$$CO_{\text{LVOT}} = SV_{\text{LVOT}} \times HR = \left(\pi r_{\text{LVOT}^2} \times VTI_{\text{LVOT}}\right) \times HR$$

Normal stroke volume is 60–100 mL per beat, and normal cardiac output is 4–8 L/min.

According to the continuity equation,

$$\text{Cardiac output at LVOT} = \text{Cardiac output at Aortic valve}$$

$$\pi r_{\text{LVOT}^2} \times VTI_{\text{LVOT}} = \text{Area}_{\text{AV}} \times VTI_{\text{AV}}$$

or,

$$\pi r_{\text{LVOT}^2} \times v_{\text{LVOT}} = \text{Area}_{\text{AV}} \times v_{\text{AV}}$$

where VTI_{LVOT} and v_{LVOT} are the velocity time integral and the velocity respectively at the LVOT and VTI_{AV} and v_{LVOT} are the velocity time integral and velocity, respectively, at the aortic valve.

Therefore;

$$\text{Area}_{\text{AV}} = \frac{\pi r_{\text{LVOT}^2} \times V_{\text{LVOT}}}{V_{\text{AV}}}$$

or,

3.

$$\text{Area}_{\text{AV}} = \frac{\pi \text{r}_{\text{LVOT}^2} \times VTI_{\text{LVOT}}}{VTI_{\text{AV}}}$$

$$\begin{aligned} SV_{\text{LVOT}} &= \pi r_{\text{LVOT}^2} \times VTI_{\text{LVOT}} \\ &= 3.14 \times (1.25) 2 \times 17.5 \text{ cm.} \\ &= 85.86 \text{ cm}^3 \text{ / beat or} 85.86 \text{mL / beat} \\ &\quad (r \text{ is half of the measured diameter } 2.5 \text{ cm} = 1.25 \text{ cm}). \end{aligned}$$

$$\begin{aligned} CO_{\text{LVOT}} &= SV_{\text{LVOT}} \times HR = 85.86 \text{ mL / beat} \times 90 \text{beats / min} \\ &= 7727.4 \text{ mL / min or } \sim 7.7 \text{L / min}. \end{aligned}$$

References

1. Darmon PL, Hillel Z, Mogtader A, et al. Cardiac output by transesophageal echocardiography using continuous-wave Doppler across the aortic valve. Anesthesiology. 1994;80:796.
2. Katz WE, Gasior TA, Quinlan JJ, Gorcsan 3rd J. Transgastric continuous-wave Doppler to determine cardiac output. Am J Cardiol. 1993;71:853.
3. Parra V, Fita G, Rovira I, et al. Transoesophageal echocardiography accurately detects cardiac output variation: a prospective comparison with thermodilution in cardiac surgery. Eur J Anaesthesiol. 2008;25:135.

Chapter 53
TEE II

Kofi B. Vandyck

A 60-year-old-patient with a history of right upper lobe lung cancer, peripheral vascular disease, and chronic bronchitis is scheduled for a transthoracic echocardiography as part of workup for lung resection. Echocardiography evaluation revealed a severely calcified aortic valve, severe left ventricular hypertrophy, and a low normal ejection fraction (EF 50%):

1. What is the etiology and pathophysiology of aortic stenosis?
2. How do you assess and grade aortic stenosis?
3. What is the natural history of patients with aortic stenosis?
4. What interventions are available for patients with aortic stenosis

---

K.B. Vandyck, MD
Department of Anesthesiology, University of Oklahoma Health Sciences Center,
750 NE 13th Street, Suite 200, Oklahoma City, OK 73104, USA
e-mail: Kofi-Vandyck@ouhsc.edu

T.D. Raj (ed.), *Data Interpretation in Anesthesia*,
DOI 10.1007/978-3-319-55862-2_53

Answers

1. Causes of aortic stenosis (AS) in adults:

   (a) Degeneration of tricuspid valve—commonest, seen after 60 years age, caused by generalized atherosclerosis
   (b) Degeneration of bicuspid valve—seen before 60, fusion of right and left cusps resulting in large anterior and small posterior cusp, associated with aortic dissection, aneurysm and coarctation
   (c) Rheumatic—commonest cause worldwide, usually associated with mitral disease as well
   (d) Outflow obstruction:

      - Subvalvular—either membrane or hypertrophic obstructive cardiomyopathy (HOCM)
      - Supravalvular—Williams syndrome

   Aortic sclerosis, defined as valve thickening without obstruction to LV outflow, is present in 25% of adults over 65 years of age. Predisposing factors common to both aortic stenosis and sclerosis are hypertension, smoking, serum low-density lipoprotein, and diabetes mellitus. Aortic sclerosis usually progresses to aortic stenosis in the presence of progressive inflammatory atherosclerosis. Ten percent of patients with aortic sclerosis progress to AS within 5 years. In the 2014 ACC/AHA guidelines on valvular disease, aortic sclerosis is considered part of the AS continuum with sclerosis assigned stage A (at risk group).

2. Diagnosis and assessment of severity of AS made on the basis of history, physical exam, and echocardiographic findings. Patients with severe aortic stenosis (AS) usually present with angina, syncope, sudden death, or heart failure. Physical exam may reveal a crescendo-decrescendo ejection murmur. ECG will show signs of left ventricular hypertrophy and left atrial enlargement.

   Two-dimensional echocardiography with Doppler evaluation (TTE or TEE) is the test of choice to confirm the diagnosis of AS and assess severity and also note the presence of coexisting diseases such as aortic regurgitation, mitral stenosis, mitral regurgitation, aortic root dilation, and coronary artery disease (Fig. 53.1).

   The peak velocity and mean pressure gradient across the aortic valve are measured by means of Doppler interrogation of the aortic valve (Fig. 53.2). Accurate Doppler measurement of aortic valve velocity (and pressure) requires a near parallel alignment of the ultrasound beam to the aortic valve. The normal aortic valve area is approximately 3.0–4.0 cm^2. The velocity and pressure gradients across the aortic valve are flow dependent. In patients with low ejection fraction, dobutamine or exercise stress echo may be needed to confirm the diagnosis. In the 2014 guidelines, severity of AS was divided into 4 stages (A, B, C, and D) based on valve anatomy, valve hemodynamics, hemodynamic consequence, and symptoms [1] (Table 53.1).

3. Patients with aortic stenosis usually present when symptoms become severe enough to disrupt normal daily activity. Prior to that, morbidity and mortality are very low. The rate of progression to severe aortic stenosis varies, but in general it has been

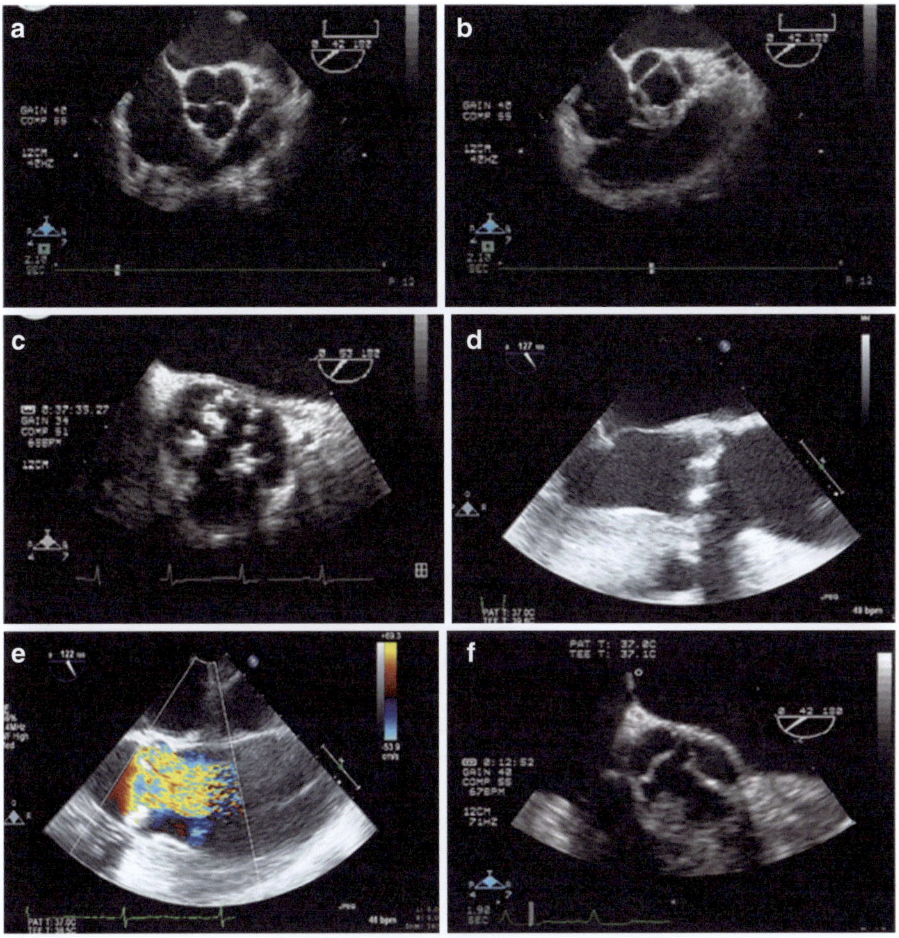

Fig. 53.1 Normal AV in ME AV SAX view (**a** and **b**), severely stenotic AV in ME AV SAX (**c**) and ME AV LAX views (**d**), color Doppler (**e**) of severely stenotic AV showing turbulent flow at the aortic valve and root. Aortic sclerosis (**f**)

shown that in patients with at least moderate aortic stenosis, jet velocity across the aortic valve increases by 0.3 m/s per year, mean gradient increases by 7 mmHg per year, and AVA decreases by 0.1 cm^2 per year [2]. Patients with symptomatic or severe aortic stenosis present with angina, dyspnea, lightheadedness, syncope, and heart failure. Sudden death is a feared complication of severe aortic stenosis, and, although rare, it has been reported to occur without symptoms. Average survival in patients with symptomatic aortic stenosis is 30–50% at 2 years. Patients with asymptomatic severe AS require close monitoring in order to detect sudden changes in symptoms. Patients with mild-to-moderate aortic stenosis will not have symptoms of the disease, but due to the unpredictable disease progression, it is mandatory for these asymptomatic patients to have regular clinical follow-up and evaluation for development of symptoms and disease progression. During these follow-ups,

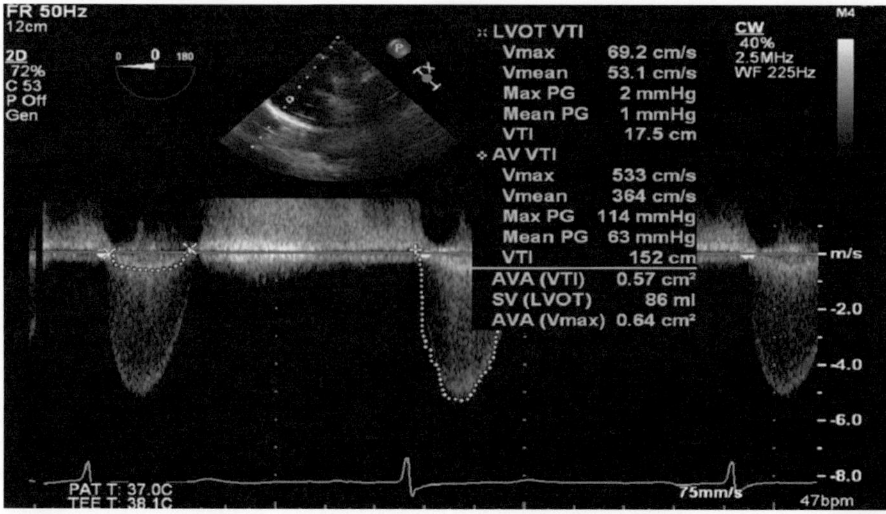

Fig. 53.2 Continous wave interrogation of stenosed aortic valve with measurement of maximum and mean pressure gradient and transvalvular velocity across aortic valve

Table 53.1 Stages of valvular aortic stenosis (Adapted from the Nishimura et al., 2014 ACC/AHA Practice Guidelines for the Management of Patients with Valvular Heart Disease)

Stage	Symptoms	Valve anatomy and hemodynamics
A	Asymptomatic but at risk	Bicuspid AV Aortic sclerosis ($v_{max} < 2$ m/s)
B	Asymptomatic but progressive	Mild-moderate leaflet calcification, some reduction in systolic motion (v_{max} 2–3.9 m/s, $P_{mean} < 20$–39 mmHg)
C	Asymptomatic severe AS	
C1	Asymptomatic severe AS	Severe leaflet calcification or stenosis with severely reduced leaflet opening ($v_{max} \geq 4$ m/s; $P_{mean} \geq 40$ mmHg, AVA ≤ 1 cm^2)
C2	Asymptomatic severe AS with LV dysfunction	Severe leaflet calcification or stenosis with severely reduced leaflet opening ($v_{max} \geq 4$ m/s; $P_{mean} \geq 40$ mmHg, AVA ≤ 1 cm^2, LVEF < 50%)
D	Symptomatic severe AS	
D1	Symptomatic severe high-gradient AS	Severe leaflet calcification or stenosis with severely reduced leaflet opening ($v_{max} \geq 4$ m/s; $P_{mean} \geq 40$ mmHg, AVA ≤ 1 cm^2, LV hypertrophy, LVEF > 50%)
D2	Symptomatic severe low-flow/low-gradient AS with reduced LVEF	Severe leaflet calcification or stenosis with severely reduced leaflet opening (Resting $v_{max} \geq 4$ m/s or $P_{mean} \geq 40$ mmHg; AVA ≤ 1 cm^2, LVEF < 50%)
D3	Symptomatic severe low-gradient AS with normal LVEF	Severe leaflet calcification or stenosis with severely reduced leaflet opening ($v_{max} < 4$ m/s or $P_{mean} < 40$ mmHg; AVA ≤ 1 cm^2 Stroke Vol Index < 35 m/m^2, LVEF $\geq$ 50%, small LV size

patients should be educated on the signs and symptoms of disease progression such as exercise intolerance, exertional chest discomfort, dyspnea, and syncope.

4. Appearance of symptoms is the most important indication for intervention in patients with aortic stenosis. There are no specific medical therapies to treat or slow the progression of aortic stenosis [1, 2]. It is recommended to treat hypertension in patients with increased risk of developing AS (stages B and C) [1, 2]. Hypertension is prevalent in patients with AS and has been shown to be a risk factor for AS and also increase the morbidity and mortality risk associated with AS [1, 3]. The treatment is started at low dose, and patients should be monitored closely by experienced cardiologist to avoid complications associated with the disease state or treatment in these high-risk patients. Angiotensin-converting enzyme (ACE) inhibitors, diuretics, and vasodilators can be used in the acute setting in patients with severe decompensated AS. The use of these medications may require invasive hemodynamic monitoring.

   Aortic valve replacement (AVR) is the only definite treatment for patient with AS. Early surgical intervention has been shown to decrease mortality in patients with severe AS [1]. Decision to operate should be based on symptoms, valve anatomy, and hemodynamics [1]. The ACC/AHA guideline recommends surgical AVR for all patients who meet an indication for AVR with low or intermediate surgical risk. Major indications for surgical AVR (class I recommendation) are severe symptomatic AS, asymptomatic severe AS with LVEF <50%, asymptomatic severe AS in patients undergoing CABG, other heart surgeries or surgery on the aorta. In patients with moderate AS undergoing other cardiac surgery, it is reasonable to perform surgical AVR if the aortic velocity is between 3 and 3.9 m/s or the mean pressure gradient is between 20–39 mmHg (class IIa recommendation). These patients are likely to have symptoms of the disease within 5 years due to the progressive nature of aortic stenosis [2].

   Transcatheter aortic valve replacement (TAVR) is a minimally invasive surgical procedure for replacing the aortic valve. At present, it is indicated in patients with severe AS who are high risk for open surgical replacement of the aortic valve. It involves placing a valve mounted on balloon at the tip of a catheter over a diseased native aortic valve. The catheter is fed through either the femoral artery or through the apex of the heart which require a small incision to be made on the left chest wall. According to the ACC/AHA 2014 guidelines on valvular disease, TAVR is recommended in AS patients with indications for AVR who have a high risk for open AVR, or a prohibitive surgical risk and a predicted post TAVR risk greater than 12 months.

References

1. Nishimura RA, Otto CM, Bonow RO, Carabello BA, Erwin III JP, Guyton RA, American College of Cardiology/American Heart Association Task Force on Practice Guidelines. American College of Cardiology/American Heart Association Task Force on Practice Guidelines, et al. 2014 AHA/ACC guideline for the management of patients with valvular heart disease: a report of the American College of Cardiology/American Heart association task force on practice guidelines. J Am Coll Cardiol. 2014;63:e57–18.

2. Saric M. Decompensated valvular disease in the cardiac care unit. In: Herzog, E. The cardiac care unit: survival guide. 1st ed. Lippincott Williams and Wilkins, Philadelphia, PA 2012.: Chapter 25. p. 253–257.
3. Vahanian A, Alfieri O, Andreotti F, Antunes MJ, Barón-Esquivias G, Baumgartner H, Borger MA, Joint Task Force on the Management of Valvular Heart Disease of the European Society of Cardiology (ESC); European Association for Cardio-Thoracic Surgery (EACTS), et al. Joint task force on the management of valvular heart disease of the European Society of Cardiology (ESC); European Association for Cardio-Thoracic Surgery (EACTS). Guidelines on the management of valvular heart disease (version 2012). Eur Heart J. 2012;33:2451–96.
4. Skubas NJ, Shernan SK, Bollen B. An overview of the American College of Cardiology/American Heart Association 2014 valve heart disease practice guidelines: what is its relevance for the anesthesiologist and perioperative medicine physician? Anesth Analg. 2015;121(5):1132–8.

Chapter 54
Echo: Doppler I

Kofi B. Vandyck

A 45-year-old Caucasian female with a recent history of breast cancer status post-chemotherapy and radiation therapy was admitted with high-grade fever, slurred speech, back pain, and petechial rash. Surveillance cultures had been inconclusive with one of three samples being positive for coagulase-negative *Staphylococcus aureus*. Transthoracic echocardiography, performed as part of initial workup, showed no valvular vegetation, preserved ejection fraction (55%), and mild aortic

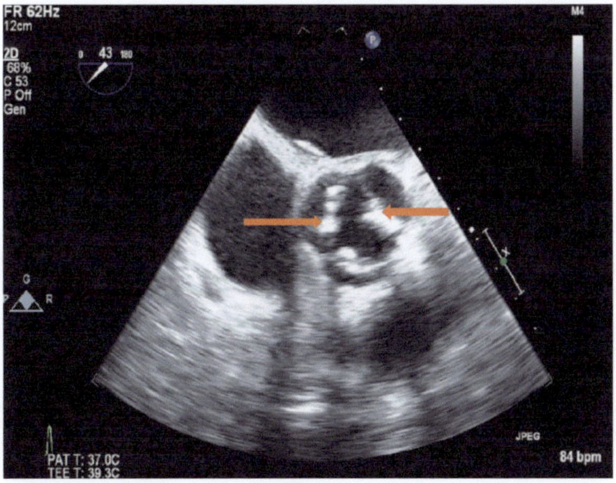

Fig. 54.1 Mid-esophageal short axis view of aortic valve showing vegetation on aortic leaflets. *Arrows* showing vegetation on aortic valve leaflets

K.B. Vandyck, MD
Department of Anesthesiology, University of Oklahoma Health Sciences Center, 750 NE 13th Street, Suite 200, Oklahoma City, OK 73104, USA
e-mail: Kofi-Vandyck@ouhsc.edu

T.D. Raj (ed.), *Data Interpretation in Anesthesia*,
DOI 10.1007/978-3-319-55862-2_54

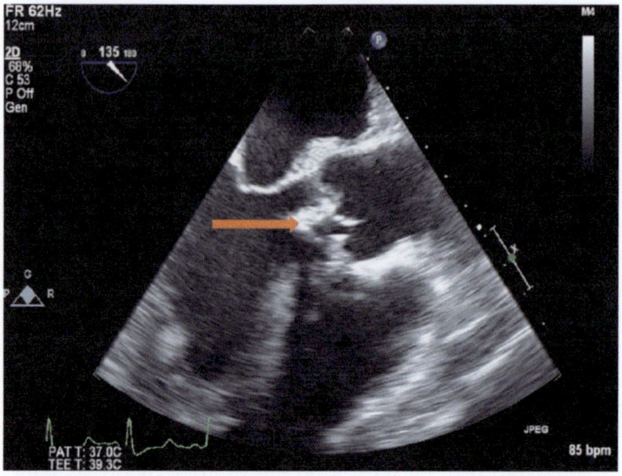

Fig. 54.2 Mid-esophageal long axis view of aortic valve showing mobile vegetation on aortic valve. *Arrow* showing vegetation on aortic valve leaflet. Valve viewed in long axis

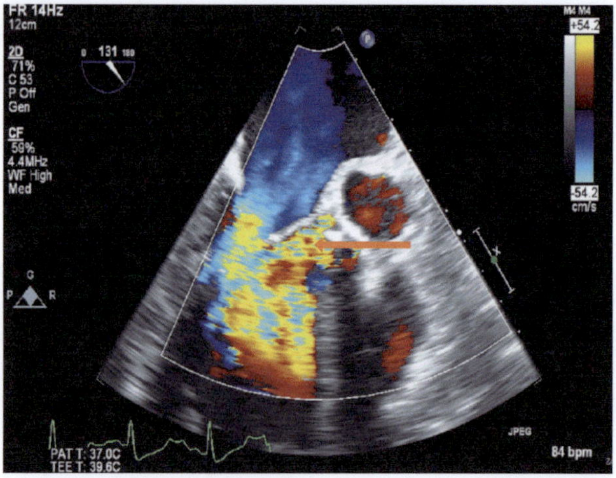

Fig. 54.3 Mid-esophageal long axis view with color Doppler in a patient with aortic valve endocarditis showing severe regurgitation at the aortic valve

regurgitation. A diagnosis of infective endocarditis was suspected, and despite treatment with antibiotics, the patient continued to have intermittent high-grade fever and signs and symptoms of congestive heart failure. Transesophageal echocardiography performed 7 days' post-presentation showed a large mobile mass on the aortic valve, severe aortic regurgitation with a depressed ejection fraction of 40% (see Figs. 54.1, 54.2, and 54.3). Therefore, cardiothoracic surgery was consulted for evaluation for possible valve replacement surgery.

Questions

1. What are the risk factors for infective endocarditis?
2. Explain the pathophysiology of infective endocarditis?
3. Describe the clinical manifestations of infective endocarditis?
4. How do you diagnose infective endocarditis?
5. What is the role of TTE and TEE in the diagnosis of infective endocarditis?
6. What are the treatment options for patients with infective endocarditis?
7. Which are the guidelines on managing high-risk patients presenting for surgery?

Answers

1. The following patients present a high risk for infective endocarditis [1–9]:
   (a) Male, elderly (age > 60)
   (b) Prior history of prior IE
   (c) Poor dental hygiene
   (d) Patient undergoing dental procedures involving gingival tissues
   (e) Patients with valvular heart disease (e.g., rheumatic valvular disease)
   (f) Patients with uncorrected or partially corrected congenital heart disease
   (g) IV drug use
   (h) Prosthetic valves
   (i) Immunosuppressed patient
   (j) Patients with history of diabetes
   (k) Patients with intracardiac devices
   (l) Patients undergoing hemodialysis

2. Pathophysiology:
   (a) IE occurs when bacteria or fungi invade sterile platelet-rich thrombus at sites of injury in the endocardium.
   (b) Sources of bacteria include the skin, oral cavity, mucosal surfaces, or sites of focal infection.
   (c) Infection results in invasion of the thrombus and destruction of the underlying valvular and endocardial tissues.
   (d) Bacteria usually resistant to the complement system of the body.
   (e) Common bacterial species: *Staphylococcus*, *Streptococcus*, *Enterococci*, and HACEK group (*Haemophilus*, *Actinobacillous*, *Corynebacterium*, *Eikenella*, and *Kingella*).

3. Infective endocarditis can affect all organ systems of the body [1–9]:
   (a) Nonspecific symptoms: fever (most common symptoms), chills, sweats, headaches, weight loss, back pain, myalgia arthralgia, cough, and pleuritic chest pain
   (b) Other symptoms highly specific for IE: cardiac murmur (85% of patients), splinter hemorrhage in nail beds, petechiae on skin and mucous membranes, Janeway lesions (nontender macules on palm and sole), Roth spots (hemorrhagic lesions on retina), and Osler nodes (tender nodules on fingers and toes)
   (c) Cardiac complications: valvular insufficiency, congestive heart failure (30–40% of IE patients), and periannular and intraventricular abscesses (can result in intracardiac fistulas), cardiac arrhythmias (usually the result of periannular abscesses)
   (d) Vascular-embolic complications: septic emboli (15–35% of IE patients), mycotic aneurysm, and vertebral osteomyelitis
   (e) Neurologic complications (mostly from vascular embolic events): brain abscess, embolic stroke, and cerebral hemorrhage
   (f) Renal complications: kidney infarct from septic emboli and glomerulonephritis (caused by immune complexes)
   (g) Pulmonary complications (commonly seen in right heart IE): septic pulmonary emboli and pyopneumothorax

4. The modified Duke Criteria is the most common guideline used in the diagnosis of infective endocarditis. Pathological and clinical information obtained during workup have been divided into major and minor criteria (adapted with permission from the ACC/AHA 2014 Guidelines for Management of Valvular Heart Disease) [8]:
   (a) Major criteria:
      - Blood culture positive for IE: at least two positive cultures of blood samples drawn >12 h apart or all three or a majority of ≥4 separate cultures of blood (with first and last sample drawn at least 1 h apart)
      - Single positive blood culture for *Coxiella Burnetii* or anti-phase 1 IgG antibody titer ≥1:800
      - Evidence of endocardial involvement
      - Echocardiogram positive for IE
   (b) Minor criteria
      - Predisposing heart condition
      - IV drug use
      - Fever (temperature > 38 °C)
      - Vascular phenomena including major arterial emboli, septic pulmonary infarcts, mycotic aneurysm, intracranial hemorrhage, conjunctival hemorrhages, and Janeway lesions
      - Immunological phenomena including glomerulonephritis, Osler nodes, Roth spots, and rheumatoid factor
      - Positive blood culture but does not meet a major criterion as noted above
   (c) The criteria further stratify the diagnosis of IE into definite, possible, or rejected based on whether a patient exhibits a set of major and/or minor clinically defined characteristics (adapted with permission from the ACC/AHA 2014 Guidelines for Management of Valvular Heart Disease):
      - Definite IE:
        Pathological criteria: culture demonstrated microorganism or histology showing intracardiac abscess
        Clinical criteria: two major criteria or one major and three minor criteria or five minor criteria
      - Possible IE:
        One major criterion and one minor criterion or three minor criteria.
      - Rejected IE:
        Firm alternative diagnosis.
        No pathological evidence of IE was found at surgery or autopsy after antibiotic therapy for 4 days or less.
        Resolution of clinical manifestations occurs after ≤4 days of antibiotic therapy.
        Clinical criteria for possible or definite infective endocarditis are not met.

5. Echocardiography is a major criterion in the diagnoses of infective endocarditis, and therefore it should be performed in all patients with suspected IE [8]:
   (a) Echocardiographic evidence of IE includes (see Figs. 54.1, 54.2, and 54.3):

- Valvular vegetation
- Associated valvular regurgitation
- Intracardiac mass
- Periannular abscess

(b) Transthoracic echocardiogram (TTE):
- Initial test of choice to identify vegetation and quantify hemodynamic effect of IE.
- Good sensitivity and specificity (75% and ~100%, respectively).
- Absence of lesions on TTE does not rule out IE when there is high suspicion of IE.
- Suboptimal TTE images may be seen in patients with chronic obstructive pulmonary disease, previous thoracic and cardiovascular surgery, and morbid obesity.

(c) Transesophageal echocardiogram (TEE):
- Generally, more sensitive for the diagnosis of TEE especially for prosthetic valves, paravalvular abscess, fistulas, and intracardiac devices.
- Specificity is slightly lower than TTE.
- Recommended as the initial test of choice when feasible.
- Recommended in cases of negative TTE but high suspicion of IE.
- Recommended for follow-up of patients with IE, small left-sided heart IE and patients who develop progressive disease despite institution of antimicrobial therapy.

6. Treatment: The mainstay of treatment for infective endocarditis is antibiotic, often over weeks, with regular surveillance to gauge effectiveness of treatment.

(a) Factors that present a challenge during antibiotic treatment:
- Focal infection with high bacterial density
- Impaired immunity in the patient
- Slow rate of bacterial growth within a biofilm
- Low microorganism metabolic activity

(b) Choice of antibiotics must be based on the knowledge of the susceptibility profile of the microorganism in the vegetation.

(c) Systemic antibiotics must be in concentrations high enough to counteract the high density of bacterial in the vegetation.

(d) An expected infectious disease must be directly treated with antimicrobials in IE patient.

(e) Valve replacement is recommended in the following cases:
- Large mobile vegetation greater than 10 mm in diameter
- Vegetation with associated regurgitation
- Paravalvular infection and/or annular abscess
- Penetrating intracardiac lesion
- Endocarditis with associated heart block and/or malignant arrhythmia
- Fungal vegetation
- Persistent bacteremia despite antibiotic treatment

7. Antibiotic prophylaxis is recommended in the following highest-risk patients only:
   (a) Prosthetic heart valve
   (b) Prior history of IE
   (c) Dental procedures involving break in oral mucosa and gingival tissue
   (d) Procedures in infected gastrointestinal and genitourinary tract
   (e) Procedures on infected skin and integument
   (f) Biopsy of the respiratory tract
   (g) Unrepaired cyanotic congenital heart disease
   (h) Repaired congenital heart disease with residual defects

Antibiotics for Recommendation for Dental Procedures [1]

(a) Patients who can take oral meds:
   - Oral amoxicillin (adults 2 g, children 50 mg/kg)

(b) Patients unable to take oral meds:
   - Ampicillin IV or IM (adults 2 g, children 50 mg/kg)
   - Cefazolin IV (adults 1 g, children 50 mg/kg)
   - Ceftriaxone IV (adults 1 g IV or IM, children 50 mg/kg)

(c) Patients allergic to penicillin (anaphylaxis, angioedema, urticaria):
   - Oral azithromycin or clarithromycin (adult 500 mg, children 15 mg/kg)
   - Oral clindamycin (adults 600 mg, children 20 mg/kg)

(d) Patients allergic to penicillin and unable to take oral medications:
   - Clindamycin IV or IM (adults 600 mg, children 20 mg/kg)
   - Vancomycin IV (adults 15 to 20 mg/kg, children 15 mg/kg)

References

1. Baddour LM, Wilson WR, et al. Infective endocarditis in adults: diagnosis, antimicrobial therapy, and management of complications. Circulation. 2015;132:1435–86.
2. Brusch J. Infective endocarditis: management in the era of intravascular devices. New York, NY: Informa Healthcare; 2007.
3. Durante-Mangoni E, Bradley S, Selton-Suty C, et al. Current features of infective endocarditis in elderly patients: results of the International Collaboration on Endocarditis Prospective Cohort Study. Arch Intern Med. 2008;168:2095.
4. Gould FK, Denning DW, Elliott TS, et al. Guidelines for the diagnosis and antibiotic treatment of endocarditis in adults: a report of the Working Party of the British Society for Antimicrobial Chemotherapy. J Antimicrob Chemother. 2012;67:269.
5. Habib G, Lancellotti P, Antunes MJ, et al. ESC guidelines for the management of infective endocarditis: the task force for the management of infective endocarditis of the European Society of Cardiology (ESC). Endorsed by: European Association for Cardio-Thoracic Surgery (EACTS), the European Association of Nuclear Medicine (EANM). Eur Heart J 2015. 2015;36:3075.
6. Michel PL, Acar J. Native cardiac disease predisposing to infective endocarditis. Eur Heart J. 1995;16(Suppl B):2.

7. Murdoch DR, Corey GR, Hoen B, et al. Clinical presentation, etiology, and outcome of infective endocarditis in the 21st century: the International Collaboration on Endocarditis-Prospective Cohort Study. Arch Intern Med. 2009;169:463.
8. Nishimura RA, Otto CM, Bonow RO, et al. AHA/ACC guideline for the management of patients with valvular heart disease: a report of the American College of Cardiology/American Heart Association Task Force on Practice Guidelines. J Am Coll Cardiol. 2014;e57:63.
9. Wilson W, Taubert KA, Gewitz M, Lockhart PB, et al. Prevention of Infective Endocarditis. Guidelines from the American Heart Association. A Guideline from the American Heart Association Rheumatic Fever, Endocarditis, and Kawasaki Disease Committee, Council on Cardiovascular Disease in the Young, and the Council on Clinical Cardiology, Council on Cardiovascular Surgery and Anesthesia, and the Quality of Care and Outcomes Research Interdisciplinary Working Group. Circulation. 2007;116:1736. Copyright © 2007 Lippincott Williams & Wilkins

Chapter 55
Echo: Doppler II

Talla A. Rousan

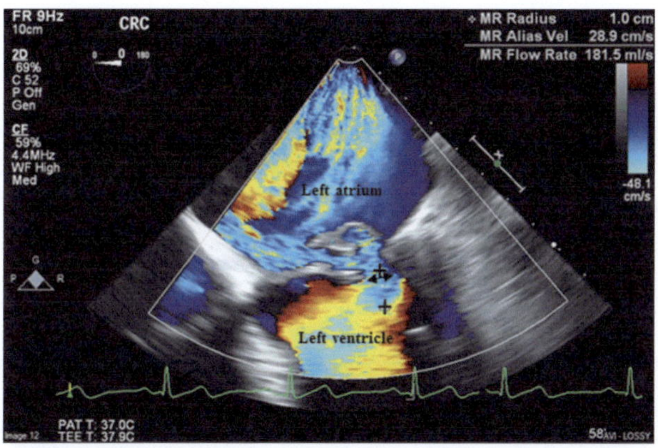

Fig. 55.1 Color flow Doppler imaging of mitral valve regurgitation from the transesophageal echocardiographic Four-chamber mid-esophageal view with zoom-in on the mitral valve. Vena contracta (black double arrow) and proximal isovelocity surface area radius (the distance between the "+" signs) are shown

Questions

1. What do Figs. 55.1, 55.2, and 55.3 represent?
2. Define color flow Doppler and its application in mitral valve regurgitation.
3. What is continuous wave Doppler?
4. Describe the different grades of mitral valve regurgitation.

T.A. Rousan, MD, FACC
Department of Medicine, The University of Oklahoma Health Sciences Center and the Veteran Affairs Medical Center, 800 Stanton L. Young Blvd, COM 5400, Oklahoma City, OK 73104, USA
e-mail: Talla-rousan@ouhsc.edu

T.D. Raj (ed.), *Data Interpretation in Anesthesia*,
DOI 10.1007/978-3-319-55862-2_55

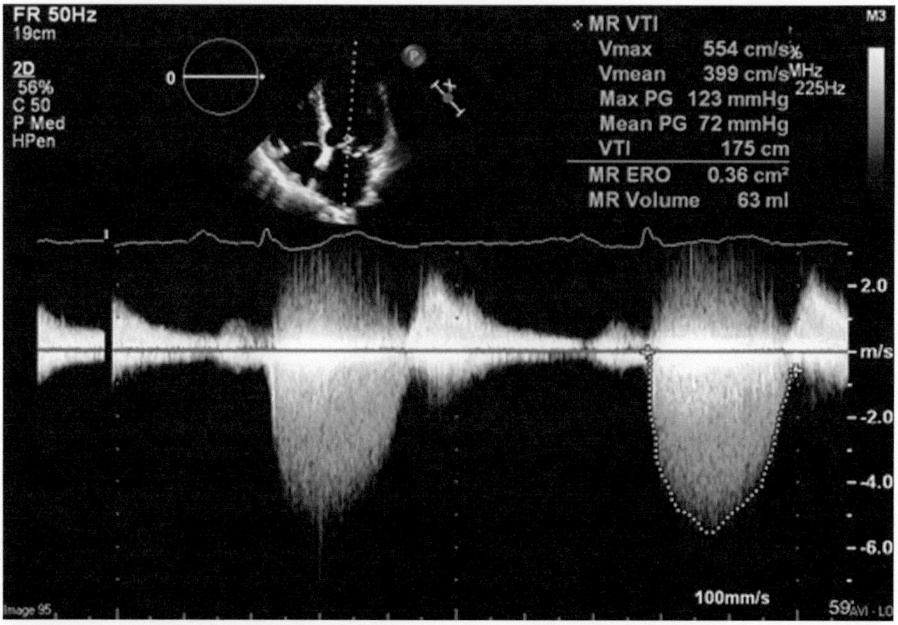

Fig. 55.2 Continuous wave Doppler sampled across the mitral valve

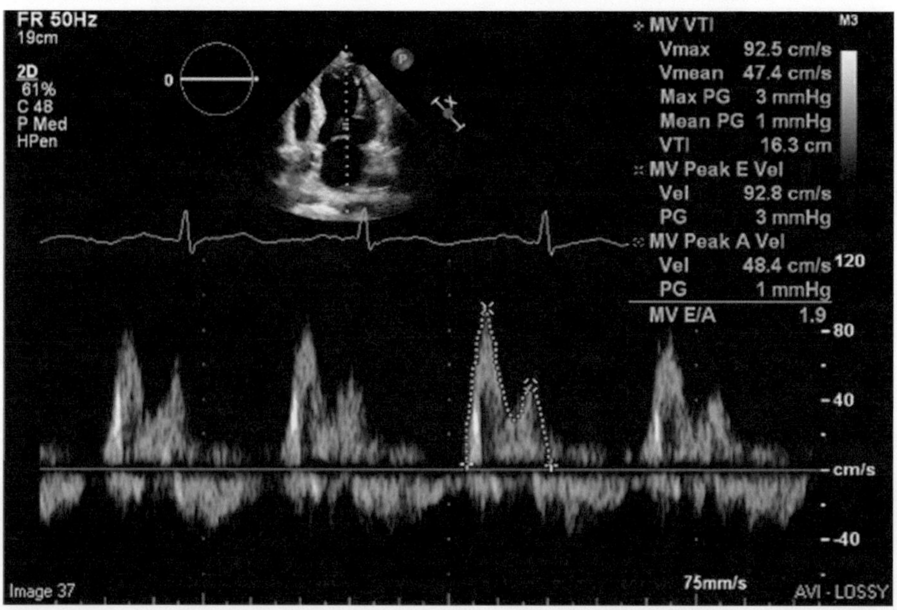

Fig. 55.3 Pulsed wave Doppler sampled at the mitral valve

Answers

1. The figures show still echocardiographic frames for a patient with mitral valve regurgitation. Figure 55.1 is color flow Doppler with transesophageal echocardiography, and Figs. 55.2 and 55.3 demonstrate continuous wave Doppler sampled across the mitral valve and pulsed wave Doppler sampled at the mitral valve using transthoracic echocardiography (TTE).

2. **Color flow Doppler** displays intracavity blood flow in colors (red, blue, green, or their combinations) depending on the velocity, direction, and extent of turbulence [1]. Color flow Doppler is a widely used method for the detection of regurgitant valvular heart disease. This technique provides visualization of the origin and width (vena contracta) of the regurgitation jet, spatial orientation of the jet area in the receiving chamber, and flow convergence into the regurgitant orifice [2]. The area of the regurgitant jet can provide a rapid quantitative assessment of the severity of the regurgitation; generally speaking, a large area may indicate a more significant regurgitation [2]. **Vena contracta** or regurgitant jet width (black double arrow in Fig. 55.1) is the narrowest portion of a jet that occurs at/or just downstream from the orifice of the valve, and it is an indirect measure of the regurgitant orifice [3]. **Proximal isovelocity surface area (PISA)** or flow convergence is another method to quantify the severity of mitral valve regurgitation. It is based on the continuity equation and the principle of flow conversation [1, 2]. As blood in the left ventricle approaches the mitral regurgitant orifice, there is convergence and flow acceleration. This is seen in hemispheric waves of decreasing area but of equal velocity (hence, the term isovelocity) [1, 2]. PISA is identified by color flow Doppler as the "red-blue" aliasing interface (PISA radius is the distance between the "+" signs in Fig. 55.1). PISA radius is used to calculate the effective regurgitant orifice area (ERO), which is the cross-sectional area of the vena contracta, and regurgitant volume (which is the volume of the blood that is leaking back to the left atrium during systole) [1]. ERO and the regurgitant volume can also be calculated using the volumetric method [1]. In the absence of significant aortic valve regurgitation, the regurgitant volume is equal to the flow across the mitral valve minus the flow across the left ventricular outflow tract (systemic stroke volume) [1]. These calculations are made by obtaining the LVOT and mitral valve diameters and LVOT and mitral valve time-velocity integral (TVI) [1]. Figure 55.3 shows pulsed wave Doppler at the mitral valve which depicts the TVI of the mitral valve.

3. Doppler echocardiography measures blood flow velocities in the heart chambers as well as in the great vessels [1]. Continuous wave Doppler measures the changes in velocities along the beam path and is used to record the highest flow velocity available [1]. Analysis of continuous wave Doppler signal by noting the shape, contour, density, and velocity of the signal can provide an insight on the severity of mitral valve regurgitation [4].

4. Mitral valve regurgitation is graded into mild, moderate, and severe. This is based on quantitative as well as qualitative assessment, and it involves the use of

Table 55.1 Grades of mitral valve regurgitation severity

Severity	Jet area (cm^2)	Jet/left atrium area (cm^2)	Regurgitant fraction	Vena contracta width (cm)	Regurgitant volume (mL/beat)	Effective regurgitant orifice area (cm^2)
Mild	<4	<20%	<30%	<0.3	<30	<0.20
Moderate	4–10	20–40%	30–49%	0.3–0.69	30–59	0.20–0.39
Severe	>10	>40%	≥50%	≥0.7	≥60	≥0.40

Doppler echocardiography. The visualization of the jet area and jet area to left atrium area ratio by color flow Doppler provides a quick assessment tool of the severity of mitral valve regurgitation [3]. This method tends to underestimate eccentric jets and overestimate the severity of mitral regurgitation in ventral jets [3]. Mitral valve regurgitation can be quantitatively assessed by measuring the vena contracta width, effective regurgitant orifice area, the regurgitant volume, and the regurgitant fraction (the ratio between the regurgitant volume and the flow across the mitral valve) [1, 3]. Table 55.1 illustrates the different grades of mitral valve regurgitation using the different variables [3]. Based on the data provided in the figures, this case represents severe mitral valve regurgitation (vena contracta 0.7 cm and regurgitant volume of 63 mL).

References

1. Oh JK, Seward JB, Tajik AJ. The echo manual. 3rd ed. Philadelphia: Lippincott Williams & Wilkins; 2007.
2. Zoghbi WA, et al. Recommendations for evaluation of the severity of native valvular regurgitation with two-dimensional and Doppler echocardiography. J Am Soc Echocardiogr. 2003;16(7):777–802.
3. Grigioni F, et al. Clinical use of doppler echocardiography in organic mitral regurgitation: from diagnosis to patients' management. J Cardiovasc Ultrasound. 2015;23(3):121–33.
4. Fadel BM, et al. Spectral Doppler interrogation of mitral regurgitation -spot diagnosis. Echocardiography. 2015;32(7):1179–83.

Chapter 56
Echo: Doppler III

Nicole T. Tran

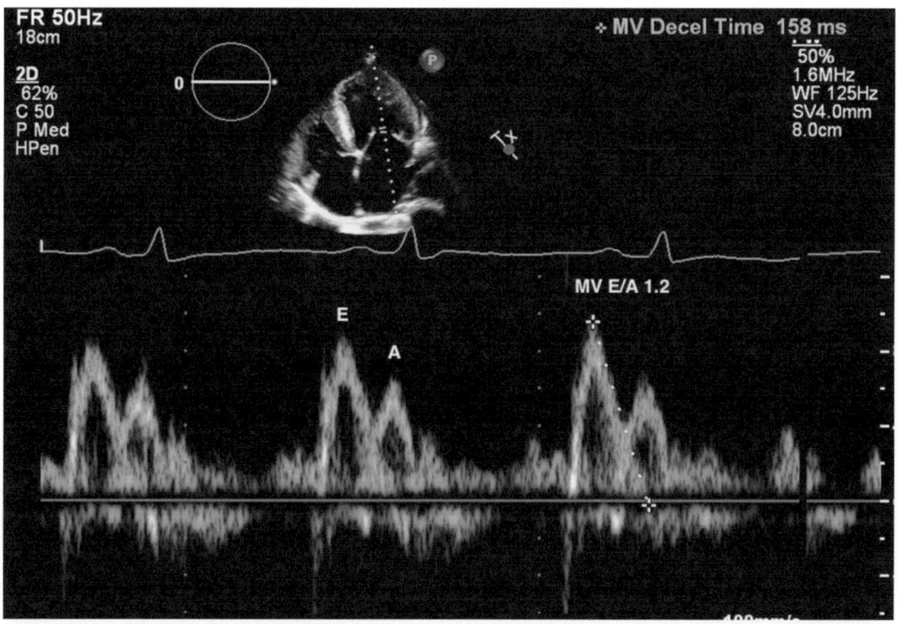

Fig. 56.1

N.T. Tran, MD
Department of Cardiology, University of Oklahoma Health Sciences Center, Oklahoma City, OK, USA
e-mail: Nicole-tran@Ouhsc.edu

T.D. Raj (ed.), *Data Interpretation in Anesthesia*,
DOI 10.1007/978-3-319-55862-2_56

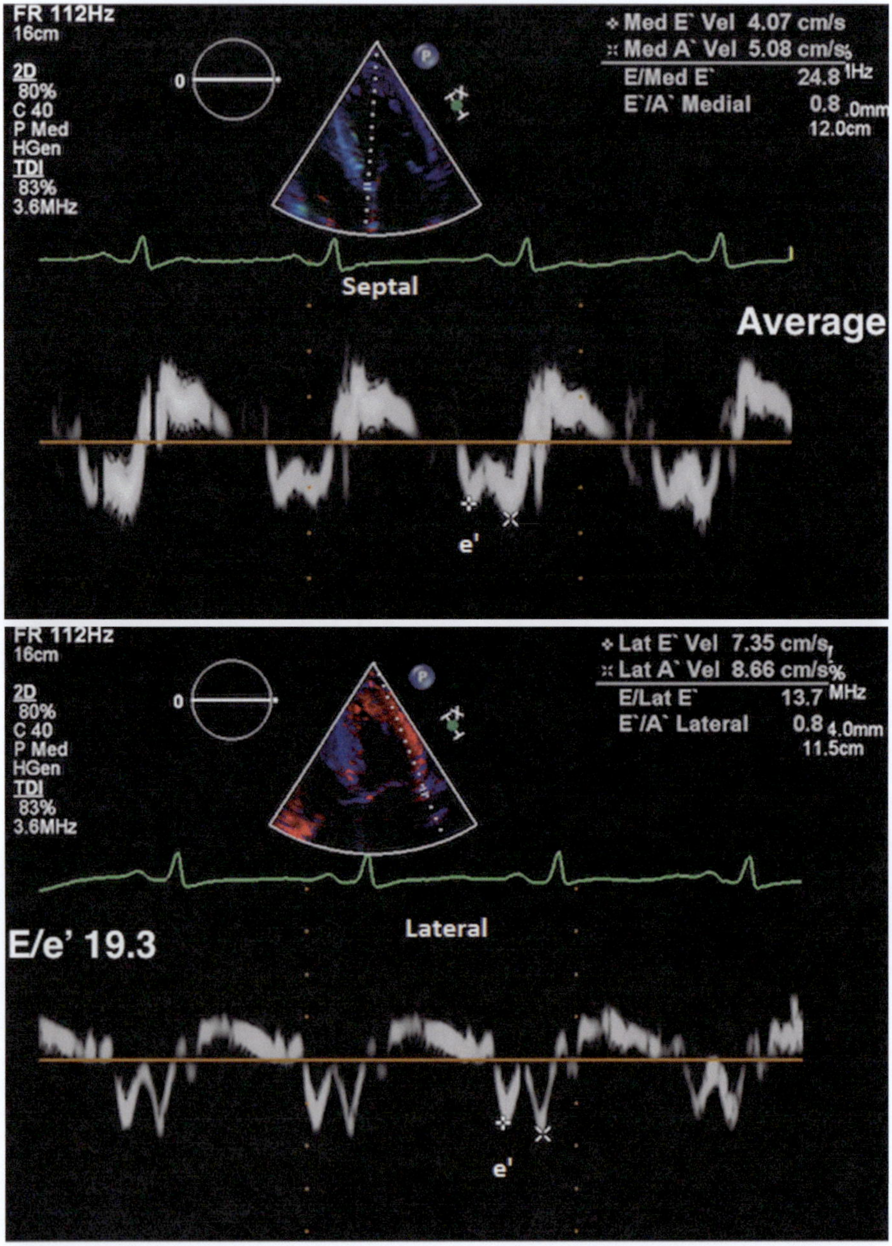
FR 112Hz
16cm
2D
80%
C 40
P Med
HGen
TDI
83%
3.6MHz
Med E` Vel 4.07 cm/s
Med A` Vel 5.08 cm/s
E/Med E` 24.8
E`/A` Medial 0.8
12.0cm
Septal
Average
e'
FR 112Hz
16cm
2D
80%
C 40
P Med
HGen
TDI
83%
3.6MHz
Lat E` Vel 7.35 cm/s
Lat A` Vel 8.66 cm/s
E/Lat E` 13.7
E`/A` Lateral 0.8
4.0mm
11.5cm
Lateral
E/e' 19.3
e'

Fig. 56.2

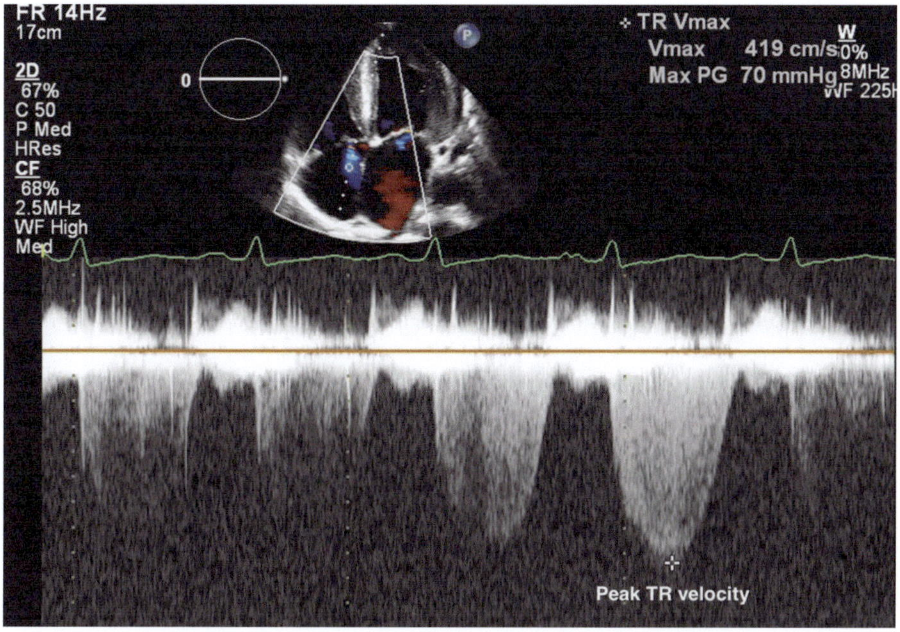

Fig. 56.3

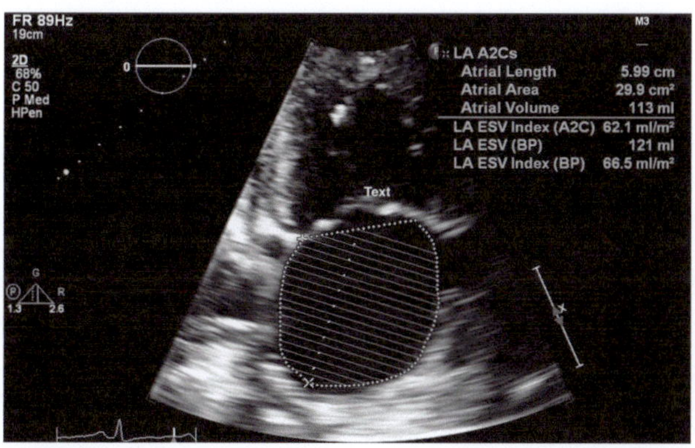

Fig. 56.4

I. A 48-year-old male with history of uncontrolled hypertension and end-stage renal disease on hemodialysis presents for TTE as part of preoperative risk stratification prior to possible renal transplant. He has NYHA Class III symptoms at baseline. 2D images show moderately to markedly increased left ventricular wall thickness. LVEF calculated by the biplane Simpson's method is 56%. The remainder of his diastolic parameters are as shown in Figs. 56.1, 56.2, 56.3, and 56.4.

Questions

1. Describe what happens in normal diastole.
2. What are the causes of diastolic dysfunction? What is the difference between diastolic dysfunction and heart failure with preserved ejection fraction (HF-pEF)?
3. How do you use echocardiography to grade diastolic dysfunction?
4. What do Figs. 56.1, 56.2, 56.3, and 56.4 show?
5. Does this patient have normal or abnormal diastolic function? How would you grade it?
6. What are the key considerations for managing diastolic dysfunction in the preoperative period?

Answers

1. Diastole is defined as the portion of the cardiac cycle between aortic valve closure and mitral valve closure. It is normally divided into four phases: isovolumic relaxation, rapid early diastolic filling, diastasis, and atrial contraction. Isovolumic relaxation occurs between aortic valve closure and mitral valve opening. Through an active, calcium-dependent process, left ventricular pressure decreases, while volume remains the same [1]. When left ventricular end-diastolic pressure falls below left atrial pressure, the mitral valve opens and rapid early diastolic filling begins. This usually accounts for 70% of left ventricular filling [1, 2]. As pressures equalize between the left atrium and left ventricle, a small amount of filling continues via passive flow from the pulmonary veins; this is diastasis. Diastasis generally accounts for 5% of left ventricular filling and is only present at slower heart rates. If the patient is in sinus rhythm, atrial systole follows diastasis. Left atrial pressure again transiently increases, and there is further filling of the left ventricle. Atrial contraction generally accounts from 25% of left ventricular filling in the normal heart. Diastolic function is influenced by volume status, properties of the left ventricle (stiffness, recoil), atrial properties, and catecholamines.
2. Aging, hypertension, diabetes, obesity, coronary artery disease, renal disease, valvular heart disease, and infiltrative processes all affect left ventricular mechanics/stiffening and thus diastolic function. In the presence of systolic dysfunction, diastolic function is always abnormal. HF-pEF is defined as the presence of diastolic dysfunction accompanied by signs/symptoms of clinical heart failure in patients with an ejection fraction of at least 50% [3].
3. In the 2016 American Society of Echocardiography/European Association of Cardiovascular Imaging guidelines, there are four main echocardiographic parameters used to assess diastolic dysfunction: mitral inflow pulse wave (PW) Doppler, annular tissue Doppler imaging (TDI), peak tricuspid regurgitant (TR) velocity, and left atrial end-systolic volume index (LAESVi).

Mitral inflow PW Doppler is measured in the apical four chamber (A4C) view with the Doppler cursor placed at the mitral leaflet tips [2, 4]. The initial wave of early diastolic filling is labeled the E wave. The second wave represents filling due to atrial contraction and is labeled the A wave (Fig. 56.1). In normal hearts the E/A ratio is typically between 0.9 and 1.5 [2]. As relaxation becomes

Table 56.1 Grading diastolic dysfunction

	Normal	Grade I	Grade II	Grade III/IV
E/A	0.9–1.5	<0.9	0.9–2.0	≥2.0
Average E/e′ ratio	<14	<14	>14	>>14
Peak TR velocity	<2.8 m/s	<2.8 m/s	≥2.8 m/s	≥2.8 m/s
LAESVi	<34 mL/m^2	<34 mL/m^2	≥34 mL/m^2	≥34 mL/m^2

impaired, but before left atrial pressures (LAP) rise, there is an increased reliance on atrial contraction to maintain diastolic filling, and the E/A ratio is <0.9 [2]. As LAP continues to rise, there is again more filling happening in early diastole due to the increased pressure gradient between the left atrium (LA) and left ventricle (LV), and the E/A ratio becomes "pseudo normal." As left ventricular compliance decreases and LAP rises further, there is initial brief filling in early diastole with relatively little filling happening during atrial contraction, and the E/A ratio increases to ≥ 2. Mitral inflow PW Doppler varies with volume status, mitral valve disease, and atrial arrhythmias.

Annular TDI velocities are measured with PW Doppler in the A4C view with the cursor placed at both the septal and at the lateral mitral annulus (Fig. 56.2). Myocardial relaxation in early diastole is labeled e′. Septal and lateral e′ velocities are normally >7 cm/s and >10 cm/s, respectively [3]. As myocardial relaxation becomes impaired, annular tissue Doppler velocities decrease. The ratio of mitral inflow during early diastolic filling (E) and tissue Doppler early myocardial relaxation (e′) has been shown to correlate with LAP. Specifically, an average E/e′ ratio > 14, a septal E/e′ ratio > 15, and a lateral E/e′ ratio > 13 are consistent with elevated LAP [2]. Annular TDI velocities are not dependent on volume status but are unreliable in the presence of significant mitral annular calcification, a mitral prosthesis, or a mitral annuloplasty ring.

The **peak TR velocity** (Fig. 56.3) also positively correlates with LAP and pulmonary capillary wedge pressure (PCWP) in the absence of pulmonary vascular or pulmonary parenchymal disease. It should be measured using continuous wave (CW) Doppler in multiple views with an attempt to get the cursor as parallel as possible to the direction of regurgitant flow. A peak TR velocity > 2.8 m/s is consistent with elevated LAP [3].

Finally, left atrial size is related to chronic elevations in LAP (in the absence of mitral valve disease, atrial arrhythmias, or post-cardiac transplant). Left atrial size is best assessed by the **left atrial end-systolic volume index (LAESVi)**, with left atrial area traced in atrially focused A4C, and apical 2-chamber (A2C) views one to two frames before mitral valve opening. Left atrial volume is calculated using either Simpson's method of disks or the area-length method $(0.85 \times A1 \times A2)/(L1–L2/2)$ and is indexed to body surface area (BSA). A LAESVi >34 mL/m^2 is consistent with chronic elevations in left atrial pressure [2].

Currently, the main purpose in grading diastolic dysfunction is to evaluate whether LAP is elevated as elevated LAP is modifiable and correlates with symptoms and outcomes. Grade I diastolic dysfunction is characterized by impaired left ventricular relaxation with normal filling pressures. There is a decrease in early diastolic filling and an increase in filling with atrial contraction. Filling pressures are elevated in grades II–IV diastolic dysfunction. In grade II diastolic dysfunction, the left atrium remodels and left atrial pressures increase to compensate for elevated left ventricular end-diastolic pressures. Grades III–IV diastolic dysfunction represent restrictive filling where left ventricular filling only occurs in the setting of markedly elevated left atrial pressures due to reduced left ventricular compliance (exaggerated change in pressure for a small change in volume). Grade III is reversible; grade IV is irreversible [1–3]. Table 56.1 summarizes the findings for each of the four key variables in grades I–IV diastolic dysfunction.

4. Figure 56.1 shows the mitral inflow PW Doppler from our patient. The 2D image (above) shows the PW Doppler cursor placed at the mitral valve leaflet tips. The Doppler waveform (below) shows left ventricular filling. E represents early diastolic filling and A represents atrial contraction. Figure 56.2 shows annular TDI with the PW Doppler cursor placed at the medial (septal) annulus (left) and lateral annulus (right). e′ (myocardial relaxation in early diastole) is labeled on the Doppler tracing below. This and the mitral inflow data from Fig. 56.1 are used to calculate the average E/e′ ratio. Figure 56.3 shows a CW Doppler TR signal. The 2D image (top) shows the Doppler sampling line going through tricuspid regurgitation (blue signal). The peak TR velocity is marked on the Doppler waveform. Figure 56.4 shows a zoomed in view of the left atrium in an A2C view. The LAESVi is shown being calculated using the Simpson's method of disks. This would be combined with the A4C tracing of the left atrium to calculate left atrial volume and then divided by BSA to get the LAESVi.

5. With our patient, the mitral inflow PW Doppler E/A ratio is 1.2 (Fig. 56.1). This is either normal or pseudo normal. Therefore, we need to assess his average E/e′ ratio, his peak TR velocity, and his LAESVi. His average E/e′ ratio is >14 at 19.3 (Fig. 56.2). His peak TR velocity is >2.8 m/s at 4.19 m/s (Fig. 56.3). His LAESVi is >34 mL/m^2 at 66.5 mL/m^2 (Fig. 56.4). As all three parameters are abnormal, LAP is elevated, and he has grade II diastolic dysfunction.

6. The data is mixed on how anesthesia affects diastolic function. It used to be thought that isoflurane and desflurane prolonged isovolumic relaxation; however, further studies have had opposite findings [5]. Ketamine can reduce left ventricular compliance, and propofol can prolong isovolumic relaxation; however, propofol can also decrease preload, which improves left atrial pressures [5]. The important thing is to recognize which patients have diastolic dysfunction as these patients will be more sensitive to changes in preload, tachycardia, and arrhythmias. Volume overload/increased preload will further increase already elevated left atrial pressures and can precipitate pulmonary edema. Atrial arrhythmias (atrial fibrillation, atrial flutter) result in loss of coordinated atrial systole. In patients with impaired relaxation who rely on atrial contraction to fill the ventricle, this can result in sudden impaired filling and elevation of LAP. Diastole is shorter at higher heart rates, and tachycardia can worsen already impaired diastolic dysfunction by further limiting diastolic filling.

References

1. Galderisi M. Diastolic dysfunction and diastolic heart failure: diagnostic, prognostic and therapeutic aspects. Cardiovasc Ultrasound. 2005;3:9.
2. Otto CM. Textbook of clinical echocardiography. 5th ed. Philadelphia, PA: Elsevier/Saunders; 2013.

3. Nagueh SF, Smiseth OA, Appleton CP, et al. Recommendations for the evaluation of left ventricular diastolic function by echocardiography: an update from the American Society of Echocardiography and the European Association of Cardiovascular Imaging. J Am Soc Echocardiogr. 2016;29:277–314.
4. Nagueh SF, Appleton CP, Gilbert TC, et al. Recommendations for the evaluation of left ventricular diastolic function by echocardiography. J Am Soc Echocardiogr. 2009;22:107–33.
5. Deng Y, John S, Mangunta V. Perioperative diastolic dysfunction for the anesthesiologist. Anesthesiology News. New York, NY: McMahon Publishing; 2016.

Chapter 57
Echo IV

German Barbosa-Hernandez

Abbreviations

BKA	Below-knee amputation
BP	Blood pressure
CVP	Central venous pressure
EKG	Electrocardiogram
HR	Heart rate
IVC	Inferior vena cava
PA-pressure	Pulmonary artery pressure
pRBC	Packed red blood cells
RA	Right atrium
RR	Respiratory rate
SO_2	Oxygen saturation
TTE	Transthoraccic echocardiography

G. Barbosa-Hernandez, MD
Department of Anesthesia, Oklahoma University Health and Science Center, 800 NE 10th Street, Oklahoma City, OK 73102, USA
e-mail: German-BarbosaHernandez@ouhsc.edu

T.D. Raj (ed.), *Data Interpretation in Anesthesia*,
DOI 10.1007/978-3-319-55862-2_57

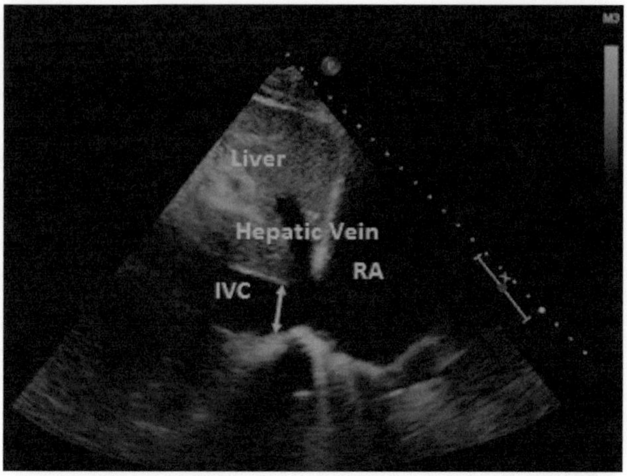

Fig. 57.1 TTE image

A 70-year-old male presents to the ED after an industrial accident causing a traumatic below-knee amputation on the right side. The patient has been obtunded and dyspneic since arrival. A total of six pRBC units and 5 L of crystalloids have been given in the last hour. You have been asked to evaluate this patient prior to operative BKA. HR, 120; BP, 90/60; RR, 35; SpO_2, 84%.

Questions

1. What is the view shown in the picture and how do you obtain it (See Fig. 57.1)?
2. Is it accurate to measure fluid status and fluid responsiveness with TTE?
3. How do you interpret the following images?
4. Would you change this patient's management, based on the ultrasound findings, and how?
5. How would you confirm your suspicion?

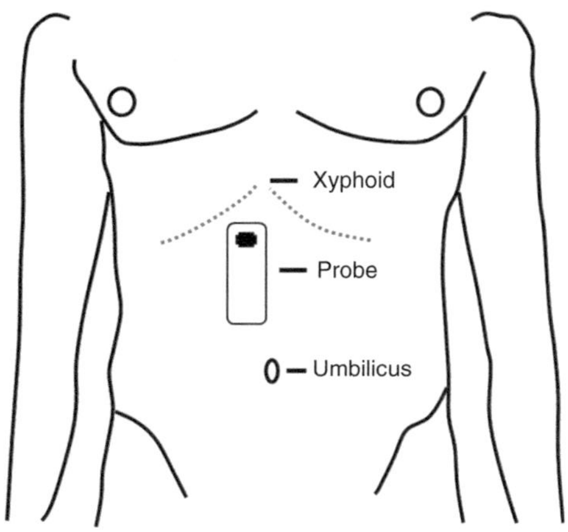

Fig. 57.1A Probe placement

Answers

1. This is a longitudinal view of the subcostal inferior vena cava.

   In the supine position, if possible with the knees bent, (relaxes abdominal wall) the probe is placed in the midline 2 or 3 cm below the xyphoid perpendicular to the abdominal wall with the orientation marker pointing toward the 3 o'clock position (See Fig. 57.1A). Focusing on the right atrium the probe is turned counterclockwise until the orientation marker is pointing toward the patient's head or until the IVC is seen merging into the RA. The IVC diameter is best-measured 2–3 cm before the IVC-RA junction, where the IVC walls are parallel [1].

2. IVC diameter and dynamic measurements of the IVC diameter have been used as surrogates for CVP, fluid status, and responsiveness to fluid therapy. Several difficulties may be encountered when using this technique. It maybe difficult to obtain the appropriate image; the liver or diaphragm may tend to splint open the IVC in the most proximal portions. Tricuspid valve dysfunction, right heart structural abnormalities, and variation in the diameter of the IVC among normal patients may also confound the matter [2].

   As recommended by the American society of echocardiography, in the context of focused cardiac ultrasound, IVC diameter and plethora are useful as surrogates of fluid status, when formal transthoracic echocardiography is not practical or readily available [3].

   The IVC diameter and respiratory variation should be used along with other indicators of volume status for clinical correlation. The interpretation of this image alone should not be used for clinical decision-making.

3. The following ultrasound images are obtained from the patient:

   Figure 57.2 shows a longitudinal view of the subcostal inferior vena cava.

   Figure 57.3 shows a longitudinal view of the subcostal inferior vena cava in M-mode measuring the IVC diameter during inspiration and expiration.

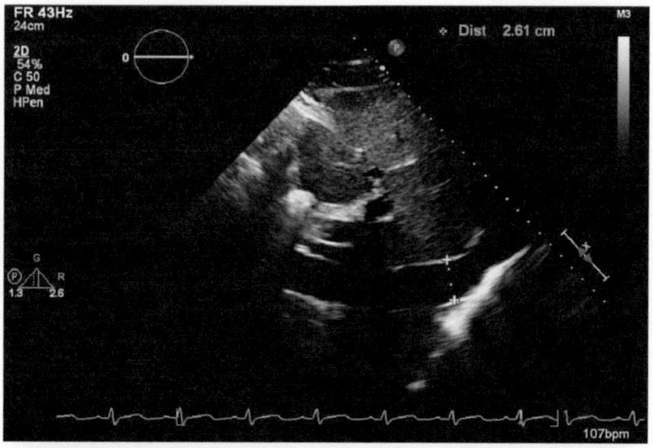

Fig. 57.2 Subcostal TTE longitudinal view of the subcostal inferior vena cava

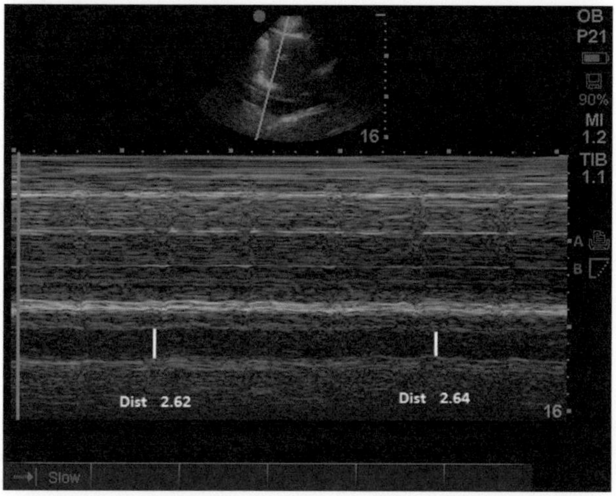

Fig. 57.3 Subcostal TTE longitudinal view of the subcostal inferior vena cava, M-mode measuring the IVC diameter at inspiration and expiration. (With permissions from American College of Emergency Physicians [4])

Ultrasound images of the IVC could be interpreted using the following criteria [1]:

(a) Hypovolemia: a reduced IVC diameter (<2.5 cm) and collapse with inspiration greater than half or complete collapse
(b) Hypervolemia: an increase in IVC diameter (>2.5 cm) and minimal collapse with inspiration.
   - Other situations that can cause this appearance are cardiac tamponade, mitral regurgitation, or aortic stenosis.

Interpretation of IVC Diameter [5]:

(a) By measuring IVC diameter (normal 1.5–2.5 cm):
   - Less than 1 cm: Very possible large blood loss necessitating blood transfusion
   - Less than 1.5 cm: Possible hypovolemia
   - More than 2.5 cm: Possible hypervolemia

(b) By measuring IVC diameter collapse with inspiration (Caval Index) preferably in M-mode as shown in Fig. 57.3:

- $$Caval\ index = \frac{(IVC\ diameter\ in\ expiration - IVC\ diameter\ in\ inspiration)}{IVC\ diamter\ in\ expiration} \times 100$$
- Caval index >50% suggests fluid responsiveness.

(c) Central venous pressure estimated by IVC imaging.

- CVP of 0–5 cm H_2O: Findings include an IVC diameter of less than 1.5 cm and a total collapse with inspiration.
- CVP of 5–10 cm H_2O: Findings include an IVC diameter between 1.5 and 2.5 cm, and a caval index of >50%.
- CVP of 11–15 cm H_2O: Findings include an IVC diameter between 1.5 and 2.5 cm, and a caval index of <50%.
- CVP of 16–20 cm H_2O: Findings include an IVC diameter larger than 2.5 cm, and a caval index of <50%.
- CVP larger than 20 cm H_2O: Findings include an IVC diameter larger than 2.5 cm, and no changes in the diameter with inspiration.

The dynamic image of the IVC ultrasound obtained in this case shows volume overload in the patient based on criteria discussed.

4. The ultrasound images (see answer to question 3) appear to show a patient that could be in acute congestive heart failure, secondary to massive transfusion of blood products/crystalloids (flash pulmonary edema).

   This finding needs to be confirmed (see answer to question 5).

   If congestive heart failure is strongly suspected continuing fluid resuscitation will worsen the situation. A more precise measurement of his fluid status and cardiac function is necessary to guide further therapy. Other supportive measures like ventilatory support, forced diuresis, and inotropic support might be necessary [6].

5. Clinical examination of the patient followed by further testing which should include EKG, chest X-Ray, and formal transthoracic echocardiography. Invasive tests include CVP and PA pressure measurement and cardiac catheterization. Laboratory tests include N-terminal pro-B-type natriuretic peptide and markers of cardiac ischemia.

References

1. Goldflam K, Lewiss R. Focus on: inferior vena cava ultrasound. Irving, TX. 2011. http://www.acep.org/Content.aspx?id=80791. Accessed 31 Mar 2016.
2. De Lorenzo RA, Morris MJ, Williams JB, Haley TF, Straight TM, Holbrook-Emmons VL, et al. Does a simple bedside sonographic measurement of the inferior vena cava correlate to central venous pressure? J Emerg Med. 2012;42(4):429–36. doi:10.1016/j.jemermed.2011.05.082.
3. Spencer KT, Kimura BJ, Korcarz CE, Pellikka PA, Rahko PS, Siegel RJ. Focused cardiac ultrasound: recommendations from the American Society of Echocardiography. J Am Soc Echocardiogr. 2013;26(6):567–81. doi:10.1016/j.echo.2013.04.001.

4. Goldflam K, Saul T, Lewiss R. Focus on: inferior vena cava ultrasound. ACEP News. June 2011.
5. Scott Moses M. Inferior vena cava ultrasound for volume status. Minneapolis-St Paul, Minnesota. 2013. http://www.fpnotebook.com/cv/rad/InfrVnCvUltrsndFrVlmSts.htm. Accessed 31 Mar 2016.
6. Chen HH, Schrier RW. Pathophysiology of volume overload in acute heart failure syndromes. Am J Med. 2006;119(12 Suppl 1):S11–6. doi:10.1016/j.amjmed.2006.09.012.

Chapter 58
Ultrasound I

German Barbosa-Hernandez

Abbreviations

PECS Pectoralis nerves

A 50 kg patient receives a supraclavicular peripheral nerve block in the preoperative area for anesthesia and postoperative pain for open reduction and internal fixation of an ulnar fracture on the left arm. The patient received a total of 20 cc of 0.5% ropivacaine during the block (See Fig. 58.1). 55 min later, the surgery starts and the patient complains of pain in the area of the surgery.

G. Barbosa-Hernandez, MD
Department of Anesthesia, Oklahoma University Health and Science Center, 800 NE 10th Street, Oklahoma City, OK 73102, USA
e-mail: German-BarbosaHernandez@ouhsc.edu

T.D. Raj (ed.), *Data Interpretation in Anesthesia*,
DOI 10.1007/978-3-319-55862-2_58

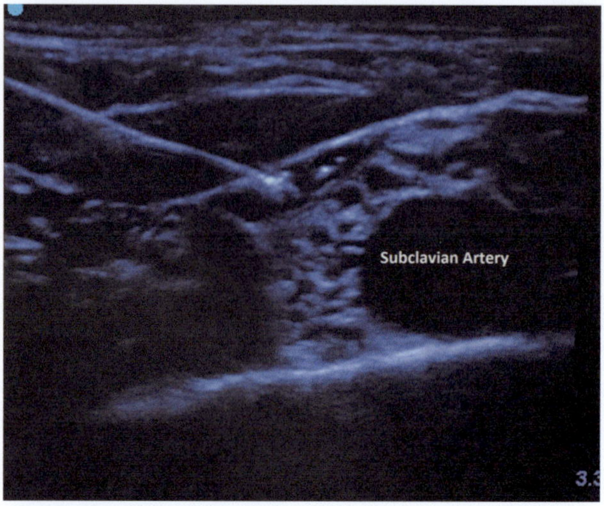

Fig. 58.1 Ultrasound image of the brachial plexus in the supraclavicular location, a needle is seen injecting a pool of local anesthetic

Questions

1. Based on the ultrasound image above what is the most likely cause of the patient's pain?
2. How would you supplement the block?
3. Are there other reasons for pain during surgery?
4. Should a continuous nerve catheter been placed?
5. Do additives in the block mixture have a role?

Answers

1. Most probably this patient experienced ulnar sparing due to poor distribution of the injection to the lower trunk [1]. This occurs commonly when the injection is made superficial to the plexus and does not cover the lower trunk (in the "eight ball corner pocket," which is the area formed by the angle between the brachial plexus and first rib).

   These patients will report adequate motor and sensory block over the median, radial, and musculocutaneous distribution; however, the area of the ulnar nerve, and medial cutaneous nerve of the forearm retain sensation and function.

2. Time permitting, the block could be supplemented by placing more local anesthetic in the "eight ball corner pocket," since the patient could safely still receive more local anesthetic [2].

   The maximum dose of ropivacaine in this patient is 150 mg (3 mg/kg). So we could safely repeat the block targeting the area of interest and inject up to another 10 cc of ropivacaine 0.5%.

   Awake patients might complaint of tourniquet pain. All patients experience neuropathic pain after a few minutes of a tourniquet being inflated to 100 mmHg above the systolic blood pressure. With enough time this manifests as pain, sometimes severe in awake patients, or a sympathetic response in patients under general anesthesia.

   Other reasons for pain are due to surgical stimulation in the area covered by the intercostobrachial nerve, the upper, inner aspect of the upper arm, which is not routinely covered by brachial plexus blocks. This area can be anesthetized with a field block of the medial side of the arm or a PECS II (pectoralis nerves) block.

3. A catheter is indicated if it's expected that the patient will require continuous analgesic coverage beyond the first 24 h after surgery, would need strenuous physical therapy, and has unresolved trauma or a chronic pain syndrome among others.

   A peripheral nerve catheter placed under ultrasound guidance has a better chance of success, with fewer complications, than the one placed with stimulation alone [3, 4]. It also prolongs the pain relief in the postoperative setting, which might contribute to better patient satisfaction and active participation in rehabilitation with selective sensory blockade [5].

   In this particular case, a catheter is not indicated since the pain of the trauma and surgery is expected to decrease after surgery; there is no need for strenuous physical therapy, and the patient has no chronic pain.

4. Some additives might have a role. The effects of these additives are:

Epinephrine: Delays the entry of local anesthetics into plasma. This effect is noted with lidocaine, mepivacaine, prilocaine, and bupivacaine, but not on ropivacaine [6].

Dexamethasone: Increases the duration of motor and sensory blockade at a recommended dose of 4–8 mg. The mechanism is unknown. It may act by increasing the activity of inhibitory potassium channels on nociceptive C fibers via glucocorticoid receptors, thereby decreasing the fibers' activity, and it appears that the same effect is achieved with intravenous use [6].

Clonidine: Prolongs motor and sensory blockade with all local anesthetics except mepivacaine. However, it might cause hypotension, sedation, bradycardia, and fainting possibly due to systemic absorption [6].

Buprenorphine: Perineural 150–300 μg of buprenorphine significantly prolongs the duration of blocks. Intravenous or intramuscular use provides only partial benefit [6].

In this case, dexamethasone would be an adequate choice as it will help prolong the duration of the block, and it has a long history of safe use in the epidural space. Patients may show modest temporary increases in blood glucose levels, especially in patients with diabetes mellitus.

References

1. Fredrickson MJ, Patel A, Young S, Chinchanwala S. Speed of onset of 'corner pocket supraclavicular' and infraclavicular ultrasound guided brachial plexus block: a randomised observer-blinded comparison. Anaesthesia. 2009;64(7):738–44. doi:10.1111/j.1365-2044.2009.05918.x.
2. Morfey DH, Brull R. Finding the corner pocket: landmarks in ultrasound-guided supraclavicular block. Anaesthesia. 2009;64(12):1381. doi:10.1111/j.1365-2044.2009.06141_17.x.
3. Liu SS, Zayas VM, Gordon MA, Beathe JC, Maalouf DB, Paroli L, et al. A prospective, randomized, controlled trial comparing ultrasound versus nerve stimulator guidance for interscalene block for ambulatory shoulder surgery for postoperative neurological symptoms. Anesth Analg. 2009;109(1):265–71. doi:10.1213/ane.0b013e3181a3272c.
4. Mariano ER, Loland VJ, Bellars RH, Sandhu NS, Bishop ML, Abrams RA, et al. Ultrasound guidance versus electrical stimulation for infraclavicular brachial plexus perineural catheter insertion. J Ultrasound Med. 2009;28(9):1211–8.
5. Axley M, Horn JL. Indications and management of continuous infusion of local anesthetics at home. Curr Opin Anaesthesiol. 2010;23(5):650–5. doi:10.1097/ACO.0b013e32833e27bc.
6. Bailard NS, Ortiz J, Flores RA. Additives to local anesthetics for peripheral nerve blocks: evidence, limitations, and recommendations. Am J Health Syst Pharm. 2014;71(5):373–85. doi:10.2146/ajhp130336.

Chapter 59
Ultrasound II

German Barbosa-Hernandez

Abbreviations

ACLS	Advanced cardiac life support
ASRA	American Society of Regional Anesthesia and Pain Medicine
CNS	Central nervous system
LAST	Local anesthetic systemic toxicity
NSAID	Nonsteroidal anti-inflammatory drugs
TENS	Transcutaneous electrical nerve stimulation

Figure 59.1 image is obtained from a patient (80yo M, 60 kg) in the PACU after a repeat femoral peripheral nerve block for postoperative pain of a knee arthroplasty. The patient received a total of 30 cc of 0.5% bupivacaine and 20 cc of 0.5% ropivacaine. Patient is complaining of persistent pain in the area of the surgery.

G. Barbosa-Hernandez, MD
Department of Anesthesia, Oklahoma University Health and Science Center, 800 NE 10th Street, Oklahoma City, OK 73102, USA
e-mail: German-BarbosaHernandez@ouhsc.edu

T.D. Raj (ed.), *Data Interpretation in Anesthesia*,
DOI 10.1007/978-3-319-55862-2_59

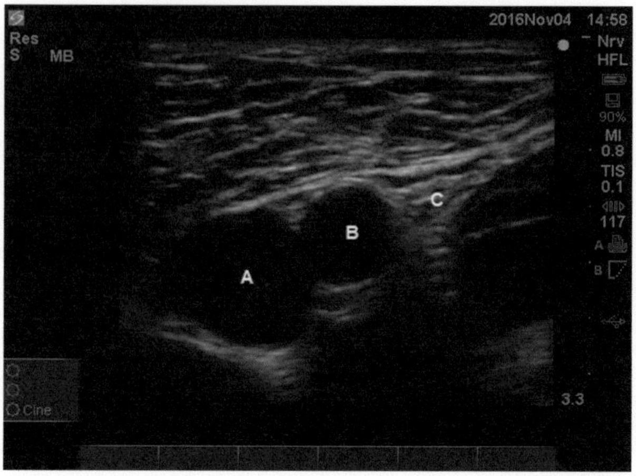

Fig. 59.1 Ultrasound view of the groin area at the level of the inguinal crease

Questions

1. What are the structures labeled a, b, and c?
2. What are the possible causes of persistent postoperative pain?
3. Would you repeat the block?
4. If the patient develops seizures how would you treat him?
5. If the patient develops hypotension and asystole how would you treat him?
6. What other options are available to treat this patient's pain?

Answers

1. a, femoral vein; b, femoral artery; c, femoral nerve.

2. Persistent pain might be due to:
   (a) Inadequate distribution of the local anesthetic in the correct plane, possibly due to difficult and distorted anatomy after multiple attempts
   (b) Lack of coverage of the sciatic nerve area on the back of the knee or the obturator nerve on the medial aspect of the thigh

3. This patient has received a large amount of local anesthetic after the two attempts; a repeat one is inadvisable as we are over the maximum safe dose for local anesthetic.

   In this patient, the maximum safe dose of ropivacaine (3.5 mg/kg) is 280 mg and bupivacaine (2 mg/kg) is 160 mg.

   In the case of combined local anesthetics, the proportional maximum dose of each agent should be calculated, and the sum should not exceed 100%.

   This patient has received 100 mg of ropivacaine and 150 mg of bupivacaine.

   The proportion of the maximum safe dose per agent is calculated as follows:

$$Proportion\ of\ the\ maximum\ dose = \frac{Dose\ given\ in\ mg}{Maximum\ safe\ dose\ in\ mg} \times 100$$

In this patient the proportion for each agent is calculated as follows:

$$Proportion\ of\ the \max\ dose\ of\ Ropivacaine = \frac{100mg}{280mg} \times 100 = 36\%$$

$$Proportion\ of\ the \max\ dose\ of\ Ropivacaine = \frac{150mg}{160mg} \times 100 = 94\%$$

   The total dose of local anesthetic in this patient exceeds the 100% (94 + 36) of the maximum safe dose. Further use of local anesthetic is unadvisable.

4. Seizures in this setting would be very suspicious for local anesthetic systemic toxicity (LAST). According to the American Society of Regional Anesthesia and Pain Medicine (ASRA), management in this setting should include [1]:
   (a) Airway management: ventilate with 100% oxygen.
   (b) Seizure suppression: benzodiazepines are preferred; avoid propofol in patients having signs of cardiovascular instability.
   (c) Alert the nearest facility having cardiopulmonary bypass capability.

(d) Lipid emulsion therapy (not propofol):
   - Bolus 1.5 mL/kg.
   - Continuous infusion at 0.25 mL/kg/min.
   - Bolus may be repeated and the infusion raised to 0.5 mL/kg/min for persistent hypotension.
   - Continue treatment for 10 min after attaining stability.
   - Maximum dose of lipid—10 mL/kg in first 30 min.

(e) Other possibilities of seizure activity in this setting are pseudo-seizures, cryptogenic, metabolic insult, toxic insult, CNS infection, stroke, brain trauma, cerebral hemorrhage, and alcohol or drug withdrawal.

5. Management of cardiovascular collapse in this setting differs from the one caused by other etiologies and current recommendations by ASRA are [1]:
   (a) Advanced Cardiac Life Support (ACLS):
   - Avoid vasopressin, calcium channel blockers, beta-blockers, or local anesthetics.
   - Reduce individual epinephrine doses to <1 mcg/kg, to avoid onset of malignant arrhythmias.

   (b) Lipid emulsion (20%) therapy:
   - Bolus 1.5 mL/kg (lean body mass) intravenously over 1 min.
   - Continuous infusion 0.25 mL/kg/min.
   - Repeat bolus once or twice for persistent cardiovascular collapse.
   - Double the infusion rate to 0.5 mL/kg/min if blood pressure remains low.
   - Continue infusion for at least 10 min after attaining circulatory stability.
   - Recommended upper limit: Approximately 10 mL/kg lipid emulsion over the first 30 min.

   (c) Consider placing the patient on cardiopulmonary bypass if prolonged resuscitation with no return of cardiac function is present.

6. Preoperatively patients should be counseled on postoperative goals and expectations of pain control; patients with medical and psychiatric comorbidities will especially benefit from preoperative optimization as well. For persistent pain, before repeating the femoral nerve block, patient assessment to determine the pain location would help in distinguishing between a failed femoral nerve block and pain in an area not covered by a femoral block. If the latter is the case, then the patient would benefit with supplementation of sciatic and obturator nerve blocks.

   Acute postoperative pain requires a multimodal approach. The patient will benefit from the use of acetaminophen, NSAIDs, antidepressants, and/or antiepileptic medications. Continuous evaluation of pain and titration of opioids, if needed, is recommended which may also be administered as a patient-controlled option [2, 3]. Other options available in the postoperative period are topical application of local anesthetics and the use of TENS.

References

1. Neal JM, Mulroy MF, Weinberg GL, American Society of Regional A, Pain M. American Society of Regional Anesthesia and Pain Medicine checklist for managing local anesthetic systemic toxicity: 2012 version. Reg Anesth Pain Med. 2012;37(1):16–8. doi:10.1097/AAP.0b013e31822e0d8a.
2. Clarke H, Bonin RP, Orser BA, Englesakis M, Wijeysundera DN, Katz J. The prevention of chronic postsurgical pain using gabapentin and pregabalin: a combined systematic review and meta-analysis. Anesth Analg. 2012;115(2):428–42. doi:10.1213/ANE.0b013e318249d36e.
3. Chou R, Gordon DB, de Leon-Casasola OA, Rosenberg JM, Bickler S, Brennan T, et al. Management of postoperative pain: a clinical practice guideline from the American Pain Society, the American Society of Regional Anesthesia and Pain Medicine, and the American Society of Anesthesiologists' Committee on Regional Anesthesia, Executive Committee, and Administrative Council. J Pain. 2016;17(2):131–57. doi:10.1016/j.jpain.2015.12.008.

Chapter 60
Lung Ultrasound

Marcos E. Gomes

An ultrasound of the chest/lung is obtained on a multi-trauma patient with chest drains and on a ventilator in the ICU.

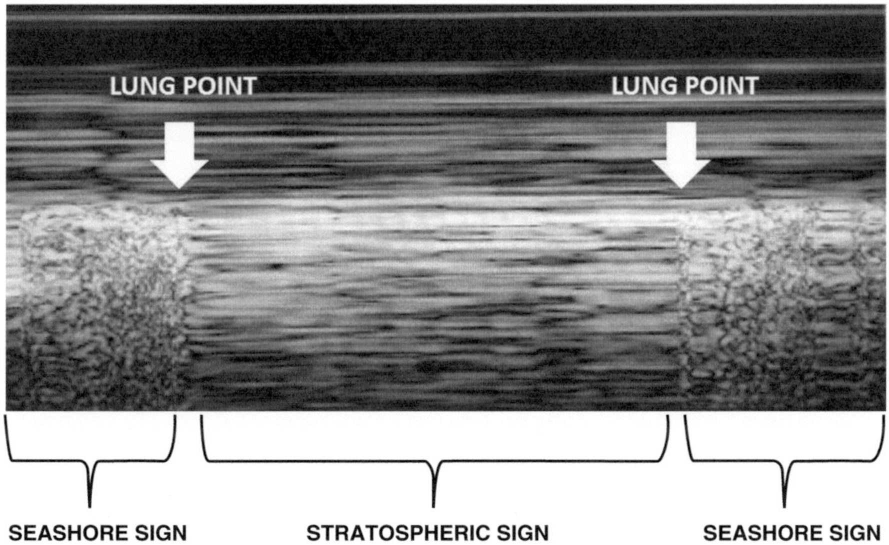

Fig. 60.1 Lung ultrasound, M-mode method

M.E. Gomes, MD
Department of Anesthesiology, University of Oklahoma Health Sciences Center, 750 NE 13th Street, Suite 200, Oklahoma City, OK 73104, USA
e-mail: mewgomes@gmail.com

T.D. Raj (ed.), *Data Interpretation in Anesthesia*,
DOI 10.1007/978-3-319-55862-2_60

Questions

1. What is lung sliding?
2. What is the difference between lung sliding and lung pulse?
3. What is the best ultrasound method to detect lung sliding?
4. What is the differential diagnosis for absence of lung sliding?
5. What is lung point?
6. Besides lung sliding, what other two common artifacts can help with differential diagnosis?

Answers

1. Lung sliding is the movement of the pleural interface in a synchronous fashion with spontaneous or mechanical ventilation. The parietal and visceral pleura constitute the pleural interface, which is a hyperechoic structure between two ribs on bidimensional ultrasound. It is maximized in the lower lung fields, as the lung descends toward the abdomen. Lung sliding identification is the most commonly used artifact in the exclusion of pneumothorax as well as in the confirmation of endotracheal intubation [2].

2. Lung pulse artifact is a small to-and-fro movement of the visceral on the parietal pleura induced by the heartbeat rather than respirations. It is more prominent on the left side, closer to the heart. In order for it to be visualized, ventilation and, consequently, lung sliding must be absent. It implies an intact pleural interface, and its presence excludes a pneumothorax.

3. M-mode ultrasound is the preferred method for lung movement imaging, producing the characteristic "seashore sign" (Fig. 60.1). This image has two portions. The superficial part (top of the figure) is typically composed of multiple horizontal lines that correspond to motionless soft tissue. It ends on the pleural line. The other portion corresponds to the motion of the normal lung. This motion generates an artifact that originates from the pleural line and looks like sand on a beach. The image on its entirety looks like water waves in the ocean touching the sand on a beach.

4. Lung sliding becomes vague in pulmonary overexpansion, parietal emphysema, pneumonia, and severe ARDS. It disappears in pneumothorax, complete atelectasis, pleural fibrosis, and apnea.

5. On two-dimensional ultrasound, lung point is the transition point between the presence and absence of a lung sliding. It represents the border of the pneumothorax and the intact pleural interface. In M-mode, the absence of lung sliding will create a series of black and white horizontal lines called the "stratospheric

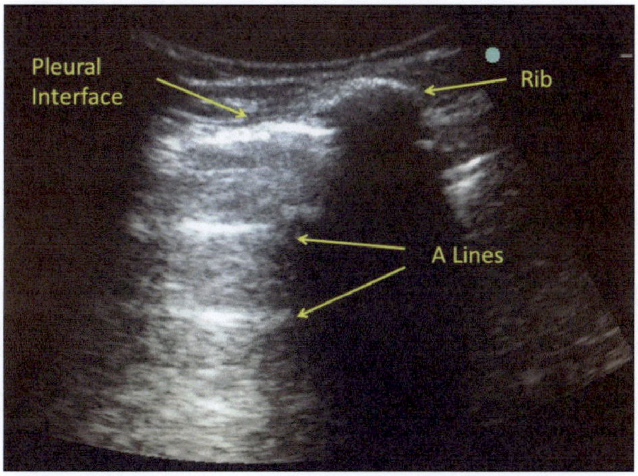

Fig. 60.2 A-lines

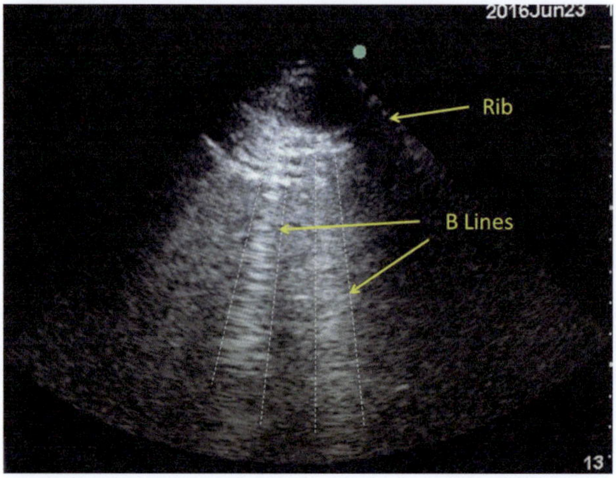

Fig. 60.3 B-lines

or barcode" sign. In this mode, the lung point can be identified by the transition of a seashore sign to a stratospheric sign (Fig. 60.1). This is a pathognomonic sign for the presence of pneumothorax, with 100% specificity [3].

6. **A-lines** are multiple horizontal regularly spaced hyperechogenic lines which represent reflections of the pleural interface. Each A line is separated by a distance equivalent to the thickness of the subcutaneous tissue between the ultrasound probe and the pleural interface (Fig. 60.2). They are present in a normal lung as well as in the presence of pneumothorax.

   B-lines, also known as comet tails or lung rockets, are artifacts created by repetitive reflections of the ultrasound wave within the lung parenchyma because of a higher concentration of physiologic or pathologic fluid. They are vertical white lines, originating from the visceral pleura and reaching the bottom of the screen (Fig. 60.3). B-lines will erase the A-lines on their passage. A few B-lines (less than 3) may be seen in a healthy lung and more so in the dependent regions. Their presence is utilized in the diagnosis of alveolar interstitial syndrome (pulmonary edema, ARDS) and exclusion of pneumothorax [4].

References

1. Barillari A, et al. Lung ultrasound: a new tool for the emergency physician. Intern Emerg Med. 2010;5:335–40.
2. Xirouchaki N, et al. Lung ultrasound in critically ill patients: comparison with bedside chest radiography. Intensive Care Med. 2011;37:1488–93.
3. Piette E, et al. Basic concepts in the use of thoracic and lung ultrasound. Curr Opin Anesthesiol. 2013;26:20–30.
4. Lichtenstein DA, et al. Relevance of lung ultrasound in the diagnosis of acute respiratory failure: the blue protocol. Chest. 2008;134:117–25.

Chapter 61
Abdominal X-Ray

Abhinava S. Madamangalam

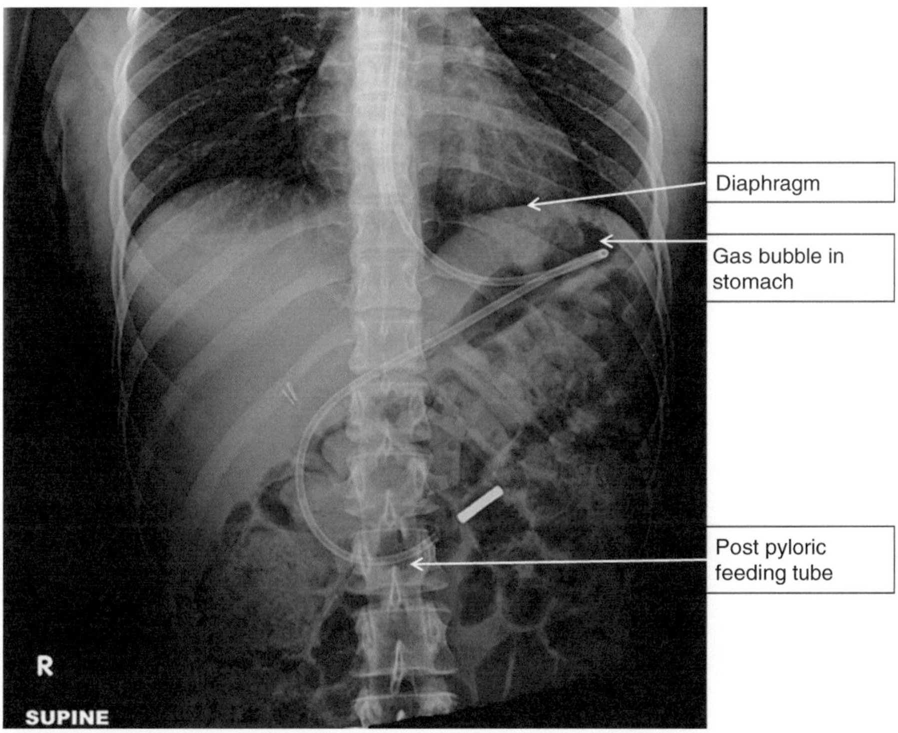

Fig. 61.1 X-ray of an appropriately placed feeding tube

A.S. Madamangalam, MBBS, MD
Department of Anesthesiology and Perioperative Medicine, Augusta University Medical Center, 1120 15th Street, BI-2144, Augusta, GA 30912, USA
e-mail: amadamangalam@augusta.edu

T.D. Raj (ed.), *Data Interpretation in Anesthesia*,
DOI 10.1007/978-3-319-55862-2_61

Questions

1. What are the indications for a feeding tube placement?
2. Name some methods available to confirm appropriate placement of a feeding tube, and what are the drawbacks of the most definite methods of confirming feeding tube placement?
3. What preconditions need to be met for placement of a feeding tube?
4. Are there complications associated with feeding tube placement?

Answers

1. Early records note that Capivacceus placed a tube to deliver nutrients into the foregut [1]. The practice became more common during the seventeenth century. The tubes are inserted to decompress the stomach or for intestinal ileus or obstruction [2, 3]. Patients that most frequently need a naso-enteric tube (NET) are in surgical intensive care settings. Other indications include prematurity, failure to thrive (or malnutrition), neurologic and neuromuscular disorders, inability to swallow, anatomical and postsurgical malformations of the mouth and esophagus, cancer and digestive disorders. The feeding tubes could be for short-term or even long-term use [2]. Feeding tubes are placed in patients either through the nose or percutaneously.

2. Appropriate placement of an NET is not always successful. Misplacement is said to occur about 13–20% in adults and in 39–55% of pediatric patients [3]. Many different methods have been used to confirm proper placement. These include:

   (a) Auscultation—injecting air into the feeding tube and listening for the rush of air over the stomach
   (b) Bubbling—placing the end of the tube under water to look for bubbling which would indicate misplacement into the tracheobronchial tree
   (c) Appearance and pH of aspirate from NET
   (d) Endoscopy and fluoroscopy—expensive and time consuming
   (e) Capnometry—to detect CO_2 from the tracheobronchial tree in misplaced NET
   (f) Detection of a copper wire in the stylet of the feeding tube with a locator device placed over the chest
   (g) The gold standard—radiography of the chest and abdomen which should visualize the entire feeding tube within the gastro intestinal tract to identify proper positioning.

   None of these methods ensure that the incidence of misplacement is reduced to zero [4].

   To date, two "gold standard" methods of confirming the appropriate placement of the feeding tube are recognized: the radiographic (or fluoroscopic) and the endoscopic method. Both these modalities provide confirmation of appropriate placement with great accuracy.

   Fluoroscopy exposes the patient to radiation, which is avoided by endoscopy. Both procedures are expensive in terms of finances and time. There is the issue of ready availability of equipment as well as the technical difficulty of interpreting the images reliably with both methods. Quite often when a method other than the radiographic method is used for the confirmation of the location of the tip of the NET, an X-ray of the abdomen is performed to additionally verify location of the tip of the NET. This further adds a cost to the process as well as exposing the patient to radiation.

3. The process of placing the NET is noted to be simple and safe. Ideally the patient is not on an anticoagulant. Patients are also required to be fasting for about 6 hours, if the feeding tube is placed percutaneously; in such situations the patient may require moderate sedation or even a general anesthetic for NET placement.

4. There are a few risks associated with the placement of the NET such as bleeding, infection, dislodgement of the tube, as well as bloating and nausea. Undetected placement of the NET in the respiratory tract may lead to pneumonia, lung puncture, pneumothorax, empyema, and even death.

References

1. Chernoff R. An overview of tube feeding: from ancient times to the future. Nut Clin Pract. 2006;21(4):408–10.
2. Kirby DF, et al. American gastroenterological association technical review on tube feeding for enteral nutrition. Gastroenetrology. 1995;108(4):1282–301.
3. Huffman S, et al. Methods to confirm feeding tube placement: application of research in practice. Pediatr Nurs. 2004;30(1):10–3.
4. Institute ECRI. Confirming feeding tube placement; old habits die hard. Pa Patient Saf Auth. 2006;3(4):23–30.

Chapter 62
Angio I

Aneesh Venkat Pakala

Fig. 62.1

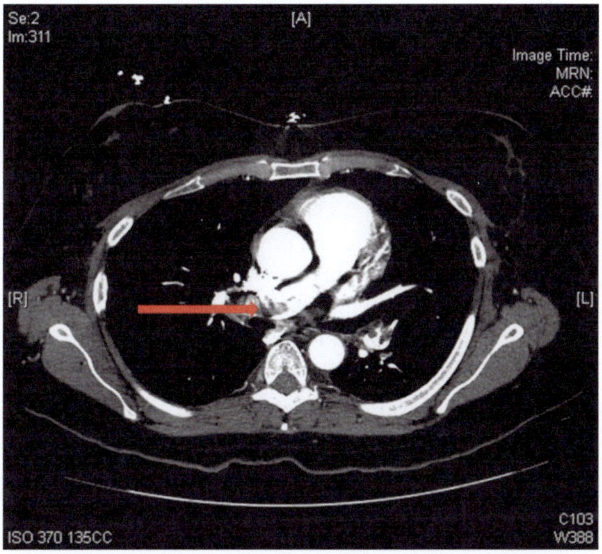

A.V. Pakala, MD
Section of Cardiovascular Disease, Department of Medicine, University of Oklahoma College of Medicine, Oklahoma City, OK, USA
e-mail: aneeshpakala@yahoo.com; Aneesh-Pakala@ouhsc.edu

T.D. Raj (ed.), *Data Interpretation in Anesthesia*,
DOI 10.1007/978-3-319-55862-2_62

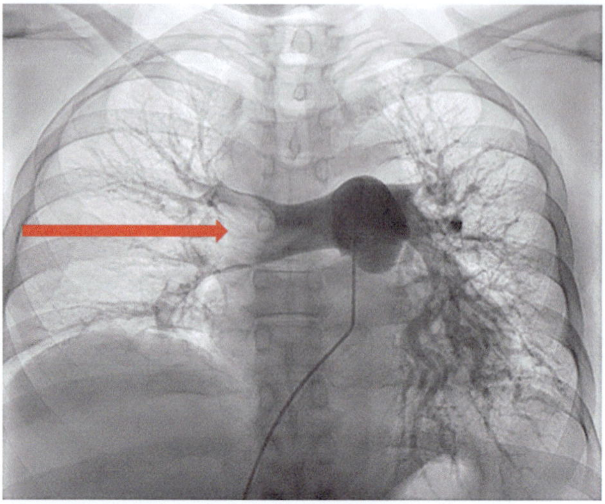

Fig. 62.2

Questions

1. What do these images show?
2. How does one assess the pretest probability for this finding?
3. How does imaging play a role in diagnosis?
4. What are the acute therapeutic options in this situation?
5. When is thrombolytic therapy used?
6. What is the role of catheter based therapy?

Answers

1. Figure 62.1 is computed tomography showing a large pulmonary embolism (PE) involving the right pulmonary artery (red arrow). Figure 62.2 is pulmonary angiography of the same patient showing the same finding.

2. Wells score (Table 62.1) is used to calculate the pretest probability of PE.

3. In patients with high pretest probability for PE, imaging is the test of choice. Pulmonary arteriography is the gold standard for diagnosis of PE. Current generation multi-detector helical computed tomography (CT) has high sensitivity and specificity, comparable to pulmonary arteriography, in detection of PE [2]. Helical CT is the most widely used modality in current clinical settings and would be the diagnostic test of choice in this case. However, in patients with high pretest probability for PE (as in our case) and a negative CT, further investigation in the form of duplex ultrasound of lower extremities or pulmonary arteriography should be considered [3].

4. In patients with high pretest probability for PE, therapeutic anticoagulation should be initiated immediately while awaiting further diagnostic testing (CT, duplex ultrasound, etc.) [4]. Treatment for PE has evolved with the introduction of novel oral anticoagulants or non-warfarin oral anticoagulants (NOAC). Treatment for acute PE can be one of the following:

   (a) Weight-based low-molecular-weight heparin (LMWH) for 5 days followed by dabigatran, edoxaban, or warfarin (NOACs)
   (b) Rivaroxaban or apixaban without initial LMWH

   The treatment for acute PE is divided into the following treatment phases: acute phase of 5–10 days, short-term phase 3–6 months, and long-term phase beyond 6 months. The duration of therapy depends on the underlying cause for the PE and the risk to benefit ratio of anticoagulation.

Table 62.1 A score of <2 indicates a low probability of pulmonary embolism

Clinical characteristic	Score
Active cancer	1
Surgery or bedridden for 3 days or more during the past 4 weeks	1.5
History of deep venous thrombosis or pulmonary embolism	1.5
Hemoptysis	1
Heart rate > 100 beats/min	1.5
Pulmonary embolism judged to be the most likely diagnosis	3
Clinical signs and symptoms compatible with deep venous thrombosis	3

A score of 2–6 indicates an intermediate probability of PE. A score > 6 indicates a high probability of pulmonary embolism [1]

Table 62.2 PESI score, a total point score for a given patient, is obtained by summing the patient's age in years and the points for each applicable predictor

Predictors	Points assigned
Age, in years	Age, in years
Altered mental status	+60
Systolic blood pressure < 100 mmHg	+30
History of cancer	+30
Arterial O_2 saturation < 90%	+20
Temp <36°C	+20
Respiratory rate > 30/min	+20
Pulse >110 bpm	+20
Male sex	+10
History of heart failure	+10
History of chronic lung disease	+10

Points' assignments correspond with the following risk classes: class 1 (very low risk), <65; class II (low risk), 65–85; class III (intermediate risk), 86–105; class IV (high risk), 106–125; class V (very high risk), >125

Outcomes in PE patients depend on the clinical presentation. Based on clinical presentation, they can be further classified into [5]:

(a) Massive PE: Acute PE with sustained hypotension (systolic BP < 90 mmHg sustained for over 15 min or requiring ionotropic support) in the absence of any other cause, pulselessness, or profound bradycardia (highest risk of adverse outcomes).
(b) Sub-massive PE: Acute PE without sustained hypotension, with signs of hypoperfusion, right ventricular dysfunction on echocardiography, elevated cardiac troponins, and elevated brain natriuretic peptide (intermediate risk of adverse outcomes).
(c) Low-risk PE: Acute PE with normal blood pressures, normal cardiac biomarkers, and normal RV function (low risk of adverse outcomes).

Further risk stratification using Pulmonary Embolism Severity Index (PESI) scores (Table 62.2), signs of cardiovascular decompensation, and signs of shock-like state allows for consideration of inpatient versus outpatient treatment setting for further management and for the consideration for advanced therapies including thrombolytic therapy [6].

5. The role of systemically administered thrombolysis in acute PE is reserved for patients with clinically massive PE who are not at risk for major bleeding. As mentioned above, massive PE is defined as PE with resulting hypotension (SBP < 90 mmHg) [7].

   In low-risk PE, antithrombotic therapy is sufficient. Thrombolytic therapy may be considered down the road in these patients if they acutely develop hypotension while on antithrombotic therapy. Thrombolysis may also be considered in those patients who were initially stable, if blood pressure decreases but is still >90 mmHg, and they develop a shock-like state along with supplemental signs of cardiac decompensation including acute right ventricular failure, elevated cardiac troponins, and brain natriuretic peptide levels (sub-massive PE) [4].

Table 62.3 Contraindications for systemic thrombolytic therapy [8]

Absolute contraindications for thrombolytic therapy
Prior intracranial hemorrhage
Known structural cerebral vascular lesion
Known malignant intracranial neoplasm
Ischemic stroke within 3 months (excluding stroke within 3 h)
Suspected aortic dissection
Active bleeding or bleeding diathesis (excluding menses)
Significant closed-head trauma or facial trauma within 3 months
Relative contraindications for thrombolytic therapy
Severe uncontrolled hypertension on presentation (SBP >180 mmHg or DBP >110 mmHg)
History of ischemic stroke more than 3 months prior
Major surgery less than 3 weeks
Recent (within two to 4 weeks) internal bleeding
For streptokinase—Prior exposure (more than 5 days ago) or prior allergic reaction to these agents
Pregnancy
Active peptic ulcer
Current use of anticoagulant (e.g., warfarin sodium) that has produced an elevated international normalized ratio (INR) >1.7 or prothrombin time (PT) >15 s

Contraindications to systemic thrombolysis are mentioned in Table 62.3. Thrombolytic agents approved by the FDA are alteplase (100 mg infusion over 2 h), urokinase (4400 U/kg as a loading dose given at a rate of 90 mL/h over a period of 10 min, followed by continuous infusion of 4400 U/kg/h at a rate of 15 mL/h for 12 h), and streptokinase (250,000 U as a loading dose over 30 min, followed by 100,000 U/h over 12–24 h).

6. Patients who are not candidates for systemic thrombolysis should be monitored closely for development of shock-like state (hypotension, worsening tachycardia, gas exchange, oliguria, mentation, etc.) [4]. If there is concern for clinical deterioration, catheter-based thrombectomy may be considered over systemic thrombolysis especially in the presence of a relative contraindication for systemic thrombolysis) [9]. Catheter-based thrombectomy consists of catheter-directed thrombolysis (reduced dose of thrombolytic administered directly to the thrombus) or mechanical thrombectomy without thrombolysis (endovascular catheter is used to mechanically disrupt the thrombus).

References

1. Kearon C, Ginsberg JS, Douketis J, Turpie AG, Bates SM, Lee AY, et al. An evaluation of D-dimer in the diagnosis of pulmonary embolism: a randomized trial. Ann Intern Med. 2006;144(11):812–21.
2. Winer-Muram HT, Rydberg J, Johnson MS, Tarver RD, Williams MD, Shah H, et al. Suspected acute pulmonary embolism: evaluation with multi-detector row CT versus digital subtraction pulmonary arteriography. Radiology. 2004;233(3):806–15.

3. Quiroz R, Kucher N, Zou KH, Kipfmueller F, Costello P, Goldhaber SZ, et al. Clinical validity of a negative computed tomography scan in patients with suspected pulmonary embolism: a systematic review. JAMA. 2005;293(16):2012–7.
4. Streiff MB, Agnelli G, Connors JM, Crowther M, Eichinger S, Lopes R, et al. Guidance for the treatment of deep vein thrombosis and pulmonary embolism. J Thromb Thrombolysis. 2016;41(1):32–67.
5. Jaff MR, McMurtry MS, Archer SL, Cushman M, Goldenberg N, Goldhaber SZ, et al. Management of massive and submassive pulmonary embolism, iliofemoral deep vein thrombosis, and chronic thromboembolic pulmonary hypertension: a scientific statement from the American Heart Association. Circulation. 2011;123(16):1788–830.
6. Jimenez D, Aujesky D, Yusen RD. Risk stratification of normotensive patients with acute symptomatic pulmonary embolism. Br J Haematol. 2010;151(5):415–24.
7. Meyer G, Vicaut E, Konstantinides SV. Fibrinolysis for intermediate-risk pulmonary embolism. N Engl J Med. 2014;371(6):581–2.
8. Kearon C, Akl EA, Comerota AJ, Prandoni P, Bounameaux H, Goldhaber SZ, et al. Antithrombotic therapy for VTE disease: antithrombotic therapy and prevention of thrombosis, 9th ed: American College of Chest Physicians Evidence-Based Clinical Practice Guidelines. Chest. 2012;141(2 Suppl):e419S–94S.
9. Kucher N, Boekstegers P, Muller OJ, Kupatt C, Beyer-Westendorf J, Heitzer T, et al. Randomized, controlled trial of ultrasound-assisted catheter-directed thrombolysis for acute intermediate-risk pulmonary embolism. Circulation. 2014;129(4):479–86.

Chapter 63
Angio II

Aneesh Venkat Pakala

A sixty-one-year-old male with known descending thoracic aortic aneurysm with Stanford-type B aortic dissection underwent thoracic endovascular aortic repair (TEVAR) due to ongoing pain and rapidly expanding aneurysm. The procedure was complicated due to significant curvature of the thoracic aorta; patient was subsequently discharged home.

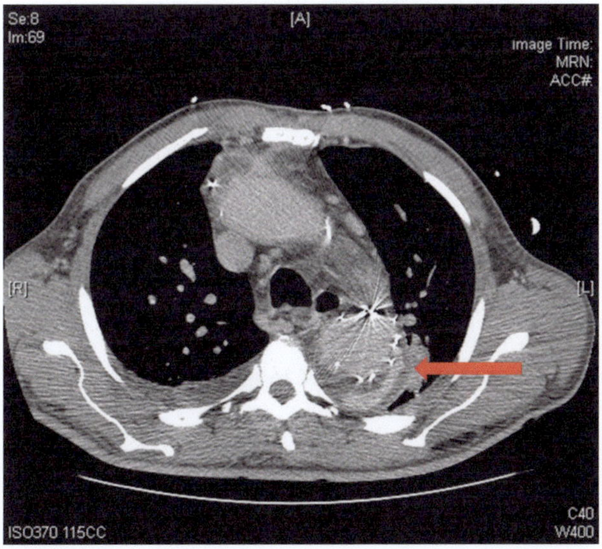

Fig. 63.1

A.V. Pakala, MD
Section of Cardiovascular Disease, Department of Medicine, University of Oklahoma College of Medicine, Oklahoma City, OK, USA
e-mail: aneeshpakala@yahoo.com; Aneesh-Pakala@ouhsc.edu

T.D. Raj (ed.), *Data Interpretation in Anesthesia*,
DOI 10.1007/978-3-319-55862-2_63

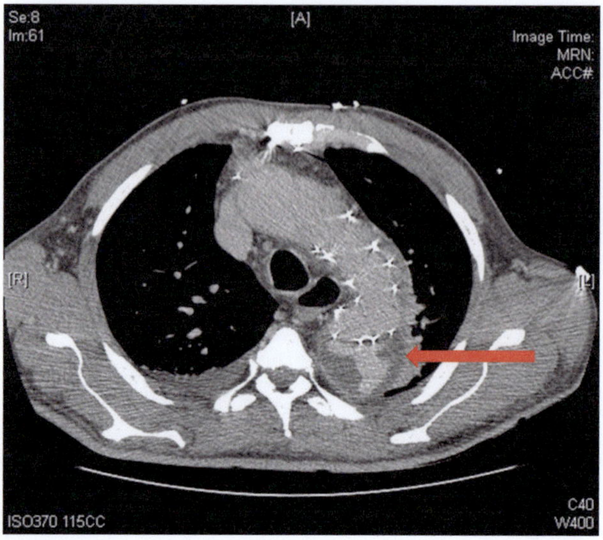

Fig. 63.2

Patient was readmitted 2 weeks later with worsening chest pain, back pain, and dizziness. At the time of presentation, patient was in distress.

Examination revealed sinus tachycardia HR 120 bpm, no obvious cardiovascular exam findings were noted, pulses were equal in all four extremities, and serum chemistry was unremarkable except for mild renal insufficiency.

Due to recent TEVAR procedure, CT angiography was obtained; images are displayed below.

Questions

1. What is seen in the images?
2. How is the above complication classified?
3. What are the treatment options?
4. What is the recommended surveillance to detect this complication?

Answers

1. Figure 63.1 is a triple phase computed tomographic image (CT) showing a type III endoleak in the descending thoracic aorta originating from the stent graft. Figure 63.2 is also a triple phase CT image of the same patient showing the extension of the type III endoleak proximally. This patient underwent a thoracic endovascular aortic repair (TEVAR) procedure for urgent repair of acute type B thoracic aortic dissection with ongoing chest pain and rapid aneurysmal expansion. TEVAR is the procedure of choice in patients with complicated type B dissections [1]. The CT images are consistent with an endoleak. Endoleak is defined as blood collection outside the stent graft but within the aneurysm sac. This is a known complication following TEVAR. According to reported data, it occurs in about 5–20% of cases [1].

2. The most widely used method classifies endoleaks depending on the mechanism of formation of the endoleak [2]:

   (a) Type I endoleak: Proximal or distal reperfusion of the aneurysmal sac. This occurs due to malapposition of the stent graft to the aortic wall. This is an early complication following TEVAR and needs urgent intervention. This is considered to be a form of treatment failure.
   (b) Type II endoleak: Retrograde reperfusion of the aneurysmal sac from branch vessels. These have a benign course and usually need surveillance only.
   (c) Type III endoleak: Leak into the aneurysmal sac due to structural damage to the stent graft in the form of tears, fractures, or junctional separation. This requires urgent intervention and is considered to be a form of treatment failure.
   (d) Type IV endoleak: Leakage into the aneurysmal sac due to endograft porosity.
   (e) Type V endoleak: Increase in the aneurysm sac in the absence of leak (endotension). This is poorly understood.

3. Type I endoleaks are caused by malapposition of the proximal or the distal end of the stent graft to the aortic wall leading to a direct communication of the luminal blood to the aneurysmal sac and potential for rupture. Treatment involves securing the proximal and distal ends of the stent graft using endovascular approach, usually with balloon angioplasty. If endovascular repair fails, open repair is recommended [3, 4]. Type III endoleaks are caused by structural damage to the stent graft leading to direct communication of the luminal blood to the aneurysmal sac, leading to expansion and rupture of the aneurysmal sac. Initial treatment strategy is endovascular stent graft placement or extension; if this fails, then open repair is recommended [3, 4].

4. Lifelong surveillance is recommended following TEVAR since complications like type III endoleaks can occur many years down the line [4]. Triple phase CT (images obtained before, during, and after contrast administration) angiography is the modality of choice in many centers. As in our case, endoleak on a triple phase CT angiography will show up as contrast outside the stent graft structure in delayed imaging after the contrast has cleared the aortic lumen [3]. Patients receive CT angiography immediately post procedure, then at 1 month, 6 month, and then yearly with clinical follow-up. Magnetic resonance imaging (MRI) can be used as an alternative modality to reduce cumulative radiation in cases where MRI compatible grafts have been used. Ultrasound is not as reliable in the setting of TEVAR due to chest wall interference. Transesophageal echocardiography as a follow-up tool has some disadvantages due to its invasive nature.

References

1. Grabenwoger M, Alfonso F, Bachet J, Bonser R, Czerny M, Eggebrecht H, et al. Thoracic Endovascular Aortic Repair (TEVAR) for the treatment of aortic diseases: a position statement from the European Association for Cardio-Thoracic Surgery (EACTS) and the European Society of Cardiology (ESC), in collaboration with the European Association of Percutaneous Cardiovascular Interventions (EAPCI). Eur Heart J. 2012;33(13):1558–63.
2. Veith FJ, Baum RA, Ohki T, Amor M, Adiseshiah M, Blankensteijn JD, et al. Nature and significance of endoleaks and endotension: summary of opinions expressed at an international conference. J Vasc Surg. 2002;35(5):1029–35.
3. Criado FJ, Abul-Khoudoud OR, Domer GS, McKendrick C, Zuzga M, Clark NS, et al. Endovascular repair of the thoracic aorta: lessons learned. Ann Thorac Surg. 2005;80(3):857–63; discussion 63.
4. Stavropoulos SW, Carpenter JP. Postoperative imaging surveillance and endoleak management after endovascular repair of thoracic aortic aneurysms. J Vasc Surg. 2006;43(Suppl A):89A–93A.

Chapter 64
Angio III

Aneesh Venkat Pakala

A 46-year-old male presents to the ER after a syncopal event. The patient developed severe precordial chest pain while lifting weights, immediately followed by syncopal event lasting 30 seconds. Currently in the ER, he continues to have chest pain that radiates to the back. He describes it as a tearing sensation. Pain does not respond to nitroglycerine. On exam patient appears in distress, diaphoretic, HR 120 bpm, BP 150/70 mmHg on right, and 120/60 mmHg on left; chest exam is within normal limits.

EKG is consistent with sinus tachycardia and ST depressions anterolaterally.

CXR reveals widened mediastinum.

Creatinine 2.0 ng/ml (0.0–0.399 ng/ml)

Troponin 0.2 ng/ml (0.0–0.399 ng/ml)

D-dimer 800

BNP 240 pg/ml (0–100 pg/ml)

Echocardiography is performed next and a couple of images are displayed below.

A.V. Pakala, MD
Section of Cardiovascular Disease, Department of Medicine, University of Oklahoma College of Medicine, Oklahoma City, OK, USA
e-mail: aneeshpakala@yahoo.com; Aneesh-Pakala@ouhsc.edu

T.D. Raj (ed.), *Data Interpretation in Anesthesia*,
DOI 10.1007/978-3-319-55862-2_64

Fig. 64.1

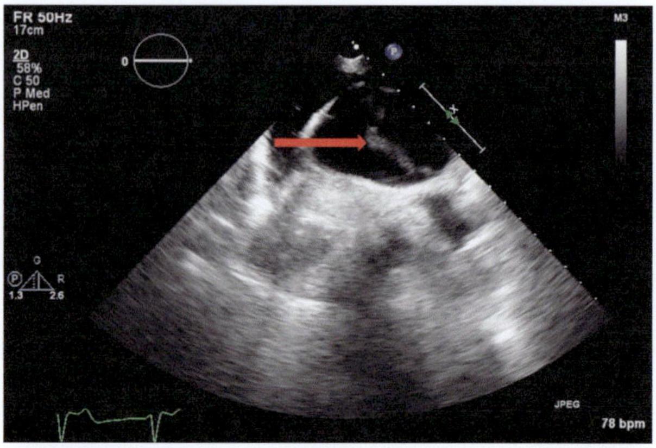

Fig. 64.2

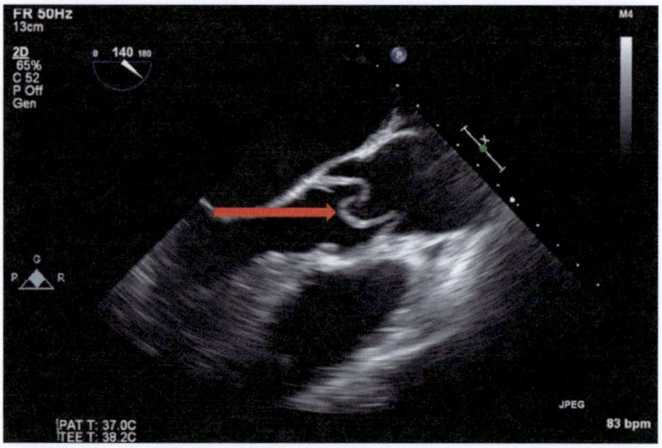

Questions

1. What do the images show?
2. How is this condition created?
3. What are the presenting features of this condition?
4. How is this condition classified?
5. What end organ complications can we expect?
6. What is the role of imaging and laboratory testing?
7. What is the treatment of choice?

Answers

1. Figure 64.1 shows a transthoracic echocardiographic image of a Stanford type A acute aortic dissection. Figure 64.2 shows a transesophageal echocardiographic image of the same patient confirming the same finding.

2. Acute aortic syndromes have very high mortality and need a very high index of suspicion for diagnosis. Acute aortic dissection, intramural hematoma, and penetrating aortic ulcer are all considered to be acute aortic syndromes [1].

   Aortic dissection is a disruption of the medial layer of the aortic wall with bleeding within or along the wall of the aorta. The blood may tear through the adventitia or back into the intima creating a dissection flap. Acute aortic dissection is rapidly fatal, 40% patients die immediately, about 20% patient die during or immediately after surgery, and only about half the patients are alive 5 years out from surgery [2, 3].

   Conditions that place extreme stress on the aortic wall (hypertension, deceleration injury, weight lifting) or lead to degeneration of the aortic media (genetic syndromes, inflammatory vasculitides, bicuspid aortic valve) can increase the risk of aortic dissection.

3. Presenting symptoms are sudden onset and severe chest, back, or abdominal pain that is described as tearing or ripping in quality [4, 5]. Some patients with acute aortic dissections may not have any chest pain at all and may present with syncope and shock like state. Patients also present with perfusion defects and end organ damage depending on the extension of the dissection flap, with resulting neurological deficits, myocardial ischemia, renal insufficiency, mesenteric ischemia, or limb ischemia.

   On physical exam, patients may demonstrate perfusion deficits in the form of a pulse deficit and systolic blood pressure deferential. Vascular examination of all four extremities should be conducted in all patients with suspected aortic dissection [6].

4. Thoracic aortic dissections are classified according to the involvement of the various segments of the thoracic aorta. Accurate classification is necessary to decide on surgical versus medical management. Two classification schema have been proposed: DeBakey and Stanford. The Stanford classification is more widely used, it classifies thoracic aortic dissections based on the involvement of the ascending aorta into:
   (a) Stanford A: involving ascending aorta (before the brachiocephalic artery). Urgent surgery is recommended.
   (b) Stanford B: involving the descending aorta only (after the left subclavian artery). Surgery usually not recommended.

Classification of Aortic Dissection

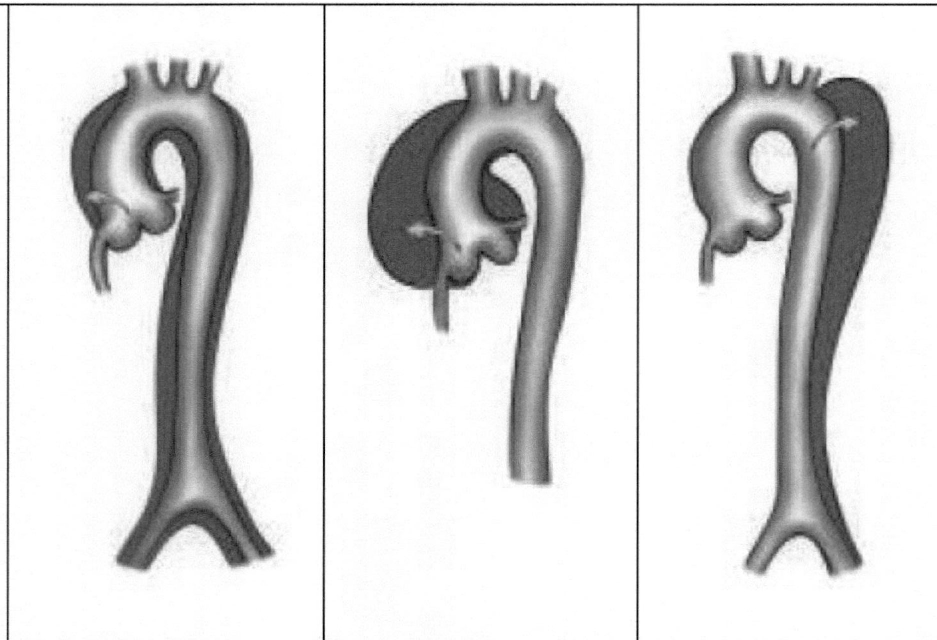

Percentage	60%	10–15%	25–30%
Type	DeBakey 1	DeBakey 11	DeBakey 111
	Stanford A (Proximal)		Stanford B (Distal)

Fig. 64.3 DeBakey and Stanford classification of thoracic aortic dissections

Table 64.1 End organ complications of acute thoracic aortic dissection [1]

Type	End-organ complication
Cardiovascular	Aortic regurgitationPericardial tamponade Coronary artery dissection Congestive heart failure
Neurological	Ischemic stroke Ischemic spinal injury
Pulmonary	Aortopulmonary fistula
Gastrointestinal	Mesenteric ischemia
Nephrology	Acute renal failure
Limb	Acute limb ischemia

The DeBakey classification:
(a) Type I: Originates in ascending aorta and propagates distally. Urgent surgery is recommended.
(b) Type II: Dissection is limited to the ascending aorta only. Urgent surgery is recommended.
(c) Type III: Originates in the descending thoracic aorta and propagates distally. Surgery is usually not recommended.

5. As mentioned previously, acute thoracic aortic dissections carry high morbidity and mortality. This is largely due to the end organ complications that arise due to obstruction to blood flow via the dissection flap. The various end organ complications are listed in (Table 64.1).

6. The role of D-dimer testing in the screening of aortic dissection has been reported in literature. In patients with low to intermediate pretest probability for aortic dissection, D-dimer test may have a role in ruling out dissection and avoiding further imaging. However, the guidelines do not recommend the use of D-dimer testing in patients with suspected aortic dissection [1, 7].

   First step in the algorithm for managing patients with suspected aortic dissection is to determine the pretest probability of aortic dissection. In patients who have a high pretest probability (severe chest pain, known risk factors, and high-risk exam features), the first step is immediate surgical consultation followed by imaging in the form of transesophageal echocardiography, computed tomography, or magnetic resonance imaging. Transesophageal echocardiography has several advantages including quick access, absence of radiation, and ability to be performed in patients who are unstable [1].

7. Stanford type A dissection is rapidly fatal due to high rate of complications. Immediate surgical consultation should be obtained. Urgent surgery is the treatment of choice in unstable patients. In patients who are relatively stable, preoperative cardiovascular evaluation and coronary angiography should be considered prior to surgery.

While awaiting surgery or in patients who are not considered surgical candidates, intravenous beta blockers should be initiated to reduce heart rate to <60 bpm. Non-dihydropyridine calcium channel blockers can be used in patients who cannot tolerate beta blockers. If blood pressure remains elevated (>120 mmHg) despite adequate heart rate control, vasodilators can be initiated.

Intraoperative transesophageal echocardiography to evaluate for acute aortic regurgitation should be performed. In presence of aortic valve involvement or significant coronary artery disease, valve replacement surgery or bypass grafting is performed in addition. The surgery involves replacing the entire dissected segment with a Dacron graft. If the aortic valve is not involved, it is resuspended onto the graft.

References

1. Hiratzka LF, Bakris GL, Beckman JA, Bersin RM, Carr VF, Casey DE Jr, et al. 2010 ACCF/AHA/AATS/ACR/ASA/SCA/SCAI/SIR/STS/SVM Guidelines for the diagnosis and management of patients with thoracic aortic disease. A Report of the American College of Cardiology Foundation/American Heart Association Task Force on Practice Guidelines, American Association for Thoracic Surgery, American College of Radiology, American Stroke Association, Society of Cardiovascular Anesthesiologists, Society for Cardiovascular Angiography and Interventions, Society of Interventional Radiology, Society of Thoracic Surgeons, and Society for Vascular Medicine. J Am Coll Cardiol. 2010;55(14):e27–e129.
2. Masuda Y, Yamada Z, Morooka N, Watanabe S, Inagaki Y. Prognosis of patients with medically treated aortic dissections. Circulation. 1991;84(5 Suppl):III7–13.
3. Crawford ES, Kirklin JW, Naftel DC, Svensson LG, Coselli JS, Safi HJ. Surgery for acute dissection of ascending aorta. Should the arch be included? J Thorac Cardiovasc Surg. 1992;104(1):46–59.
4. Januzzi JL, Eagle KA, Cooper JV, Fang J, Sechtem U, Myrmel T, et al. Acute aortic dissection presenting with congestive heart failure: results from the International Registry of Acute Aortic Dissection. J Am Coll Cardiol. 2005;46(4):733–5.
5. Miller DC, Stinson EB, Oyer PE, Rossiter SJ, Reitz BA, Griepp RB, et al. Operative treatment of aortic dissections. Experience with 125 patients over a sixteen-year period. J Thorac Cardiovasc Surg. 1979;78(3):365–82.
6. Yagdi T, Atay Y, Engin C, Mahmudov R, Tetik O, Iyem H, et al. Impact of organ malperfusion on mortality and morbidity in acute type A aortic dissections. J Card Surg. 2006;21(4):363–9.
7. Marill KA. Serum D-dimer is a sensitive test for the detection of acute aortic dissection: a pooled meta-analysis. J Emerg Med. 2008;34(4):367–76.

Chapter 65
CXR: Pediatric I

Frederic J. Sage and Frederick van Damme

Fig. 65.1 Normal pediatric chest X-ray

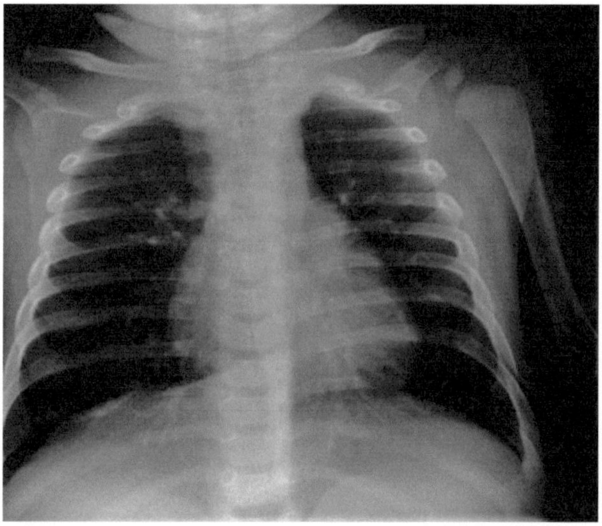

F.J. Sage, MD, FRCA, FFICM (✉) • F. van Damme, MB, ChB (Stell), FRCA
Department of Anaesthesia, East Surrey Hospital, Canada Avenue,
Redhill, RH1 5RH, UK
e-mail: frederic.sage@sash.nhs.uk

T.D. Raj (ed.), *Data Interpretation in Anesthesia*,
DOI 10.1007/978-3-319-55862-2_65

Questions

1. How do pediatric chest X-rays differ from those of an adult?
2. Consider this normal chest X-ray of an infant (Fig. 65.1). Is there a system for interpreting the image?
3. What points do you look for?
4. What is specific to each age group?
5. What should you not expect to see on an infant chest X-ray?
6. Do not forget?

Answers

1. Pediatric chest X-Ray differ from those of adults because:
   (a) They are difficult to obtain as cooperation is limited [1].
   (b) Chest X-rays change with age.
   (c) Children present with different conditions.
   (d) There are specific areas to review when interpreting a pediatric chest X-ray.
   (f) The thymus can cause confusion.

2. There are many ways of reading a CXR [2]. Adopt a method that suits you and stick to it. Here is an example:
   (a) Check ID and quality
   (b) Bone structure
   (c) Tracheobronchial tree and mediastinum
   (d) Heart silhouette
   (e) Contours of thorax
   (f) Lung fields
   (g) Abdomen
   (h) Soft tissues
   (i) Lines, tubes, and artefacts

3. Points to look for:
   (a) Check ID and quality:
      - Age will guide you in your interpretation.
      - Quality of the picture: rotation, inspiration, and exposure [2]. Over- or underexposed films will impair your judgement on parenchymal density and vascularity.
      - Position: AP, PA, and supine. Particularly important in neonates where lung mechanics are different such as the angle of the ribs. This can be affected by poor positioning of the child.
      - Also, ensure the orientation markers are correct (R and L). This is an opportunity to detect situs inversus or dextrocardia.

   (b) Bone structure:
      - Check skeleton integrity. Premature neonates have an absence of humeral head ossification [3].
      - Is the spine visible behind the mediastinum reflecting correct exposure?
      - Rotation can be excluded if the clavicles are symmetrical either side of the midline.
      - Ribs direction will vary with age. Flatter in neonates. Rib notching of coarctation is not usually visible until the age of 5.
      - Trauma of delivery: shoulders and clavicles. Non-accidental injuries (NAI) in older children: fractured ribs, upper limbs, etc.
      - In infants, a higher proportion of the skeleton is visible including head and neck, upper limbs, pelvis, and hips. These should all be checked.

(c) Tracheobronchial tree and mediastinum:
- Position and integrity of trachea and main bronchi.
- Presence of a foreign body either directly visible or indirectly by its effect on ventilation.
- The thymus is routinely visible until the age of 3. It is readily identifiable but can make the heart shadow difficult to analyze.
- Some lines should be visible within the mediastinum in particular the esophagus. Look for possible esophageal atresia if the nasogastric tube curls up before reaching the stomach.
- There are some common mediastinal tumors in children including lymphomas, neurogenic tumors (ganglioneuromas), thymomas, teratomas, and lipoblastomas.

(d) Heart silhouette and hila:
- This area can provide a number of clues in cases of cardiovascular malformations. A clinical suspicion is likely and it is useful to know if the child has a cyanotic or non-cyanotic condition.
- Points to consider are heart size, shape, and position.
- Special attention needs to be given to the lung vasculature from the pulmonary vessels in the hila to the overall vascularity of the lung fields up to the periphery of the thoracic cavity. Do the lungs appear hypo- or hypervascularized? Correct X-ray exposure is crucial [1].

(e) Contours of the thorax:
- A systematic review of all the peripheral regions of the thoracic cavity is necessary.
- Check the apices for pneumothoraces but remember that the child could be supine.
- Inspect the margins of the mediastinum and heart silhouette, the costodiaphragmatic angles, and the position and shapes of the two hemidiaphragms. Note the fissures if visible.

(f) Lung fields:
- Compare symmetrically: lung translucency, inflation, parenchyma, vascularization, and lung markings. Diaphragmatic hernias usually occur on the left side [1].
- A good quality X-ray is needed to identify and distinguish parenchymal disease or abnormal vasculature. You need to decide whether the pathology involves the lung or the cardiovascular system. If it is unilateral, a local process may be involved. A bilateral symmetrical aspect is more likely due to a systemic condition whether respiratory or cardiac.

(g) Abdomen:
- This must be included in the neonatal X-ray [1]. Look for the presence of air in the bowel. In esophageal atresia, air will be absent unless there also is a tracheoesophageal fistula (TOF) below the level of the atresia.
- In older children, check the size of solid organs: grossly enlarged liver, spleen, and kidneys can be visible.
- Check for free air under the diaphragm from trauma or ruptured viscus.

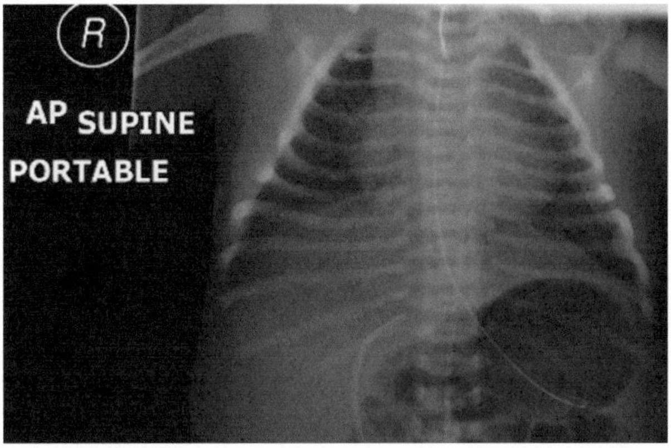

Fig. 65.2 Chest X-ray of a neonate. *Note*: the presence of ET tube, NG tube and well positioned umbilical arterial catheter. The umbilical vein catheter is not deep enough with its tip below the diaphragm

(h) Soft tissues:
- Check body fat (absent in premature children), edema (hydrops fetalis), or surgical emphysema.

(i) Artefacts:
- Children in PICU or NICU will have a number of lines inserted which need to be checked for correct position (Fig. 65.2): umbilical artery or vein catheters, central venous catheter, PICC, nasogastric (NG) tube, endotracheal (ET) tube, shunts, and drains [3].
- Artifacts include umbilical clips, skin folds, monitoring equipment, cots, or ventilator parts.

4. In every case, knowledge of the clinical presentation should guide the interpretation [2]. Furthermore, some pathologies will be more common at different ages.

For example, the following conditions should be sought in the chest X-ray of:

A premature baby or a neonate:

Remember X-ray will be AP and supine. Check fetal maturity—ossification of humeral heads. Check lines and tubes [1].

Look for acute cardiopulmonary conditions—respiratory distress in premature babies, transient tachypnea of the newborn, and meconium aspiration. Congenital malformations, cardiovascular anomalies, and hypoperfusion of the lung fields.

Rarer anomalies include:

Diaphragmatic hernia: abdominal content in the chest cavity.

Esophageal atresia: NG tube curling up and absence of intraabdominal gas unless TOF is also present [1]. Dextrocardia: check that labelling has been correctly done.

Infants: respiratory tract infections, NAI, tumors: mediastinal but also chest wall and metastatic tumors. Foreign bodies. Rib notching of coarctation (not in under 5).

Children: trauma, NAI, and infections.

5. A tension pneumothorax: this is a life-threatening condition which should be managed clinically without X-ray confirmation.
6. Do not forget: the elephant in the room [2].

   If something is obvious and appears important, notice and mention it early. It is then up to you to prioritize your interpretation according to the clinical situation.

References

1. Arthur R. The neonatal chest X-ray. Paediatr Respir Rev. 2001;2:311–23.
2. Radiologymasterclass.co.uk. http://www.radiologymasterclass.co.uk/. Accessed 25 Dec 2016.
3. Radiopaedia.org. https://radiopaedia.org/. Accessed 25 Dec 2016.

Chapter 66
CXR: Pediatric II

Frederick van Damme and Frederic J. Sage

An 11-month-old boy presented to our emergency department (ED) with a history of choking on a biscuit he was eating. He had one episode of cyanosis on choking. In the ED, he had episodes of coughing and his observations were as follows:

HR 145/min, RR 45/min, SpO_2 93% on air, SpO_2 99% on high flow oxygen (O_2).

No FB was apparent on the CXR shown below. After discussion with the otorhinolaryngologist and pediatricians, it was decided to admit this boy for observation.

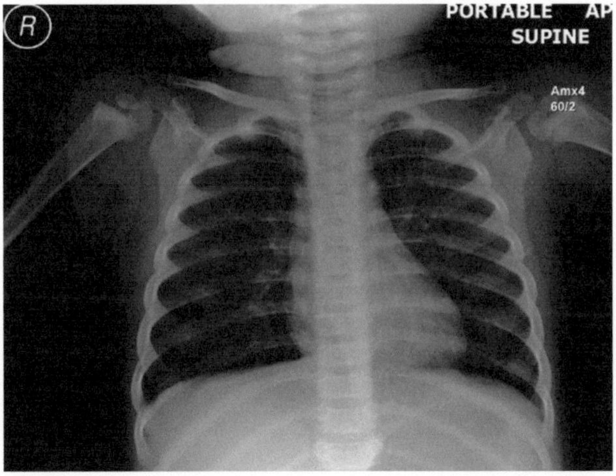

Fig. 66.1 CXR of our patient

F. van Damme, MB, ChB (Stell), FRCA • F.J. Sage, MD, FRCA, FFICM (✉)
Department of Anaesthesia, East Surrey Hospital,
Canada Avenue, Redhill, RH1 5RH, UK
e-mail: fsage@tiscali.co.uk

T.D. Raj (ed.), *Data Interpretation in Anesthesia*,
DOI 10.1007/978-3-319-55862-2_66

Questions

1. What is the initial prehospital management of a choking child? [1]
2. Describe the presentation of a foreign body (FB) aspiration in a child? [2–5]
3. What does the CXR in our patient show?
4. What is the management of aspirated and ingested FB? [1–6]
5. What is the incidence and complication rate of FB in children? [2, 6]

Answers

1. Assess severity of choking episode [1].

   (a) Effective cough (crying or verbal response to questions, loud cough, able to breath before coughing, normal GCS)
   - Encourage cough—unless patient deteriorates or until obstruction is relieved.
     Transport to ED if indicated!

   (b) Ineffective cough (unable to breath, cyanosis, decreasing GCS, unable to vocalize) [1]
   - Conscious—blind oropharyngeal finger sweep is not recommended. Alternating five back blows with five chest thrusts (infants) or five abdominal thrusts (child >1 year). Repeat until object comes out or child becomes unconscious.
   - Unconscious—start CPR.

2. **History** of aspiration from a witness (not always available).

   Presentation can range from **complete obstruction** with hypoxia and cardiac arrest to **partial obstruction** with symptoms described below to being **asymptomatic** and presenting later [2].

   Symptoms: coughing, choking, stridor or wheezing, drooling, vomiting, chest discomfort, difficulty in swallowing, reduced appetite or refusal to eat, and gagging on eating and drinking.

   Signs: tachypnea, intercostal muscles retraction, use of accessory muscles, nasal flaring, or cyanosis.

   Sometimes **asymptomatic** with no physical signs even with a reliable history of aspiration. Sometimes the presentation is with repeated pneumonias or lung abscesses.

   Physical examination:

   Persistent stridor—high-pitched inspiratory stridor usually a result of supraglottic obstruction.

   Biphasic stridor: indicates an obstruction at glottic or subglottic region.

   Expiratory stridor: indicates a tracheal or bronchial obstruction.

   Decreased breath sounds and wheezing can be indicative of an aspirated FB.

   X-rays: AP (Antero Posterior) and lateral x-rays of the chest including the neck must be obtained. Inspiratory and expiratory films will help in lateralizing (radiolucent) FB by emphasizing air trapping. Left and right lateral films are used in young, uncooperative children (the side with the FB will not deflate when placed dependent). Over 50% of X-rays are normal within 24 hours of aspiration.

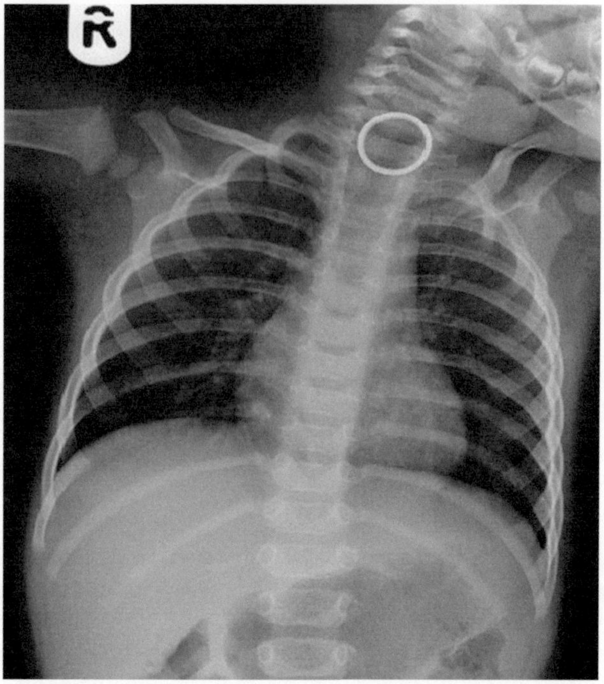

Fig. 66.2 FB (ring) at level of thoracic inlet

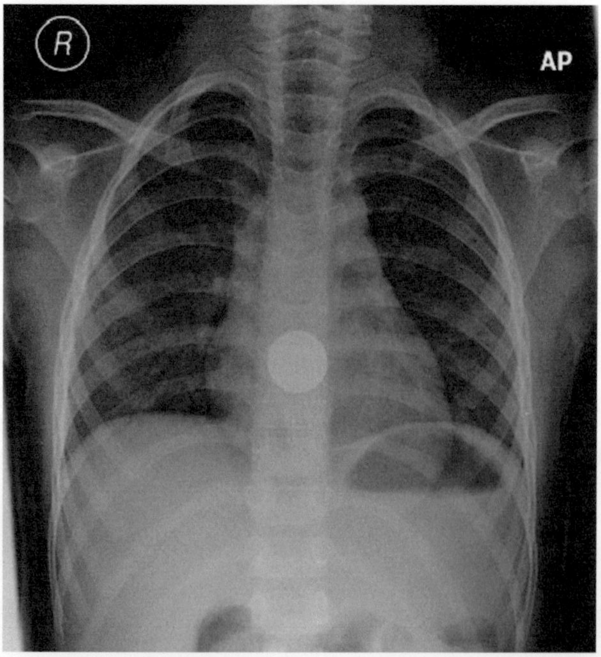

Fig. 66.3 FB (coin) in mid esophagus

Radiopaque FB:

It is important to distinguish between a battery/magnet and simple coin. Battery will have a double halo on X-ray and should be removed as a matter of urgency if stuck in the esophagus [5].

Radiolucent FB:

The following indirect signs **can** be present:

Normal or air trapping with air bronchograms.
Atelectasis and partial or total collapse of affected lung.
Hyperinflation of affected lung +/− mediastinal shift.
Pneumothorax or air in the mediastinum.
Consolidation.

3. Hyperinflated right lung with increased translucency, flattened right hemidiaphragm, wider spaced right ribs, and mediastinal shift to the left are the radiological features of obstruction.

4. Management of these cases should involve a multidisciplinary team (MDT) approach and good communication between the team members. The need for special equipment, specialized skills with a pediatric otorhinolaryngologist, a pediatric anesthesiologist, and a pediatric intensivist would warrant transfer of these patients to a facility that can provide them.

   (a) **Esophageal FB.** [2]
   Several techniques have been described in the literature for the removal of FB. Rigid and flexible esophagoscopy requires a general anesthetic (GA). Balloon retrieval and bougienage of esophageal FB does not require a GA [4]. Bougienage relies on the rationale that if you push the coin into the stomach, it will pass down the gastrointestinal tract. GA requires a rapid sequence induction and intubation to prevent aspiration. A repeat esophagoscopy is performed after removal of the FB to assess any mucosal injury.

   (b) **Button battery ingestion.** [2]
   We will consider this as a separate topic as the potential for significant esophageal injuries is very high within 2 hours of ingestion of the battery.

   Ingestion of the newer lithium button batteries are of great concern as the generation of hydroxide radicals in the esophageal mucosa result in a caustic injury from the high pH. This can lead to esophageal perforation, mediastinitis, tracheoesophageal fistula or aorto-enteric fistulas, and life-threatening bleeding. The most common battery that raises concern is the 3 V, 20/22 mm lithium button battery (CR 2032) [2].

   Ingested esophageal batteries should be removed as a matter of urgency for the reasons mentioned above. Asymptomatic gastric batteries are allowed to pass naturally but should be monitored with follow up X-rays. Symptomatic gastric batteries or simultaneous ingested magnets should be removed urgently. Children at greatest risk are those younger than 5 years of age and those with ingested battery size >20 mm and multiple battery ingestions [3].

(c) **Tracheal or bronchial FB.**

The procedure planned may be a diagnostic flexible bronchoscopy (in cases where the diagnosis is not certain) or a rigid bronchoscopy for FB retrieval in symptomatic children.

As the surgeon and anesthesiologist share management of a potentially obstructed airway, a clear communication of a detailed anesthetic and surgical plan and good cooperation between the two teams is essential.

Anesthetic Technique:

Preoperative assessment should determine where the FB has lodged, the nature of the FB, and the time it occurred. FB in the trachea means there is a risk for complete airway obstruction, and the risk is less if it is lodged beyond the carina.

There are three main anesthetic issues—method of induction, ventilation, and maintenance of anesthesia.

The optimal method of **induction** is not definitely established but maintaining spontaneous ventilation during the induction of a patient with a proximal FB is commonly practiced [2]. While spontaneous and controlled ventilation are feasible for FB removal, positive pressure ventilation down the bronchoscope with intermittent apnea while manipulating the object may be more suitable for distal FB retrieval. Airway trauma and rupture are significant and potentially fatal complications; hence, it is essential to avoid coughing and bucking secondary to the intense stimulation from a rigid bronchoscope. Movement can be prevented with neuromuscular blockade or deep anesthesia. In theory, there is a risk of positive pressure ventilation causing air trapping due to a ball-valve effect but the literature does not support this concern. **Maintenance** can be with inhalational agents or a total IV technique with propofol and remifentanil infusions with the advantage of a constant level of anesthesia irrespective of ventilation [4, 6]. **Ventilation**—spontaneous, controlled, and manual jet ventilation (with the ventilation catheter inserted separately from the bronchoscope) has been used and in one series, the incidence of intraoperative hypoxemia was less with manual jet ventilation.

To facilitate removal of the FB through the larynx, the vocal cords should be well relaxed which can be achieved with a small dose of neuromuscular blocker or propofol. If the FB occludes the trachea and cannot be removed, it can temporally be pushed down the left or right main bronchus to allow one-lung ventilation. Rarely, a tracheostomy or a thoracotomy might be needed [4].

Once the procedure is finished, a tracheal tube is inserted if a full stomach is a problem and the patient is woken up and extubated on return of protective reflexes.

The patient in our case report suffered several episodes of respiratory distress and cyanosis and was rapidly transferred to the operating room for an emergency rigid bronchoscopy. Adequate intravenous access was in situ (two cannulas minimum). Anesthesia was induced with 100% O_2 and sevoflurane after a period of

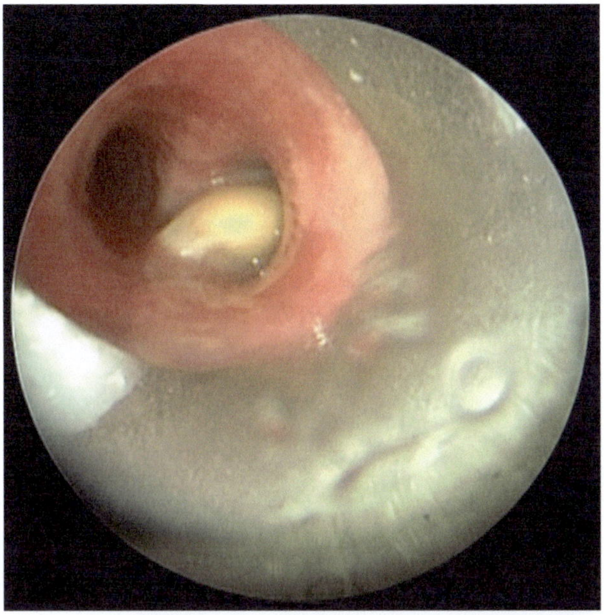

Fig. 66.4 Bronchoscopic view—FB in right main bronchus

preoxygenation with 100% O_2. Once the patient was anesthetized and the airway maintained, a rigid bronchoscope was inserted to examine the airways. The FB (an orange pip) was located at the origin of the right main bronchus (Fig. 66.4). After many difficulties, including transient occlusions of the lower trachea, the pip was removed with a rigid sucker.

All secretions and FB material were removed and the underlying mucosa was evaluated (Fig. 66.5). The child was allowed to slowly emerge from general anesthesia and was closely observed for laryngo-/bronchospasm. After a period of observation in post-anesthetic recovery area, the patient was allowed back to the pediatric ward for further observation.

5. Asphyxiation due to FB is a leading cause of death in the pediatric population aged 0–3 years in the European Union (EU) and in the United Status. During 2000, ingestion or aspiration of a foreign body (FB) was responsible for more than 17,000 emergency department visits in children younger than 14 years in the United States with a preponderance in males. In the United States, FB aspiration was responsible for about 4800 deaths in 2013, or about 1 death per 100,000 children [5], aged 0 to 4 years. Estimates in the EU show 50,000 incidences [5, 7]a year with a 10% fatality rate.

   26% of FB are food objects such as bones, nuts, or seeds. The remaining 74% are non-food objects: coins, marbles, and toys. Coins make up 15% of FB. Acute and chronic complications seem to occur in almost 15% of patients [2, 5, 7].

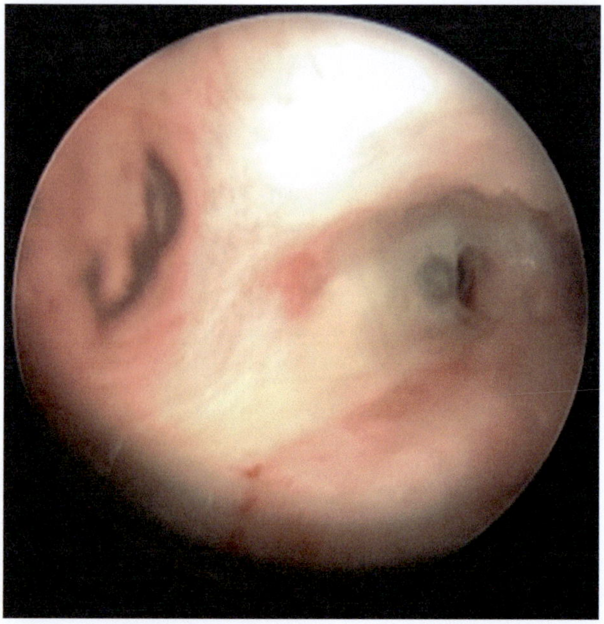

Fig. 66.5 Bronchoscopic view—FB removed. Edema and secretions visible, right main bronchus

Complications: Complete obstruction can lead to cardiac arrest and death if not treated promptly. In children in whom the diagnosis was delayed, most common complications included croup, pneumonia, pneumothorax, atelectasis, stricture, and perforation. Less commonly, perforation of the bronchial tree and fistula formation into surrounding structures can happen [2, 5].

Complications rate from rigid endoscopy and bronchoscopy is low (0.2–5%) and mortality is less than 0.2% [2].

Acknowledgment Thanks to Robert Bunting and the X-ray department at East Surrey Hospital, Redhill, United Kingdom, for providing the CXR's and to Mr. Kapoor, Consultant ENT surgeon, for the bronchoscopic images.

References

1. Resuscitation council (UK) – Paediatric Guidelines – Choking Child.
2. Berdan EA, Sato TT. Pediatric airway and esophageal foreign bodies. Surg Clin North Am. 2017 Feb;97(1):85–91.
3. Fortran F, Ballali S, et al. Foreign bodies in the airways: a meta-analysis of published papers. Int J Pediatr Otorhinolaryngol. 2012;76:S12–9.

4. Heinzerling NP, Christensen MA, Swedler R, et al. Safe and effective management of esophageal coins in children with bougienage. Surgery. 2015;158(4):1065–70.
5. Connors GP. Pediatric Foreign body ingestion. In Medscape. http://emedicine.medscape.com/article/801821-overview#a4. Accessed 1 Dec 2016.
6. Fidkowski CW, et al. The anesthetic considerations of tracheobronchial foreign bodies in children: a literature review of 12,979 cases. Anesth Analg. 2010;111:1016–25.
7. Susy Safe Working Group. The Susy Safe project overview after the first four years of activity. Int J Pediatr Otorhinolaryngol. 2012;76(Suppl 1):S3–11.

Chapter 67
ECHO: 3D

Nicole T. Tran

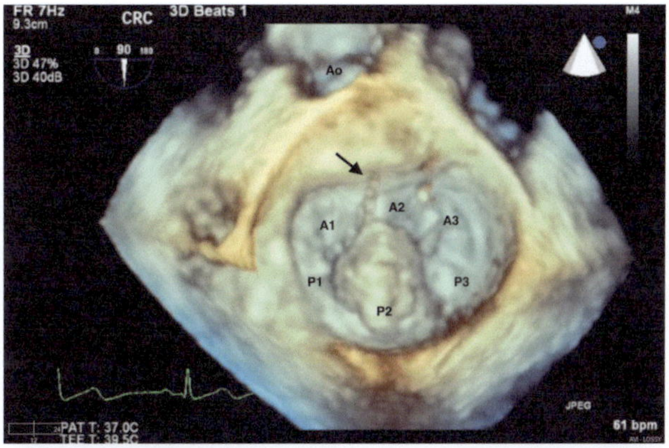

Fig. 67.1 Mitral valve systole

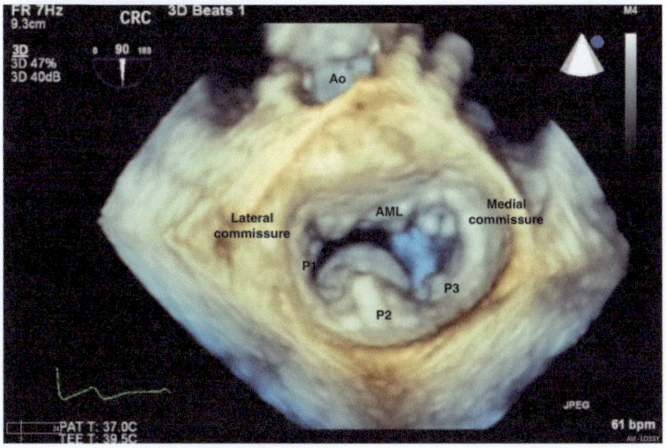

Fig. 67.2 Mitral valve diastole

N.T. Tran, MD
Department of Cardiology, University of Oklahoma Health Sciences Center, Oklahoma City, OK, USA
e-mail: Nicole-tran@Ouhsc.edu

T.D. Raj (ed.), *Data Interpretation in Anesthesia*,
DOI 10.1007/978-3-319-55862-2_67

I. A 70-year-old male with long-standing history of a cardiac murmur presents for evaluation of decreased exertion tolerance. He has no other significant past medical or surgical history. He previously was very active and walked 2–3 miles daily but recently has had to cut back to one mile due to fatigue and dyspnea. Physical exam is notable for a 3/6 holosystolic murmur located at the apex and radiating to the axilla, a laterally displaced apical impulse and an early diastolic rumble. A transthoracic echocardiogram (TTE) is obtained which prompts a transesophageal echocardiogram (TEE) for further evaluation.

Questions

1. What is the normal anatomy of the mitral valve?
2. What do Figs. 67.1 and 67.2 demonstrate?
3. How is mitral regurgitation classified?
4. What is the role of 3D TEE in the evaluation of mitral regurgitation?
5. What are the advantages and disadvantages of three-dimensional (3D) echocardiography compared to two-dimensional (2D) echocardiography?
6. What are the indications for surgical treatment of mitral regurgitation?

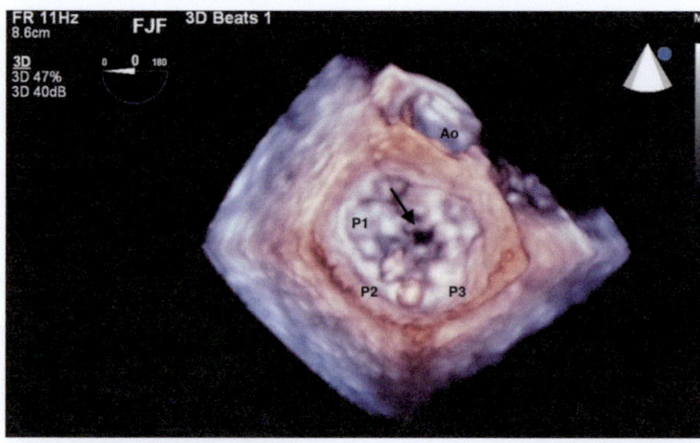

Fig. 67.3 Mitral valve systole

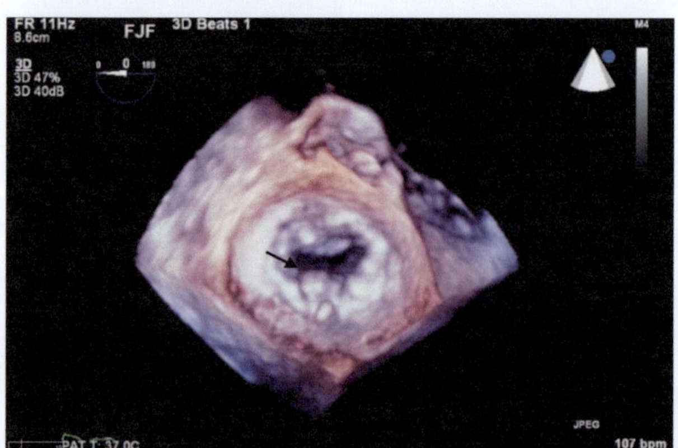

Fig. 67.4 Mitral valve diastole

Fig. 67.5 Mitral regurgitation

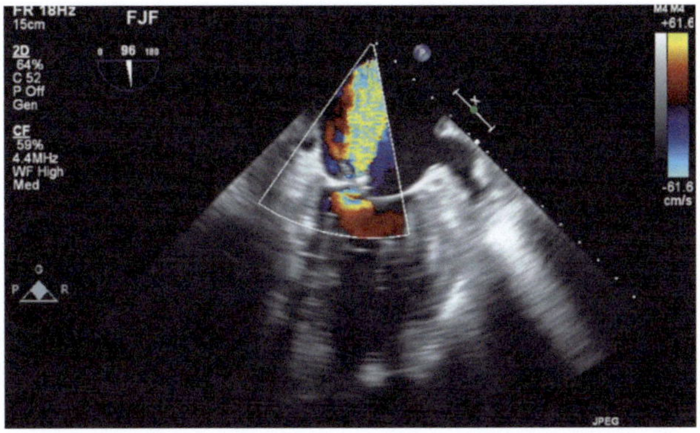

II. A 40 year old female with hypertension, diabetes, and end-stage renal disease on hemodialysis presents to the emergency room complaining of a 2 week history of fevers, chills, night sweats and a 1 day history of rapidly progressive shortness of breath. She is sitting upright, in moderate distress and appears dyspneic. Temperature is 38.4°C. 2/2 blood cultures grow *S. aureus*. Physical exam reveals an S3 and an early diastolic flow rumble.

Questions

7. What do Figs. 67.3, 67.4, and 67.5 demonstrate?
8. Using the Carpentier classification, what is the mechanism of mitral regurgitation?
9. What are additional key echocardiographic findings in the evaluation of this condition?

Answers

1. The mitral valve is the left atrioventricular (AV) valve. It is a bileaflet valve composed of anterior (aortic) and posterior (mural) leaflets. The anterior mitral valve leaflet (AML) occupies 1/3 of the mitral annulus but is broader and occupies 2/3 of the surface area of the valve. It is in fibrous continuity with the left and non-coronary cusps of the aortic valve. The posterior mitral valve leaflet (PML) occupies 2/3 of the mitral annulus but only accounts for 1/3 of the surface area of the valve [1]. It is divided into three scallops which Carpentier labeled P1, P2 and P3 going laterally to medially. By convention, the AML is similarly divided into three segments (A1, A2, A3 from lateral to medial) which correspond to the PML scallops. The mitral annulus is fibrous anteriorly, muscular posteriorly, and changes shape during the cardiac cycle. The muscular posterior portion is more prone to dilatation and calcification. On the ventricular aspect of the mitral valve, there are three layers of chordae tendinae (primary, secondary and tertiary) which attach to the papillary muscles. There are classically two papillary muscles: posteromedial and anterolateral. The posteromedial papillary muscle is connected via cords to the medial 1/2 of the mitral valve and the anterolateral papillary muscle gives cords to the lateral 1/2 of the mitral valve. With normal mitral valve function, there is a zone of coaptation where the leaflets close, as well as a 4–5 mm zone of apposition where the two leaflets overlap.

2. Figures 70.1 and 70.2 show the classical 3D TEE surgeon's view of the mitral valve in systole (Fig. 67.1) and diastole (Fig. 67.2). In the surgeon's view, the left atrium has been opened and you are looking down at an en face view of the mitral valve. The aortic valve by convention is at the top of the image. In this view, the lateral commissure and left atrial appendage are to the left of the image, and the medial commissure and tricuspid valve apparatus are to the right of the image. PML scallops are labeled by the Carpentier convention, lateral to medial, P1, P2 and P3. The adjacent segments of the AML are labeled A1, A2, A3 from lateral to medial. These images show a flail P2 segment due to a ruptured cord (arrow). A flail segment is defined as the tip of the leaflet pointing towards the left atrium in systole and the left ventricle in diastole.

3. Mitral regurgitation (MR) is typically described by the Carpentier Classification (adapted from Tsang et al.) [2]. This patient's mitral regurgitation would be described as type II (likely due to fibroelastic disease) with isolated flail P2 segment due to a ruptured cord (Table 67.1).

4. Echocardiographic evaluation of MR should seek to identify the origin of regurgitation (is it primary? secondary?), the specific lesion responsible for the regurgitation, which aspects of the mitral valve apparatus are affected (leaflets? annulus? chordae tendinae? papillary muscles?), the severity of the MR, and the downstream effects of the MR. This complete evaluation aids in surgical planning [2, 3]. TEE is indicated preoperatively or intraoperatively (class I recommendation) or when surgery is being considered (class IIa recommendation) to "establish the anatomic basis of severe MR and to assess the feasibility of and guide

Table 67.1 Carpentier classification of mitral regurgitation (inserted with answer 3)

Type	Leaflet motion	Mechanism of MR
I	Normal	Perforation Cleft Dilated annulus without leaflet tethering
II	Excess motion	Fibroelastic disease[a] Barlow's disease[b]
IIIa	Restricted motion in systole and diastole	Rheumatic/post-inflammatory
IIIb	Restricted motion in systole only	Due to symmetric or asymmetric (ischemic) ventricular dysfunction

[a]Fibroelastic disease usually characterized by a single prolapsing segment with prolapse due to focal cord elongation or rupture
[b]Barlow's disease is due to classic myxomatous changes of both leaflets and multiple segments and both leaflets may be involved. Leaflets are often thickened (>5 mm)

surgical repair" [4]. TEE is also indicated when TTE is technically inadequate or non-diagnostic in the evaluation of severe MR (class I recommendation).

5. 3D TEE provides anatomic information from a typical surgeon's viewpoint which can be critical in communicating findings in an operative setting. It is superior to 2D imaging in correctly identifying affected scallops. Changes in annular size or adjacent anatomy can result in misidentification of scallops on typical 2D TEE views. 3D TEE eliminates this source of error [5, 6]. 3D TEE is also more sensitive and specific than 2D echocardiography for the identification and characterization of commissural lesions. It provides additional information on annular size and geometry as well as on adjacent anatomic structures without necessitating mental 3D reconstruction. As a result, it is less operator dependent than 2D TEE. Current 3D probes have the ability to do X-plane imaging (imaging of simultaneous orthogonal planes), live (real-time) 3D imaging, 3D full volume imaging (4–7 heartbeats are averaged to obtain a large volume image), and 3D full color volume imaging, which with newer technology is useful in the quantification of mitral regurgitation. The main limitations of 3D TEE are the need for an adequate acoustic window, the need to minimize respiratory artifact and translational motion when obtaining full-volume imaging to minimize stitch artifacts, and the decrease in temporal resolution when compared to 2D TEE.

6. Surgery is indicated for severe acute MR (class I recommendation) [4]. For primary mitral valve pathology, surgery is indicated for chronic, severe, *symptomatic* MR as long as left ventricular ejection fraction (LVEF) is 30% or greater and left ventricular end-systolic dimension (LVESD) is less than or equal to 55 mm (class I recommendation). Surgery is indicated for chronic, severe, *asymptomatic* MR if the LVEF is between 30 and 60% and the LVESD is at least 40 mm (class I recommendation). It is reasonable to send an asymptomatic patient with chronic, severe MR, an LVEF >60%, and LVESD <40 mm for repair with an experienced surgeon if the likelihood of successful repair is >90% (class IIa recommendation). It is also reasonable to refer patients with chronic severe MR and either new onset Atrial Fibrillation or pulmonary hypertension (pulmonary

artery systolic pressure > 50 mm Hg at rest or >60 mm Hg with exercise) for surgery (class IIa recommendation). It should be noted that if at all possible, mitral valve repair is preferred over mitral valve replacement. Patients should be referred to a surgical center with expertise in mitral valve repair, where the likelihood of successful repair is at least 90% (class I recommendation). It is recommended that mitral valve surgeons do at least 25 repairs per year, and mitral valve centers of excellence do at least 50 repairs per year. Isolated P2 prolapse is the most easily repaired lesion. Repair success rates decrease with anterior or multi-segment prolapse, mitral annular calcification, and significant billowing/ excess leaflet tissue.

7. These images show a 3D TEE surgeon's view of the mitral valve in systole (Fig. 67.3) and diastole (Fig. 67.4). The aortic valve is labeled at the top of the screen (Ao). The lateral commissure is on the left by the left atrial appendage; the medial commissure is on the right by the tricuspid valve (TV) apparatus. On the atrial aspect of the P2 scallop of the PML, there is an irregular, shaggy, echogenic mass (arrow in Fig. 67.4) which involves the mitral valve annulus and is associated with local destruction of the P2 scallop. The regurgitant orifice is marked with an arrow in Fig. 67.3. Figure 67.5 shows the color doppler mitral regurgitation through the perforated leaflet. The patient has positive blood cultures for a typical organism (*S. aureus*), suggestive echocardiographic findings, and is febrile. She has two major and one minor Duke criteria which is diagnostic for infective endocarditis [7]. TEE confirmed severe MR which was likely acute given her clinical presentation. Her lack of murmur is explained by rapid equilibration of left atrial and left ventricular diastolic pressures. If present, the murmur of acute severe MR occurs in early systole and terminates in early to mid-systole. An S3 is often present due to acute left ventricular volume overload and a diastolic rumble flow murmur may be heard [8].

8. In this patient, mitral valve leaflet motion is normal. The mechanism of MR is due to leaflet perforation from infective endocarditis (IE) (Carpentier class I) (Table 67.1).

9. In this situation, 3D TEE was used to confirm the location and size of the vegetation (P2 scallop with extension into the muscular annulus), to evaluate for any other associated valvular disease (in this case leaflet perforation), to evaluate the shape/size of the mitral valve annulus for surgical planning, and to evaluate for extension into adjacent structures. The anterior mitral valve leaflet is in fibrous continuity with the left and non-coronary cusps of the aortic valve as well as the right and left fibrous trigones. With IE involving the anterior mitral leaflet, it is important to carefully examine for perivalvular or aortic valvular extension. Perivalvular extension of IE is an indication for surgical intervention. It is also important to accurately quantify the degree of regurgitation as severe, symptomatic regurgitation due to IE is an indication for surgical intervention. Large vegetations (>10 mm in size) associated with embolic phenomena, or recurrent embolic phenomenon are also indications for surgical management of IE [9].

References

1. McCarthy KP, Ring L, Rana BS. Anatomy of the mitral valve: understanding the mitral valve complex in mitral regurgitation. Eur Heart J Cardiovasc Imaging. Dec 2010;11(10):3–9.
2. Tsang W, Lang RM. Three-dimensional echocardiography is essential for intraoperative assessment of mitral regurgitation. Circulation. 2013;128:643–52.
3. Chandra S, Salgo IS, Sugeng L, et al. Characterization of degenerative mitral valve disease using morphologic analysis of real-time three-dimensional echocardiographic images: objective insight into complexity and planning of mitral valve repair. Circ Cardiovasc Imaging. 2011;4:24–32.
4. Bonow RO, Carabello BA, Chatterjee K, et al. ACC/AHA 2008 focused updated incorporated into the ACC/AHA 2006 guidelines for the management of patients with valvular heart disease: a report of the American College of Cardiology/American Heart Association Task Force on Practice Guidelines developed in collaboration with the Society of Cardiovascular Anesthesiologists endorsed by the Society for Cardiovascular Angiography and Interventions and the Society of Thoracic Surgeons. J Am Coll Cardiol. 2008;52(13):e1–e142.
5. Zekly SB, Nagueh SF, Little SH, et al. Comparative accuracy of two-and three-dimensional transthoracic and transesophageal echocardiography in identifying mitral valve pathology in patients undergoing mitral valve repair: initial observations. J Am Soc Echocardiogr. 2011;24:1079–85.
6. Pepi M, Tamburini G, Maltagliati A, et al. Head-to-Head Comparison of two- and three-dimensional trans thoracic and transesophageal echocardiography in the location of mitral valve prolapse. J Am Coll Cardiol. 2006;48:2524–30.
7. Durack D, Lukes AS, Bright DK, et al. New criteria for diagnosis of infective endocarditis: utilization of specific echocardiographic findings. Duke Endocarditis Service. Am J Med. 1994;96(3):200–9.
8. Stout KK, Verrier ED. Acute valvular regurgitation. Circulation. 2009;119:3232–41.
9. Prendergast BD, Tornos P. Surgery for infective endocarditis: who and when? Circulation. 2010;121:1141–52.

Part IV
Physiologic Studies

Chapter 68
Pulmonary Function Testing

John B. Carter

Forty-two-year-old female is 61 inches and 98 lbs and has shortness of breath. Figure 68.1 is her spirogram. FVC is 94% of predicted. FEV_1 is 46% but post bronchodilator increases to 66%. FEV_1/FVC was 39%.

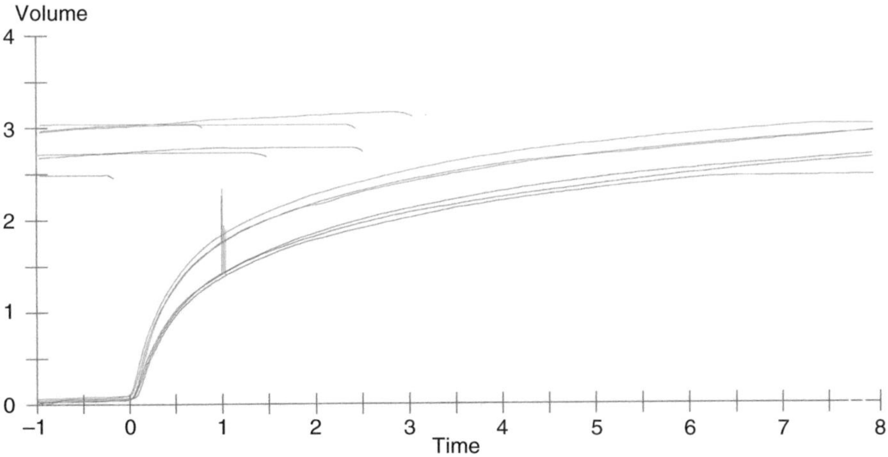

Fig. 68.1 Patient's spirometry, red curve after bronchodilator

J.B. Carter, MD
Department of Respiratory Therapy, Oklahoma University Medical Center Hospital, 750 NE 13th Street, OAC 200, Oklahoma City, OK 73104, USA
e-mail: John-b-carter@ouhsc.edu

T.D. Raj (ed.), *Data Interpretation in Anesthesia*,
DOI 10.1007/978-3-319-55862-2_68

Questions

1. How is spirometry performed and what information does it provide?
2. When is spirometry indicated?
3. Describe normal and abnormal spirometry curves.
4. Describe spirometry in COPD.
5. What is bronchodilator reversibility testing?
6. How would you interpret this patient's spirometry?

Answers

1. Spirometry: the patient inhales until the lungs are full and rapidly and forcefully exhales. The test is dependent on patient effort, so it must be properly performed. The test is repeated until three acceptable and consistent results are obtained.

   (a) Forced vital capacity or FVC. This is the total exhaled volume in liters exhaled after full inspiration, typically in the first 6 s.
   (b) Forced expiratory volume in liters during the first second or FEV_1.
   (c) The ratio of the FEV_1/FVC as a fraction. Normal is between 0.7 and 0.8.
   (d) The forced expiratory flow rate in the midportion of the FEV_1, the FEF_{25-75}.
   (e) Normal values are obtained from tables, obtained in normal controls, and vary by height, gender, and ethnicity. These data provide objective measurements to determine the severity and follow the course of the pulmonary disease [1].
   (f) These measurements are based on flow over time. Flow volume loops are flow rates plotted against volume and are discussed in a separate chapter.

2. Spirometry can confirm the presence and severity of obstructive and restrictive lung disease. The response to bronchodilator can assist to differentiate asthma from COPD. It can be useful to assess progression and response to therapy. Spirometry is not routinely necessary in preoperative testing for non-thoracic surgery. In patients evaluated for lung resection, simple spirometry, FVC, and FEV_1 should be obtained. The predicted postoperative FEV_1 is calculated as $ppoFEV_1 = \text{preop } FEV_1\% \times (1-\% \text{ functional lung removed}/100)$. A $ppoFEV_1 < 40\%$ indicates a higher risk of postoperative complications; these patients may need additional testing, and/or a $ppoFEV_1 < 30\%$ may require post-op ventilation [2].

3. Figure 68.2 is a normal spirometry curve. Figure 68.3 demonstrates abnormal spirometry curves. Three basic patterns are:

   (a) Normal: FEV_1 and FVC are >80% of predicted.
      FVC_1/FVC is >0.7.
   (b) Obstructive: $FEV_1 < 80\%$ of predicted
      FVC normal or reduced, usually decreased to a lesser degree than FEV_1
      $FEV_1/FVC < 0.7$. (Fig. 68.3)
   An obstructive pattern is usually seen in COPD or asthma.
   (c) Restrictive: FEV_1 is normal or slightly reduced.
      FVC < 80% of predicted.
      $FEV_1/FVC > 0.7$. (Fig. 68.4)

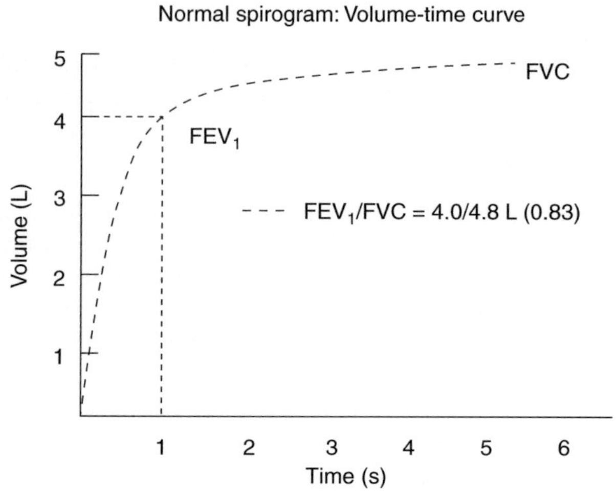

Fig. 68.2 Normal spirometry curve (with permission from Global Initiative for Chronic Obstructive Lung Disease. http://www.goldcopd.org)

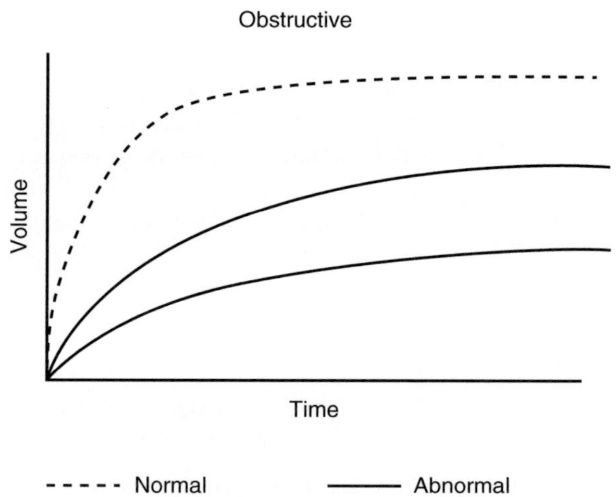

Fig. 68.3 Obstructive pattern (with permission from Global Initiative for Chronic Obstructive Lung Disease. http://www.goldcopd.org)

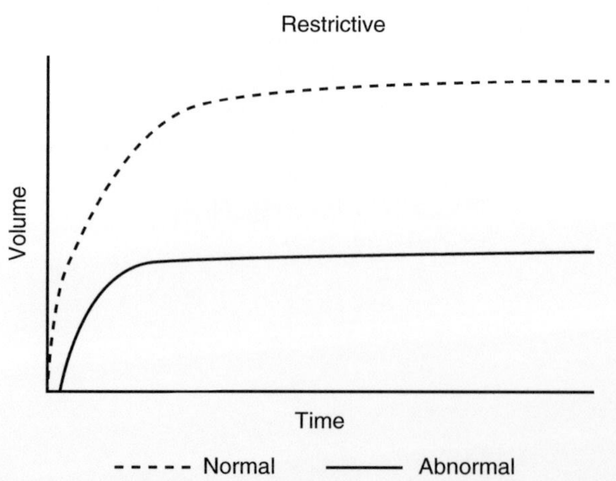

Fig. 68.4 Restrictive pattern (with permission from Global Initiative for Chronic Obstructive Lung Disease. http://www.goldcopd.org)

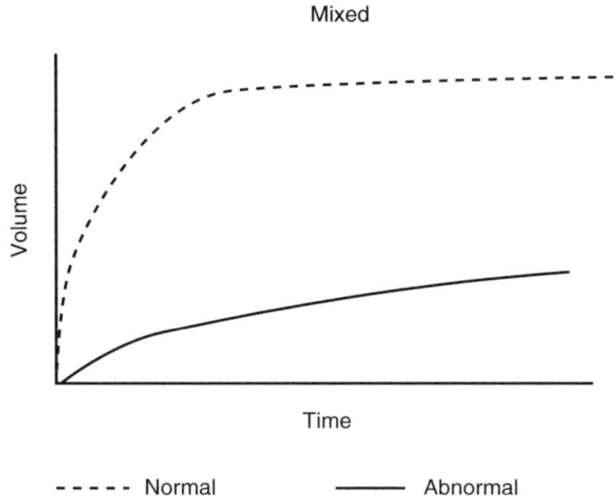

Fig. 68.5 Mixed pattern (with permission from Global Initiative for Chronic Obstructive Lung Disease. http://www.goldcopd.org)

Restrictive pattern is seen in parenchymal disease such as pulmonary fibrosis. Extraparenchymal causes include chest wall deformity such as scoliosis, obesity, pleural effusion, and neuromuscular disorder. Further pulmonary testing with CO diffusion capacity may help in the diagnosis.

If both FEV_1 and FVC are reduced, the patient may have a mixed restrictive and obstructive disorder (Fig. 68.5). Another possibility is that severe obstruction may lead to air trapping. Measuring total lung capacity and residual volume will show increased residual volume in air trapping [3].

4. Chronic obstructive lung disease COPD is common. Causes include cigarette smoking, occupational exposure to particulates such as in coal miners, and α_1 antitrypsin deficiency [4]. There is a progressive airflow limitation that is not fully reversible. This is due to loss of elastic recoil in emphysema and airway narrowing by secretions or inflammatory changes. Clinical features include productive cough, progressing dyspnea, and prolonged expiration [5].

GOLD spirometric criteria for COPD severity

I. Mild	$FEV_1/FVC < 0.7$ $FEV_1 \geq 80\%$ predicted	May be asymptomatic
II. Moderate	$FEV_1/FVC < 0.7$ $50\% \leq FEV_1 < 80\%$ predicted	Dyspnea on exertion
III. Severe	$FEV_1/FVC < 0.7$ $30\% \leq FEV_1 < 50\%$ predicted	Activity limited by SOB Exacerbations begin
IV. Very severe	$FEV_1/FVC < 0.7$ $FEV_1 < 30\%$ predicted or $FEV_1 < 50\%$ predicted and chronic respiratory failure	Impaired quality of life Exacerbations may be severe

5. Bronchodilator testing demonstrates reversibility of obstruction, indicating benefit from bronchodilator therapy, primarily beta$_2$ agonists. FVC and FEV_1 are measured at baseline and after inhaled bronchodilator.
   (a) FEV_1 increases of at least 12% or 200 ml from baseline is considered significant. This supports the diagnosis of asthma.
   (b) Some patients with COPD respond to bronchodilators.
   (c) In general spirometry that returns to normal after bronchodilator is not COPD [1].
6. This patient's spirometry has an FVC of >80%; thus, a restrictive component is not present.

The marked decreased FEV_1 at 46% predicted and FEV_1/FVC of 39% indicate an obstructive component that is severe. She shows responsiveness to bronchodilators. The diagnosis of either COPD or asthma is based on the history and physical in addition to spirometry.

References

1. Spirometry for health care providers. Global Initiative for Chronic Obstructive Lung Disease. Goldcopd.org.
2. Slinger P, Darling G. Preanesthetic assessment for thoracic surgery. In: Slinger P, editor. Principles and practice of anesthesia for thoracic surgery. New York: Springer; 2011. p. 19.
3. Feyrouz A, Reena M. Interpreting pulmonary function tests. Cleveland Clin J. 2003;70:866–81.
4. Al-Ruzzeh S, Kurup V. Stoelting's Anesthesia and Co-existing Disease, Chapter 9, 6th ed. 2012.
5. West J. Pulmonary pathophysiology the essentials. Philadelphia: Lippincott Williams & Wilkins; 2003.

Chapter 69
Stress Test

Aneesh Venkat Pakala

Sixty-five-year-old lady awaiting Whipple surgery presents to the preoperative clinic. She has a past medical history of ischemic heart disease with percutaneous coronary intervention in the past, prior ischemic stroke with left-sided hemiparesis, diabetes mellitus well controlled on metformin, essential hypertension, and hyperlipidemia. Patient stated that she started noticing chest pressure over left precordium with moderate exertion over the past 3 months. She is partially dependent. Due to suspicion of ischemic heart disease and elevated risk surgery, cardiology clinic referral is made, and surgery is postponed. Cardiologist orders a stress test. Results are displayed below.

A.V. Pakala, MD
Section of Cardiovascular Disease, Department of Medicine, University of Oklahoma College of Medicine, Oklahoma City, OK, USA
e-mail: aneeshpakala@yahoo.com; Aneesh-Pakala@ouhsc.edu

T.D. Raj (ed.), *Data Interpretation in Anesthesia*,
DOI 10.1007/978-3-319-55862-2_69

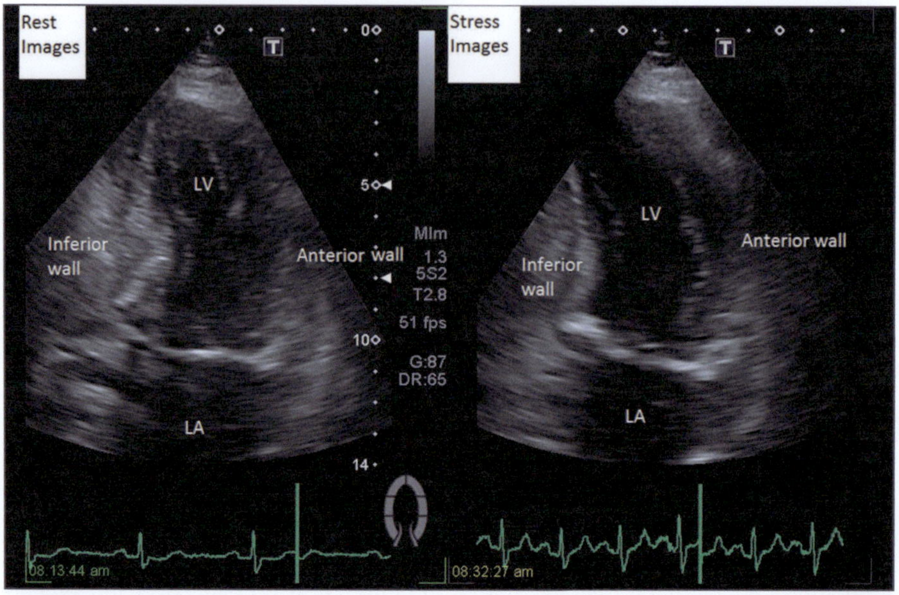

Fig. 69.1

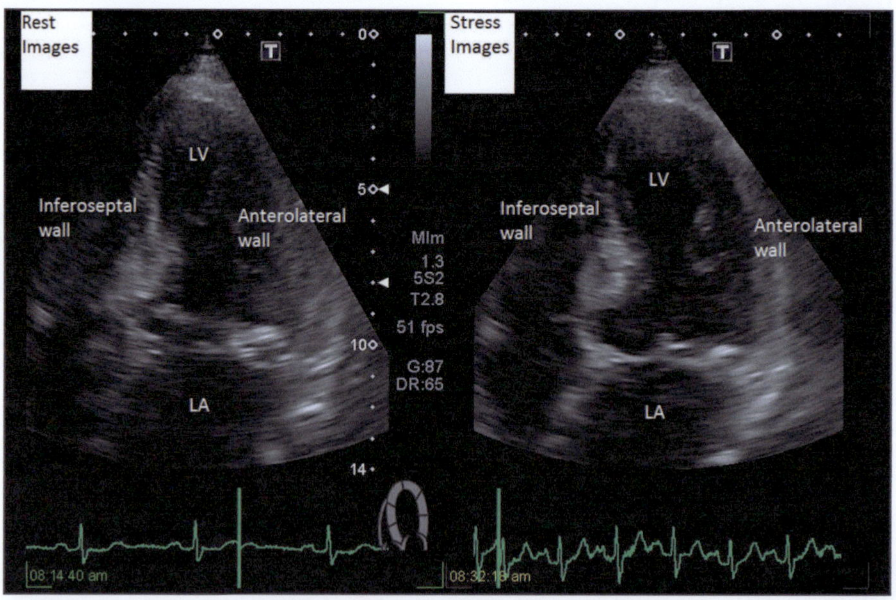

Fig. 69.2

Questions

1. What do the images demonstrate?
2. What is the pathophysiologic basis of stress testing?
3. What factors influence the choice of stress testing?
4. What is the role of stress testing in the preoperative setting?

Answers

1. Patient underwent a dobutamine stress echocardiogram. Figures show still frames of the left ventricle in end systole, at rest, and at peak stress (Figs. 69.1 and 69.2). Findings are consistent with stress-induced wall motion abnormality involving the left anterior descending coronary artery distribution (anterior and anterolateral myocardium).

2. Functional stress testing is the test of choice for detecting myocardial ischemia. Stress testing is based on the principle of "the ischemic cascade"; according to which, as the severity of ischemia increases, the ischemic manifestations worsen progressively from diastolic dysfunction, reduced epicardial perfusion, regional wall motion abnormalities, global systolic dysfunction, and finally EKG changes [1].

   The aim of a stress test is to activate the ischemic cascade with either exercise or drugs and demonstrate the resulting ischemic manifestations via EKG, echocardiography, myocardial perfusion imaging (MPI), or magnetic resonance imaging.

   Exercise stress is preferred over pharmacological stress because of the higher physiological stress levels achieved via exercise. Exercise stress also provides additional prognostic information like functional capacity. However, not all patients are candidate for exercise stress testing, especially those who have significant disabilities or disabling comorbidities.

3. The sensitivity and specificity of a stress test depend upon the pretest probability of ischemic heart disease (IHD); sensitivity of the stress test to detect disease increases in patient populations with high pretest probability of IHD (65-year-old male with typical chest pain); on the other hand the specificity of the stress test to detect the absence of disease increases in populations with low pretest probability of IHD (35-year-old female with atypical chest pain). The clinical utility of a stress test in diagnosing or ruling out IHD is best in those with intermediate pretest probability of IHD (45-year-old male with atypical chest pain).

   The choice of stress testing depends on patient's ability to exercise, body habitus, and baseline EKG. According to the ACC-AHA guidelines, exercise stress EKG testing is recommended in symptomatic patients with intermediate pretest probability for ischemic heart disease (IHD), moderate functional capacity, and interpretable EKG at baseline. Exercise stress with MPI or echocardiography is recommended in symptomatic patients with intermediate to high pretest probability of IHD, moderate functional capacity, and uninterpretable EKG at baseline. Pharmacological stress MPI or echocardiogram is recommended for symptomatic intermediate to high pretest probability patients who have limited functional capacity and are not able to exercise [1].

4. Routine stress testing for IHD in the preoperative setting is not recommended. For patients who are scheduled for elevated risk surgery (>1% risk of major adverse cardiovascular events) and have excellent functional capacity (METS > 10), it is reasonable to proceed with surgery without stress testing. Even in patients with intermediate functional capacity (METS 4–10), proceeding with surgery without stress testing may be considered [2].

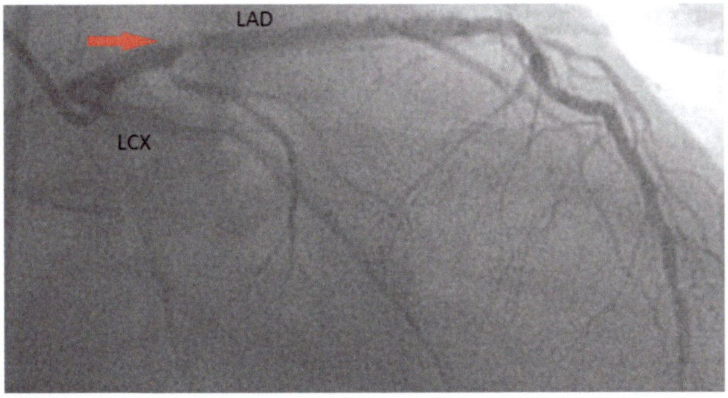

Fig. 69.3 Coronary angiogram showing the left anterior descending (LAD) coronary artery and left circumflex coronary artery (LCX) with severe stenosis in the proximal segment (*red arrow*)

Patients who are scheduled for elevated risk surgery and have poor functional capacity (<4 METS) or if functional capacity cannot be determined, stress testing may be considered if results of the stress test would change preoperative management. In our patient scheduled for elevated risk surgery, functional status estimation is not possible due to hemiparesis and partially dependent status. As per the ACC-AHA guidelines, stress testing may be considered as mentioned above.

More importantly however, our patient should be scheduled for stress testing independent of surgical status due to the fact that she has high pretest probability for ischemic heart disease and is currently symptomatic. High-risk stress features (as shown in this case) suggest a high ischemic burden which would benefit with revascularization. Our patient underwent coronary angiogram that revealed significant stenosis of the left anterior descending (LAD) coronary artery (Fig. 69.3). After discussions between the patient, surgeon, anesthesiologist, and cardiologist, multidisciplinary decision was made to postpone Whipple surgery to allow for percutaneous coronary intervention with bare metal stent and dual antiplatelet therapy for 30 days.

References

1. Fihn SD, Blankenship JC, Alexander KP, Bittl JA, Byrne JG, Fletcher BJ, et al. ACC/AHA/AATS/PCNA/SCAI/STS focused update of the guideline for the diagnosis and management of patients with stable ischemic heart disease: a report of the American College of Cardiology/American Heart Association Task Force on Practice Guidelines, and the American Association for Thoracic Surgery, Preventive Cardiovascular Nurses Association, Society for Cardiovascular Angiography and Interventions, and Society of Thoracic Surgeons. Circulation. 2014;130(19):1749–67.
2. Fleisher LA, Fleischmann KE, Auerbach AD, Barnason SA, Beckman JA, Bozkurt B, et al. ACC/AHA guideline on perioperative cardiovascular evaluation and management of patients undergoing noncardiac surgery: a report of the American College of Cardiology/American Heart Association Task Force on practice guidelines. J Am Coll Cardiol. 2014;64(22):e77–137.

Chapter 70
Flow Volume Loops

Edward Kosik

A 48-year-old male patient presents to the preanesthesia clinic to prepare for a knee arthroscopy procedure. The patient has a history of COPD and is a 40-pack-year smoker.

Vitals are HR 72, BP 140/74, SpO_2 93% on room air, and temp 36.6, with height of 64 inches and weight of 88 kilograms.

Pulmonary function tests, including a flow volume loop, were present in the patient's medical records from an outside hospital.

E. Kosik, DO
Department of Anesthesiology, University of Oklahoma Health Sciences Center, 750 NE 13th Street, OAC 200, Oklahoma City, OK 73104, USA
e-mail: Edward-kosik@ouhsc.edu

T.D. Raj (ed.), *Data Interpretation in Anesthesia*,
DOI 10.1007/978-3-319-55862-2_70

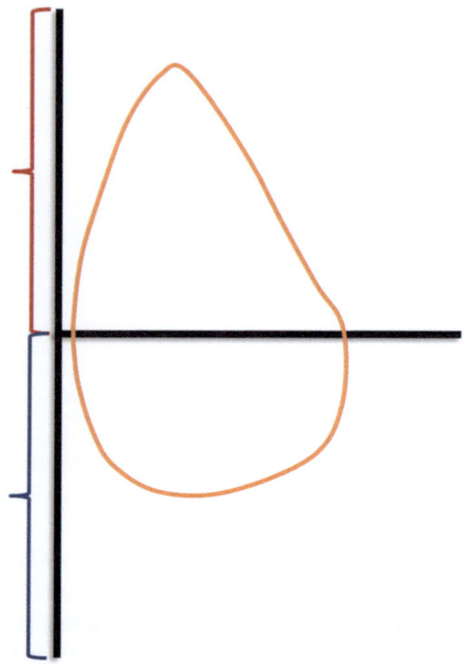

Fig. 70.1 A normal FVL

Questions

1. Draw a normal flow volume loop. Label the x- and y-axes. Where is the residual volume and total lung capacity located? Show where expiration and inspiration are represented.
2. Regarding patient effort, what is required from the patient for a flow volume loop to be accurate? What type of patients might have difficulty with a FVL?
3. Where is the peak expiratory flow rate (PEFR) located on the FVL? What are the normal values for PEFR for adult females and males? Besides a respiratory problem, what are major influences on the PEFR?
4. Where does an FVL start? What direction does the FVL follow?
5. Draw an FVL for a patient with mild COPD. Describe some key characteristics. Explain what happens to the FVL whenever there is severe COPD.
6. Draw an FVL for a patient with vocal cord paralysis.
7. Explain what an FVL for a patient with a fixed obstruction such as a goiter looks like.
8. What does an FVL typically look like for restrictive lung disease?

Answers

1. Refer to Fig. 70.1a. The y-axis represents the flow rate. On this same axis exhalation is found in the area **above** the x-axis, and inhalation is represented **below** the x-axis. The lung volume is plotted on the x-axis and the value decreases from left to right. In other words, the x-axis starts at total lung capacity at the left end, and the volume decreases progressively until residual volume is reached at the far right.
2. A flow volume loop requires the patient to provide maximal ventilatory effort. This might be difficult to obtain in pediatric patients and patients who might be in acute respiratory distress.
3. A normal peak expiratory flow rate (PEFR) is located at the highest point on a flow volume loop. A PEFR averages between 440 and 740 L/min in men and 340 and 530 L/min in women. Age and height are the major influences on PEFR [1].

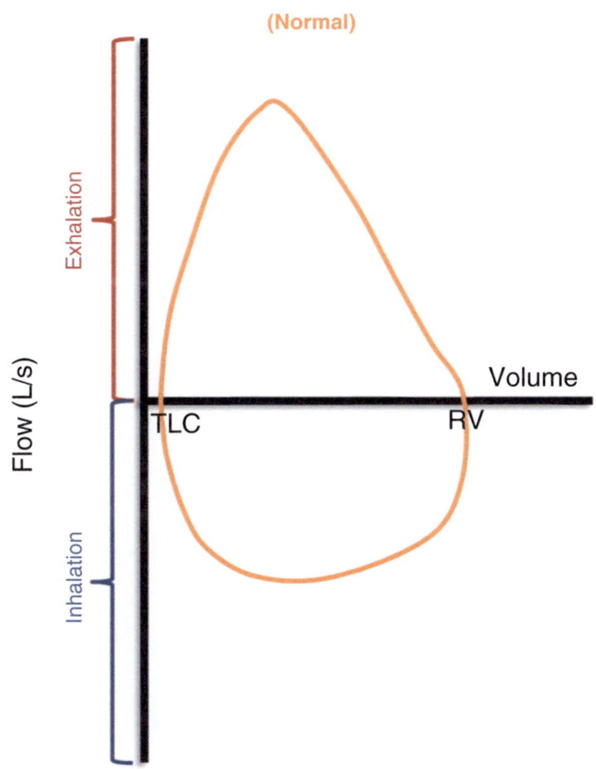

Fig. 70.1a Normal flow volume loop with labels

4. The flow volume loop begins on the left of the x-axis and follows a clockwise direction.

5. In mild COPD, the PEFR usually decreases slightly so that the initial expiratory flow is not affected significantly (Fig. 70.2). Instead of the almost linear decrease in expiratory flow, there is a "scooping" of the loop soon after the PEFR. This scooping represents the decreased amount of flow secondary to difficulty in expelling the volume of gases left in the distal airways.

   In severe COPD, the PEFR is affected more drastically. The expiratory flow does not come close to the flow of a normal subject.

6. This FVL depicts a paralyzed vocal cord adducting during inspiration resulting in decreased airflow, but expiration is not affected (Fig. 70.3).

7. The peak flow of the FVL will be decreased during exhalation and inhalation. Exhalation and inhalation flows will typically mirror each other. Since the patient is providing maximal effort, residual lung volume and total lung volume remain the same (Fig. 70.4) [2].

8. While there are many variations for FVLs representing restrictive lung diseases, typically the TLC and RV are decreased. However, the peak flows remain almost normal although for a shorter time (Fig. 70.5).

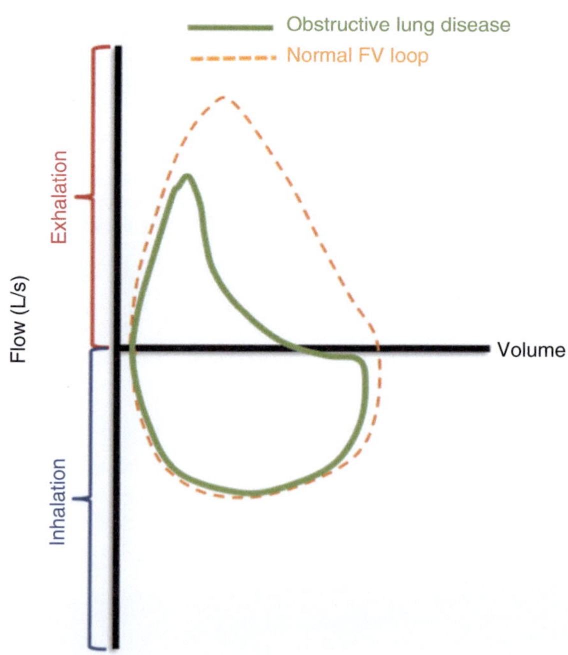

Fig. 70.2 Significant obstructive lung disease

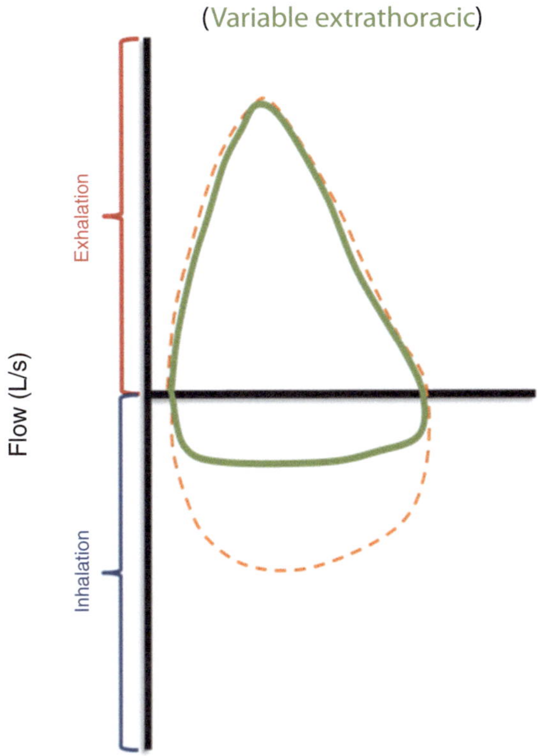

Fig. 70.3 Variable extra-thoracic obstruction

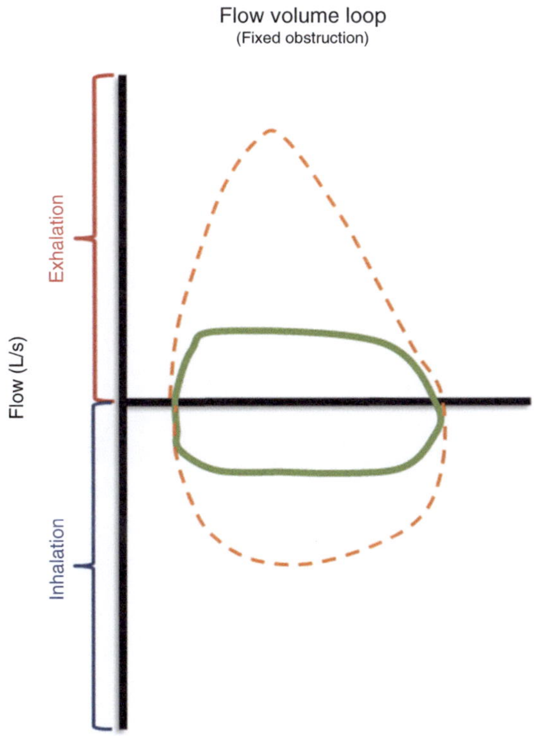

Fig. 70.4 Fixed obstruction

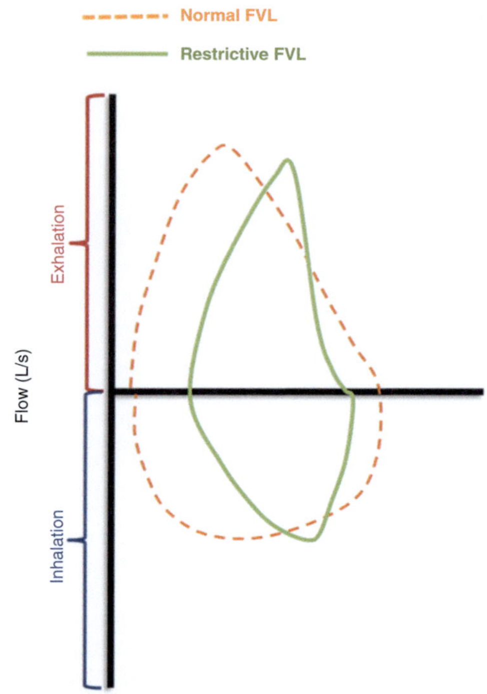

Fig. 70.5 Restrictive lung disease

References

1. Leiner GC, Abramowitz S, Small MJ, et al. Expiratory peak flow rate. Standard values for normal subjects. Use as a clinical test of ventilatory function. Am Rev Respir Dis. 1963;88:644.
2. Miller RD, Hyatt RE. Evaluation of obstructing lesions of the trachea and larynx by flow-volume loops. Am Rev Respir Dis. 1973;108(3):475–81.

Chapter 71
Cath Report

Talla A. Rousan

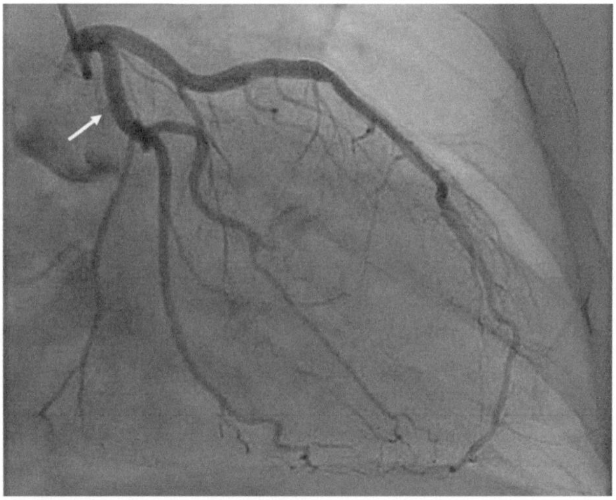

Fig. 71.1 Coronary angiogram of the left coronary artery with caudal angulation showing the left anterior descending artery and the left circumflex coronary artery (arrow)

T.A. Rousan, MD, FACC
Department of Medicine, The University of Oklahoma Health Sciences Center and the Veteran Affairs Medical Center, 800 Stanton L. Young Blvd, COM 5400, Oklahoma City, OK 73104, USA
e-mail: Talla-rousan@ouhsc.edu

T.D. Raj (ed.), *Data Interpretation in Anesthesia*,
DOI 10.1007/978-3-319-55862-2_71

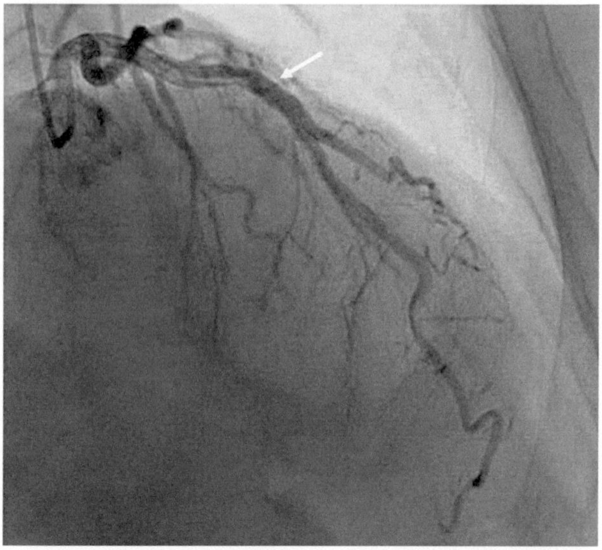

Fig. 71.2 Coronary angiogram of the left coronary artery with cranial angulation showing the left anterior descending artery (arrow) and the left circumflex coronary artery

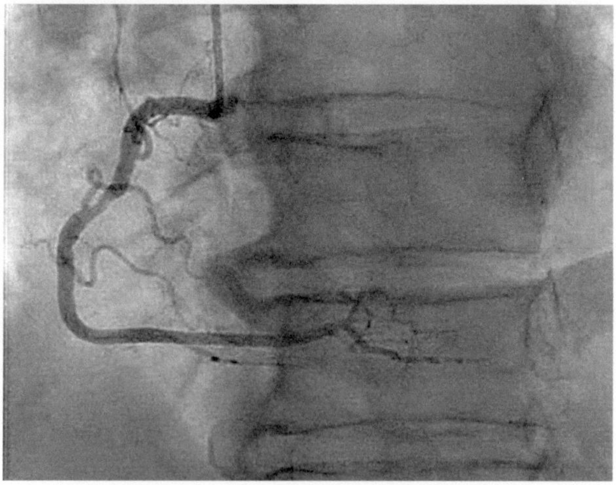

Fig. 71.3 Coronary angiogram of the right coronary artery

Questions

1. What do Figs. 71.1, 71.2, and 71.3 show?
2. Describe the normal coronary anatomy.
3. List some indications and contraindications for cardiac catheterization.
4. What are the complications of cardiac catheterization?
5. What are the determinants of myocardial demand and supply?
6. What defines a significant stenosis?
7. What are the main components of a “cath report”?

Answers

1. The images represent coronary angiography in different angiographic angulations. Coronary angiography is defined as the radiographic visualization of the coronary arteries after the injection of radiopaque iodinated contrast media [1]. This procedure is typically performed as a part of the cardiac catheterization procedure which may also include hemodynamic assessment or imaging of other cardiac chambers (usually the left ventricle). Coronary angiography is performed of both the left and right coronary arteries and bypass grafts, if present, using specialized catheters. Images are obtained in different angulations to accurately delineate the coronary anatomy. Figures 71.1 and 71.2 delineate the anatomy of the left coronary system. Figure 71.1 is a caudal angulation and best shows the left circumflex artery and its branches (arrow). Figure 71.2 is a cranial angulation view, and it best shows the left anterior descending artery and its branches (arrow). Figure 71.3 shows the right coronary artery.

2. There are two major epicardial arteries: the left main and the right coronary arteries originating typically from the left and right sinuses of Valsalva at the base of the ascending aorta [2]. The left main coronary artery further divides to the left anterior descending (LAD) and the left circumflex (LCX) coronary arteries. In some instances, the left main coronary artery also gives a third branch termed the ramus intermedius artery. The LAD and LCX further subdivide to diagonal and obtuse marginal arteries. The dominance of the coronary circulation is determined based on the origin of the posterior descending artery (PDA) which supplies the posterior part of the interventricular septum. The PDA arises from the right coronary artery in 70% of the patients rendering the circulation right dominant and from the left circumflex artery in 15% of the cases which makes the circulation left dominant. In the remainder of the cases, the PDA arises from both the right coronary and the left circumflex arteries, in which cases the circulation is termed codominant [3].

   The nomenclature of the different segments of the coronary artery tree has been described by the Bypass Angioplasty Revascularization Investigation (BARI) group, and detailed description is beyond the scope of this chapter [4]. Table 71.1 summarizes the main branches of the coronary arteries.

3. The main indication of cardiac catheterization in adults is to delineate the coronary anatomy and the severity of stenoses for suspected coronary artery disease. The procedure may be performed on elective or urgent basis [5]. Table 71.2 summarizes the main indications of coronary angiography. There are no absolute contraindications (apart from patient refusal) for cardiac catheterization. Table 71.3 summarizes the major relative contraindications.

4. Cardiac catheterization is a relatively safe procedure; however, there are a number of complications that may be associated with it, and the patient needs to be well informed about them prior to proceeding with this invasive procedure. The main complications [5, 6] encountered in this procedure are summarized in Table 71.4.

Table 71.1 The main branches of the coronary arteries (in a right dominant system)

1. Left main coronary artery
(a) Left anterior descending artery • Diagonal arteries • Septal perforator arteries
(b) Left circumflex artery • Obtuse marginal artery • Left posterolateral artery • Left posterior descending artery[a]
(c) Ramus intermedius artery[b]
2. Right coronary artery
(a) Sinus node artery[c] (b) Conus artery[d] (c) Acute marginal arteries (d) Posterior descending artery[e] (e) Posterolateral arteries

[a]Arises from the left circumflex artery in a left- or mixed-dominant coronary circulation (30% of the cases)
[b]Not present in all cases
[c]Arises from the proximal right coronary artery in 50–70% of the cases
[d]Arises from a separate ostium close to the right coronary artery ostium in 30–50% of the cases
[e]Arises from the right coronary artery in a right- or mixed-dominant coronary circulation

Table 71.2 Indications of cardiac catheterization

1. Suspected coronary artery disease (a) Stable angina (b) Unstable angina (c) Abnormal stress test
2. Acute myocardial infarction (a) ST segment elevation myocardial infarction (b) Non-ST segment elevation myocardial infarction
3. History of resuscitated sudden cardiac death
4. Valvular heart disease
5. Congenital heart disease
6. Cardiomyopathy
7. Cardiac transplant (initial assessment or follow-up)

5. The balance and interrelation between myocardial oxygen demand and supply is complex and is governed my multiple factors. The determinants of myocardial oxygen demand include the heart rate, myocardial contractility, preload (end-diastolic pressure or volume), afterload (arterial impedance), and muscle mass. The main determinants of myocardial oxygen supply include coronary blood flow and arterial oxygen content [7]. Coronary blood flow is directly proportional to coronary perfusion pressure (aortic diastolic pressure—left ventricular end-diastolic pressure) and inversely proportional to microvascular resistance (left ventricular wall tension). If demand exceeds supply, myocardial ischemia ensues with its deleterious effects.

6. A significant coronary artery stenosis is defined as an angiographic stenosis of 70% or more in a major epicardial artery. An angiographic stenosis of 50% or more

Table 71.3 Contraindications to cardiac catheterization

1. Renal failure (acute of chronic)
2. Active gastrointestinal bleeding
3. Bleeding diathesis
4. Severe anemia
5. Infection or fever
6. Recent stroke (less than 1 month)
7. Severe electrolyte imbalance
8. Severe uncontrolled hypertension
9. Severe decompensated heart failure
10. Documented allergy (anaphylactoid reaction) to iodinated contrast media
11. Uncooperative patient
12. Pregnancy

Table 71.4 Complications of cardiac catheterizations (incidence)

1. Stroke (<0.05%)
2. Myocardial infarction (<0.07%)
3. Death (<0.2%)
4. Serious ventricular arrhythmia (<0.5%)
5. Contrast-induced nephropathy (incidence varies based on baseline kidney function)
6. Contrast allergic reaction (<5%)
7. Vascular injury (<1%)
8. Access-related complications
(a) Pseudoaneurysm (0.5–9%) (b) Arteriovenous fistula (0.2–2%) (c) Arterial occlusion (0.8%) (d) Hemorrhage (hematoma (5–23%); retroperitoneal bleeding (0.1%)) (e) Infection (0.1%)

of the left main coronary artery is considered to be significant. In many instances, the stenosis does not reach the cutoff of angiographic significance, and further testing is needed. There are multiple modalities that can be used to assess the significance of an intermediate angiographic stenosis including fractional flow reserve (FFR) and intravascular ultrasound (IVUS). FFR is defined as the maximal blood flow to the myocardium in the presence of a stenosis in the supplying coronary artery, divided by the *theoretical* normal maximal flow in the same distribution [8]. A value of 0.80 or less indicates that a stenosis is hemodynamically significant and thus may be a cause of ischemia and would benefit from revascularization [9]. IVUS can be used to image the coronary artery and better characterize a stenosis. An area of less than 4.0 mm^2 (this value varies based on the different studies) in an epicardial artery or 6.0 mm^2 in the left main coronary artery is considered to be significant [10].

7. At the conclusion of cardiac catheterization, a comprehensive report is key to help in the management of the patient and for future reference. Table 71.5 summarizes the key components of the report.

Table 71.5 Components of the cardiac catheterization report

1. Patient's demographics
2. Operator(s)
3. Indication(s) of the procedure
4. Procedure(s) performed
5. Detailed narrative of the procedure including: (a) Coronary anatomy (b) Hemodynamics (c) Description of intervention (if done) (d) Medications used • Sedation • Anticoagulants • Contrast media volume
6. Complications
7. Estimated blood loss
8. Final impression
9. Recommendations

References

1. Scanlon PJ, Faxon DP, Audet AM, Carabello B, Dehmer GJ, Eagle KA, et al. ACC/AHA guidelines for coronary angiography. A report of the American College of Cardiology/American Heart Association Task Force on practice guidelines (Committee on Coronary Angiography). Developed in collaboration with the Society for Cardiac Angiography and Interventions. J Am Coll Cardiol. 1999;33(6):1756–824.
2. Angelini P. Normal and anomalous coronary arteries: definitions and classification. Am Heart J. 1989;117(2):418–34.
3. Allwork SP. The applied anatomy of the arterial blood supply to the heart in man. J Anat. 1987;153:1–16.
4. Protocol for the Bypass Angioplasty Revascularization Investigation. Circulation. 1991;84(6):1–27.
5. Kern MJ. The cardiac catheterization handbook. 5th ed. Kern MJ, editor. Philadelphia: Elsevier; 2011.
6. al. A-FMe. Arterial and venous access in the cardiac catheterization lab. 1st ed. M. A-F, editor. New Jersey: Rutgers University Press; 2016.
7. Burkhoff D, Naidu SS. The science behind percutaneous hemodynamic support: a review and comparison of support strategies. Catheter Cardiovasc Interv. 2012;80(5):816–29.
8. Pijls NH, De Bruyne B, Peels K, Van Der Voort PH, Bonnier HJ, Bartunek JKJJ, et al. Measurement of fractional flow reserve to assess the functional severity of coronary-artery stenoses. N Engl J Med. 1996;334(26):1703–8.
9. Kern MJ, Lerman A, Bech JW, De Bruyne B, Eeckhout E, Fearon WF, et al. Physiological assessment of coronary artery disease in the cardiac catheterization laboratory: a scientific statement from the American Heart Association Committee on Diagnostic and Interventional Cardiac Catheterization, Council on Clinical Cardiology. Circulation. 2006;114(12):1321–41.
10. Jasti V, Ivan E, Yalamanchili V, Wongpraparut N, Leesar MA. Correlations between fractional flow reserve and intravascular ultrasound in patients with an ambiguous left main coronary artery stenosis. Circulation. 2004;110(18):2831–6.

Chapter 72
CIED: Interrogation

Ranganathan Govindaraj

Fig. 72.1

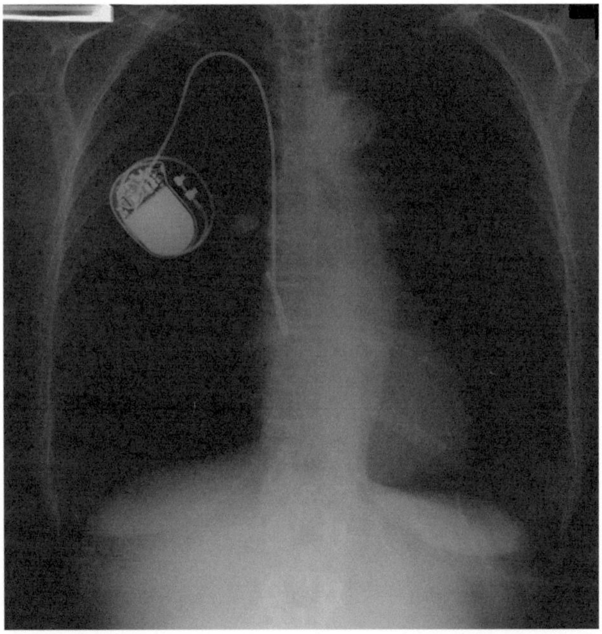

R. Govindaraj, MD, FRCA
Associate Professor for Anesthesia and Pain, Department of Anesthesiology,
UTMB, Galveston, TX 77555, USA

Director for Ultrasound Guided Regional Anesthesia, Galveston, TX 77555, USA
e-mail: gorangan@utmb.edu

T.D. Raj (ed.), *Data Interpretation in Anesthesia*,
DOI 10.1007/978-3-319-55862-2_72

You are contacted about a 61-year-old female patient who is starting a course of electroconvulsive therapy (ECT) for depression the following day. She has been a nursing home resident for the prior 2 years, has not seen a cardiologist in that time, and is a poor historian. Her comorbidities include hypertension and coronary artery disease treated with angioplasty and stents 5 years ago. A chest X-ray was done 2 days prior to rule out pneumonia and is shown below. No other information is available and there is no family.

1. What does the X-ray demonstrate?
2. What needs to be done next?
3. What is the information that needs to be communicated with the CIED team?
4. What information does the CIED team communicate with the anesthesiologist?
5. Name some sources of electromagnetic interference (EMI).
6. What are the adverse effects of EMI on CIED?
7. Is it necessary to interrogate this device? If so, why?
8. What is the effect of ECT on CIED?
9. How is anesthesia managed?

Answers

1. The chest X-ray shows what appears to be a pacemaker device over the right chest with a single lead in the right atrium. Pacemakers have one or two thin leads, and the tip of the lead can be in the atrium, right ventricle, and/or left ventricle as opposed to an ICD which will have two radiodense shock coils with one in the SVC area and the second in the right ventricle.

2. Apart from the routine pre-anesthesia assessment, the CIED needs to be addressed. ECT is an elective procedure and is a source of electromagnetic interference (EMI). As per the guidelines, before an **elective procedure**, the patient's cardiologist, if known, is contacted for recommendations. If not known, then the CIED team (cardiologist, cardiac electrophysiologist, device clinic nurses and staff) from the same or a neighboring hospital is involved.

3. Information that need to be communicated with the CIED team [1, 4]:
   (a) Intended surgical procedure and its anatomic location
   (b) Location of the pulse generator
   (c) Patient position during the procedure
   (d) Type of electrocautery to be used whether monopolar or bipolar
   (e) Presence of other sources of EMI
   (f) Cardioversion or defibrillation during the procedure
   (g) Venue for the procedure
   (h) Postoperative plan: Day case/inpatient with telemetry bed
   (i) Surgical procedure that can cause mechanical damage the leads to CIED

4. Information that the CIED team communicates with the Anesthesiologist [1, 4]:
   (a) Details of the settings in the CIED and their functioning status.
   (b) Date of last device interrogation (should be 6 months for AICD and 1 year for pacemaker).
   (c) Device type, manufacturer, and model
   (d) Indication for device placement.
   (e) Life of the battery.
   (f) Age of the leads (should be >3 months).
   (g) Current programming mode.
   (h) Is the patient pacemaker dependent?
   (i) Response of the device to magnet placement.
   (j) Any alert status on the device.
   (k) Pacing threshold on the last occasion.
   (l) Individualized prescription or perioperative recommendation based on patient information, device characteristics, and surgical factors.

5. Sources of EMI in a hospital setting [2]:
   (a) Electrocautery (especially monopolar electrocautery).
   (b) Evoked potential monitors.
   (c) Nerve stimulators.
   (d) Fasciculations.

   (e) External defibrillation.
   (f) Magnetic resonance imaging (MRI).
   (g) Radiofrequency ablation.
   (h) Extracorporeal shock wave lithotripsy (ESWL).
   (i) Electroconvulsive therapy (ECT).
   (j) Other sources of interference include large tidal volumes and shivering.

Sources of EMI in daily life [3]:
   (a) Digital music players
   (b) Magnets in stereo speakers, headphones, toys, jewelries, and some clothes
   (c) Metal detectors
   (d) Tasers
   (e) Cellular phones
   (f) Portable home phones
   (g) Auto engines
   (h) Arc welding equipment
   (i) Cockpits
   (j) RFID equipment
   (k) High-voltage power coils

6. Adverse effects of EMI [1, 4]:
   (a) Damage to the CIED circuitry.
   (b) Failure to pace, defibrillate, or both.
   (c) Asynchronous pacing.
   (d) Arrhythmia detection and AICD shocks.
   (e) Rate-adaptive sensor activation.
   (f) Electrical reset is a very rare occurrence that can happen when an energy surge directly contacts the CIED generator and results in major hardware/software failure. The reset mode is a safety backup, and depending on the manufacturer, the device will go to a preset rate and then has to be reprogrammed or replaced. The most common cause is therapeutic ionizing radiation rather than electrocautery or cardioversion.
   (g) EMI could produce enough current to flow from the generator to the pacing electrode and damage the tissue-lead interface. Acute injury may lead to loss of sensing and pacing.

7. For reasons mentioned in answer 4 and as there has not been a cardiology consultation in 2 years, this device needs to be interrogated/checked.

8. In ECT, a brief electrical current (duration 1–2 s), although sometimes a more prolonged stimulus, is delivered to the head triggering a seizure. Transient ECG changes such as increased P wave amplitude, altered QRS shape, and ST-T wave abnormalities may occur. The physiological stresses of ECT which include bradycardia, hypotension followed by tachycardia, and hypertension may provoke cardiac failure in patients with marginal cardiac function. With the brief shocks, hemodynamically significant pacing inhibition is unlikely. Similarly, with ICDs on standard programming, inappropriate shocks from this brief electrical therapy

are also unlikely. If a more prolonged stimulus is used, then there is a potential for significant bradycardia and ICD shocks. A prolonged, intense seizure may cause myopotential inhibition of the device in pacemaker-dependent patients [1].

9. Monitoring should include continuous ECG and continuous peripheral pulse. In pacemaker-dependent patients, a magnet is placed over the generator, and in others it is made available. For an AICD, a magnet is kept handy. It is also advisable to know the ICD tachycardia detection rate and be prepared to use the magnet if the heart rate, post-ECT, approaches that level. Temporary pacing systems and external cardioversion devices should be made available. Postoperatively, if the device was programmed pre-procedure, then the patient should not leave a monitored area until reprogramming and device function have been restored. Otherwise, recommendation for the follow-up assessment and reprogramming needed after surgery and the timing of postoperative CIED evaluation are based on the CIED recommendations [1, 4].

References

1. Crossley GH, Poole JE, Rozner MA, et al. The Heart Rhythm Society (HRS)/American Society of Anesthesiologists (ASA) expert consensus statement on the perioperative management of patients with implantable defibrillators, pacemakers and arrhythmia monitors: facilities and patient management. Heart Rhythm. 2011;8(7):1114–54. PMID: 21722856. doi:10.1016/j.hrthm.2010.12.023.
2. Stone ME, Salter B, Fischer A. Perioperative management of patients with cardiac implantable electronic devices. Br J Anaesth. 2011;107(Suppl 1):i16–26. doi:10.1093/bja/aer354.
3. Beinart R, Nazarian S. Effects of external electrical and magnetic fields on pacemakers and defibrillators: from engineering principles to clinical practice. Circulation. 2013;128(25):2799–809.
4. American Society of Anesthesiologists. Practice advisory for the perioperative management of patients with cardiac implantable electronic devices: pacemakers and implantable cardioverter-defibrillators. An updated report by the American Society of Anesthesiologists Task Force on perioperative management of patients with cardiac implantable electronic devices. Anesthesiology. 2011;114:247–61.

Chapter 73
Pressure–Volume Curves

Marcos E. Gomes

The image below is a snapshot of a pressure–volume curve of a patient on a ventilator in the ICU.

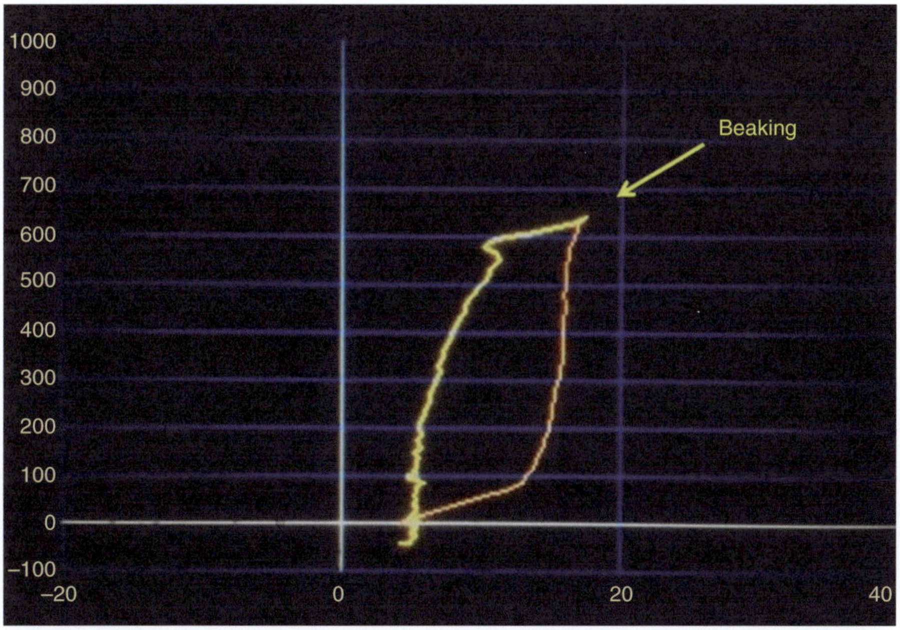

Fig. 73.1 Dynamic pressure–volume curve showing "beaking"

M.E. Gomes, MD
Department of Anesthesiology, University of Oklahoma Health Sciences Center,
750 NE 13th Street, Suite 200, Oklahoma City, OK 73104, USA
e-mail: mewgomes@gmail.com

T.D. Raj (ed.), *Data Interpretation in Anesthesia*,
DOI 10.1007/978-3-319-55862-2_73

1. What does pressure–volume (P–V) curve describe?
2. What is the goal of using P–V curves?
3. Does it improve outcome?
4. What are inflection points on the P–V curve?
5. How can one select appropriate PEEP?
6. What are the benefits of adequate PEEP?

Answers

1. Pressure–volume curves describe the mechanical behavior of the lungs and chest wall during inspiration and expiration, giving the clinician a sense of the patient's lung and chest wall compliance (Fig. 73.1). It has been studied in many disease states but most extensively in patients with ARDS. Different than static pressure–volume curves, dynamic pressure–volume curves are obtained during actual gas flow through the respiratory cycle, and add the variable of airway resistance to the equation [1]. Many ICU and OR ventilators currently come with the built-in capability to record constant flow dynamic pressure–volume curves.

2. The reason clinicians initiated the analysis of pressure–volume curves in different disease scenarios was to assess individual patient's respiratory mechanics and possibly customize the ventilator settings according to their findings. Ultimately, the goal was to optimize the ventilator settings for each patient and improve compliance, thus protecting them from ventilator-induced lung injury.

3. Despite the initial enthusiasm and excitement that the use of P–V curves could improve morbidity and mortality, it has not been borne out in studies. Difficulties in measurements and improper use of the information may have been contributors to the lack of evidence and have raised questions about the clinical usefulness of this method. Since the development of new ventilators with the built-in capacity to measure dynamic pressure–volume curves, promising research has been ongoing and hopefully will result in the initially desired clinical outcomes.

4. Lower inflection point (LIP) represents the lung volume at which some alveoli close (closing capacity). The upper inflection point (UIP) represents the start of overdistension or the stop of recruitment. Both lower and upper inflection points can be identified on a static respiratory system compliance curve (static pressure–volume curve, Fig. 73.2). In theory, the lungs should be ventilated between these two inflection points, although no outcome study has shown significant benefit with this approach. In fact, studies have considered the LIP to be the

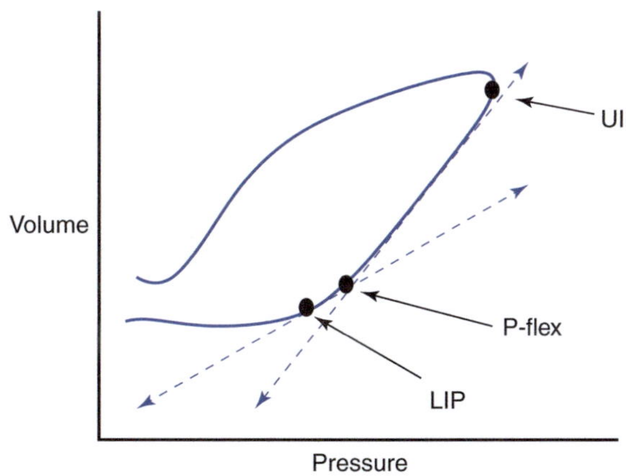

Fig. 73.2 Graphic representation of static pressure–volume curve showing the P-flex point

minimal pressure above which mechanical ventilation should take place in ARDS. Similarly, LIP is proposed as the starting point for PEEP titration in that setting. Gattinoni et al. suggested that the calculation of what they called "P-flex" could result in the optimal PEEP for a given patient. P-flex is the intersection point between the slopes of the low-compliance segment and high-compliance segment (Fig. 73.2) and corresponds roughly to the lower inflection point. Static pressure–volume curves are difficult to obtain in routine care; therefore, dynamic compliance curves, available in most ventilators, are being used instead (Fig. 73.1). Typically, inflection points are not easily identified on dynamic curves, but when visible, the presence of a lower inflection point may indicate insufficient PEEP because it represents a sudden increase in lung volume at a certain pressure. In an optimized and recruited lung, achieving a given pressure should not be required to open several alveoli at once, which makes LIP more visible. Instead, alveoli should be gradually, slowly, and uniformly opened, making LIP less visible. In Fig. 73.3, it is easier to identify the LIP and understand how recruitment (change in tidal volume) only happens after 10 cmH_2O of pressure is applied to the airway. This high pressure requirement in order to promote a change in volume implies insufficient PEEP. On the other hand, the presence of an upper inflection point may indicate excessive PEEP, over inflation, or overall excessive pressure in the respiratory system. The latter is termed "beaking" (Fig. 73.1) [2, 3].

5. The importance of selecting an adequate level of PEEP stems from the goal of not only lung recruitment for improved compliance and oxygenation but also optimization of respiratory mechanics and avoidance of the development of ventilator-induced lung injury. This type of injury can occur from different mechanisms: barotrauma (high alveolar pressure), volutrauma (alveolar overdis-

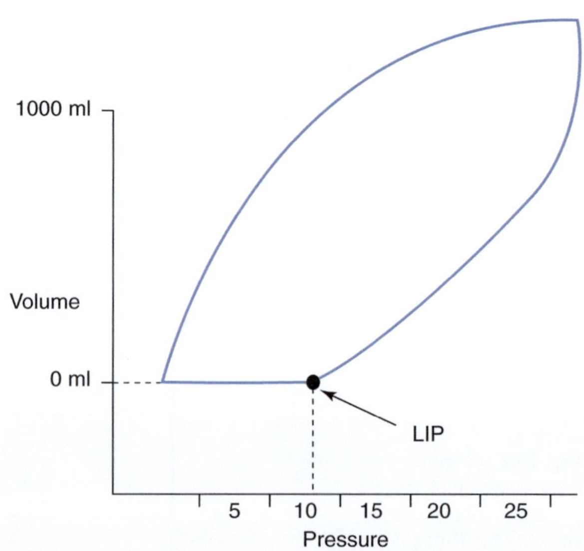

Fig. 73.3 Graphic representation of a dynamic pressure–volume curve showing easy visualization of the LIP, suggesting insufficient PEEP

tension), atelectotrauma (cyclic opening/closing of alveoli), and biotrauma (release of inflammatory mediators). Ideal ventilator settings imply a combination of PEEP and small tidal volume that causes the least insult to the lung. The only ventilator setting that has been associated with improved outcome is avoiding a plateau pressure above 30 cmH_2O. Stepwise algorithms for PEEP increments and other methods suggesting specific PEEP values for certain clinical scenarios have been questioned by investigators, mostly due to lack of benefit in survival statistics. Examples of such methods are staircase recruitment maneuver, adjusting according to FiO_2 requirements, adjusting higher than the lower inflection point on a pressure–volume curve, adjusting to maximize static compliance (TV/Pplat-PEEP), adjusting to maintain plateau pressure of 28–30 cmH_2O, and adjusting by measurement of transpulmonary pressures with esophageal balloon, titration to lowest intrapulmonary shunt (highest SvO_2) [3].

6. Adequate PEEP increases FRC, recruits atelectatic and collapsed lung areas, optimizes ventilation/perfusion ratio, reduces right to left shunt, and avoids end-expiratory alveolar collapse. Potential disadvantages are reduction of cardiac output by diminished venous return, reduction of renal/hepatic/splanchnic circulations, overdistension/rupture of alveoli, and increase of intracranial hypertension.

References

1. Jonson B, et al. Pressure–volume curves and compliance in acute lung injury. Am J Respir Crit Care Med. 1999;159:1172–8.
2. Harris S. Pressure–volume curves of the respiratory system. Respir Care. 2005;50(1):78–99.
3. Pestana D, et al. Adjusting positive end-expiratory pressure and tidal volume in acute respiratory distress syndrome according to the pressure–volume curve. Acta Anaesthesiol Scand. 2003;47:326–34.

Part V
Conceptual Images

Chapter 74
Dissociation Curve

Raghuvender Ganta and Tilak D. Raj

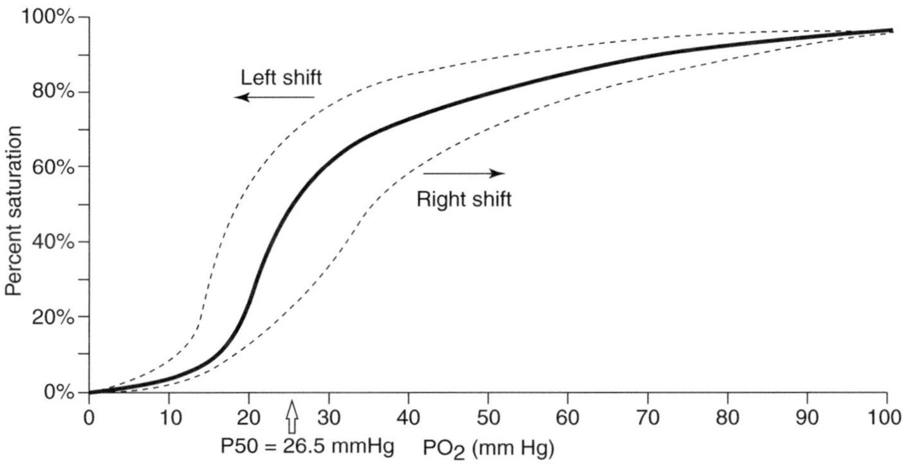

Fig. 74.1

1. What does the above image in Fig. 74.1 depict?
2. What is P_{50}?
3. How do you determine the oxygen content?
4. At what point can cyanosis be detected?

R. Ganta, MD, FRCA (✉)
Department of Anesthesiology, VA Hospital, OUMC,
921 NE 13th Street, Oklahoma City, OK 73104, USA
e-mail: raghuvender-Ganta@ouhsc.edu

T.D. Raj, MD, MRCP, FRCA
Department of Anesthesiology, Alliance Health Midwest, Midwest City, OK, USA
e-mail: tilakdraj@gmail.com

T.D. Raj (ed.), *Data Interpretation in Anesthesia*,
DOI 10.1007/978-3-319-55862-2_74

5. What variables shift the curve to the left and to the right and how does that affect oxygen transport?
6. What is Fick equation?
7. What is Bohr effect?
8. What is Haldane effect?

Answers

1. This is the oxyhemoglobin dissociation curve which demonstrates the measured relationship between the partial pressure of oxygen (PO_2) on the x-axis and the oxygen saturation (SaO_2) on the y-axis. The graph is sigmoid or S shaped. Initially, in the steep portion of the curve, the hemoglobin's affinity for oxygen increases with maximum O_2 loading, and then the graph levels off around PO_2 of 60 mmHg with little change even when the PO_2 is increased significantly.

2. P_{50} is the oxygen tension at which hemoglobin is 50% saturated which is typically around 26 mm Hg and is a measure of hemoglobin's affinity for oxygen.

3. The blood oxygen content (CaO_2) is calculated as the sum of the oxygen bound by hemoglobin (Hb) and the oxygen dissolved in the plasma.

   O_2 content = oxygen bound to hemoglobin + oxygen dissolved in blood.

   $CaO_2 = (1.39 \times Hb \times SaO_2/100) + (PaO_2 \times 0.003)$.

   For example, if Hb is 15 g/dL, SaO_2 is 100%, and PaO_2 is 100 mm Hg, then

   $CaO_2 = (15 \times 1.39 \times 1) + (100 \times 0.003)$

   $= 20.85 + 0.3$

   $= 21.15$ mL/dL.

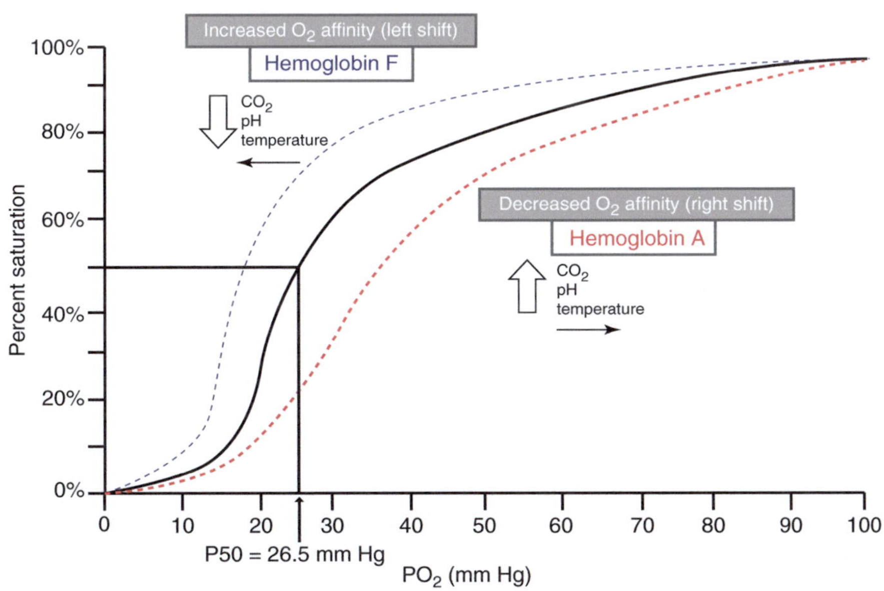

Fig. 74.2 Factors that shift the oxyhemoglobin dissociation curve

Left shift	Right shift
Alkalosis	Acidosis
Hypothermia	Hyperthermia
Decreased 2,3-DPG	Increased 2,3-DPG
Abnormal hemoglobin (fetal)	Abnormal hemoglobin
Carboxyhemoglobin	Increased CO_2
Methemoglobin	

4. Cyanosis can be detected at an SaO_2 of approximately 80%. Clear cyanosis can appear at an SaO_2 of approximately 67%. The appearance is also affected by skin perfusion, skin pigmentation, and hemoglobin concentration.

5. Variables shifting the oxyhemoglobin dissociation curve.

Diseases or other conditions (Fig. 74.2) could shift the dissociation curve either to the right (increasing P_{50}) or to the left (decreasing P_{50}). A rightward shift indicates that a higher PO_2 is required for the same 50% Hb saturation. This means lower oxygen affinity. This is seen in the peripheral tissues where oxygen "unloading" happens. Conversely, a leftward shift increases hemoglobin's affinity for oxygen [1, 2]. This is seen in the lungs where oxygen "loading" happens.
Five variables affect tissue oxygenation [3]:

1. Hemoglobin concentration.
2. Hemoglobin oxygen saturation (SaO_2).
3. Hemoglobin affinity for oxygen (P_{50}).
4. Cardiac output.
5. Tissue oxygen consumption.

6. The Fick equation expresses the relationship between oxygen consumption (VO_2), arteriovenous oxygen content difference ($CaO_2 - CvO_2$), and cardiac output (QT):

   Fick equation: $VO_2 = QT \times (CaO_2 - CvO_2)$

   CaO_2 = arterial oxygen content = 20 m/dL

   CvO_2 = mixed venous oxygen content = 15 mL/dL

   $CaO_2 - CvO_2$ = normal extraction for oxygen = 5 mL/dL

   The arteriovenous difference is a good measure of the overall adequacy of oxygen delivery.

   With a normal oxygen consumption of approximately 250 mL/min and a cardiac output of 5000 mL/min, the normal arteriovenous difference by this equation is 5 mL O_2/dL blood. Note that the normal extraction ratio for oxygen $(CaO_2 - CvO_2)/CaO_2$ is 5 mL/20 mL or 25%; thus, the body normally consumes only 25% of the oxygen carried on hemoglobin.

7. The Bohr effect is a physiological phenomenon, and it describes the inverse relationship of the hemoglobin's affinity for oxygen to acidity and to the concentration of carbon dioxide. An increase in CO_2 (which reacts with water to form carbonic acid) increases acid and lowers pH which leads to O_2 unloading by

hemoglobin. This effect facilitates the oxygen transport as hemoglobin binds to oxygen in the lung (less CO_2 and acid) and releases it in the tissues (more CO_2 and acid).

8. Oxygenated hemoglobin has a reduced capacity for CO_2, and conversely reduced Hb has an increased capacity. This is known as Haldane effect, which is of physiologic importance in governing CO_2 transport [4]. Reduced Hb in the tissues facilitates CO_2 "pickup," and in the oxygen-rich capillaries of the lung, this property promotes dissociation of CO_2 from the Hb and thereby elimination.

References

1. Morgan GE Jr. Clinical anesthesiology. 3rd ed. New York: Lange Medical Books/McGraw-Hill Medical Publishing Division; 2002.
2. Collins J-A, Rudenski A, Gibson J, et al. Relating oxygen partial pressure, saturation and content: the haemoglobin-oxygen dissociation curve. Breathe. 2015;11:194–201.
3. Faust RJ. Anesthesiology review. 4th ed. New York: Churchill Livingston; 2014.
4. Linda CS. Physiology. 5th ed. Philadelphia: Saunders/Elsevier; 2014.

Suggested Reading

Lumb AB. Nunn's applied respiratory physiology. 5th ed. Boston: Butterworth-Heinemann; 2000.
West JB. Respiratory physiology—the essentials. 6th ed. Philadelphia: Lippincott Williams & Wilkins; 2000.

Chapter 75
Frank-Starling Curve

Deepinder Mann

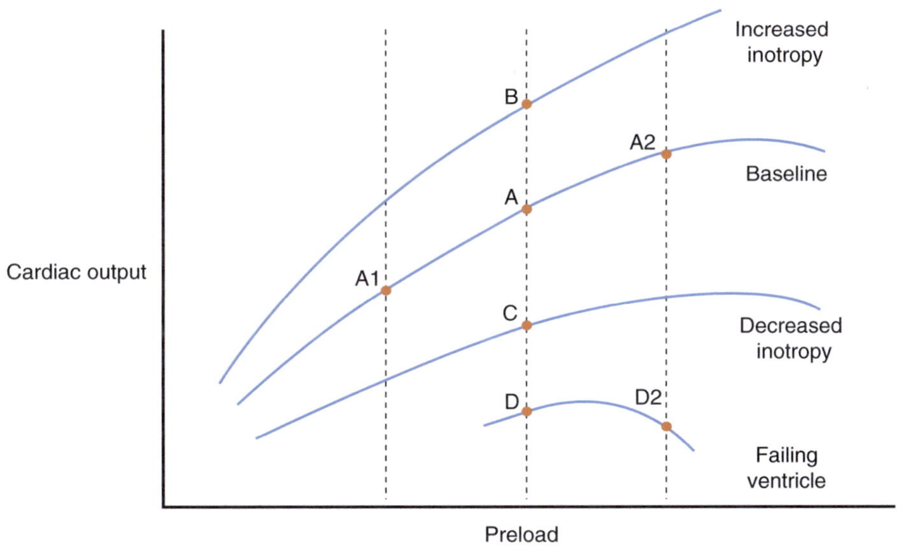

Fig. 75.1

Depicted above is a family of cardiac function curves representing a ventricle under various conditions. Point A represents baseline cardiac function with normal preload; points A1 and A2 show states of decreased and increase preload, respectively. After reviewing this figure, please answer the following questions.

D. Mann, DO
Department of Anesthesiology, University of Texas Medical Branch,
301 University Blvd, Galveston, TX 77555, USA
e-mail: dsmann@utmb.edu

T.D. Raj (ed.), *Data Interpretation in Anesthesia*,
DOI 10.1007/978-3-319-55862-2_75

Questions

1. What is Frank-Starling mechanism? Intracellularly, how can it cause a more forceful contraction?
2. For the Frank-Starling curves depicted in Fig. 75.1, what are other parameters that can be substituted for the cardiac output label on the y-axis?
3. What parameters can replace preload on the x-axis?
4. What physiological changes might cause the system to move from:
   (a) Point A to A2
   (b) Point A to A1
   (c) Point A to B
   (d) Point A to D
5. Graphically, which direction(s) will adding a beta-blocker shift a ventricle on Fig. 75.1?
6. Following a premature ventricular contraction in a normal ventricle, how will the force generated by the next contraction change?
7. After a single bolus dose of phenylephrine, what effect can be expected on cardiac output?
8. If starting at point D2 on Fig. 75.1, would a fluid bolus be expected to increase cardiac output? If not, what interventions could increase output?

Answers

1. The Frank-Starling mechanism describes a relationship where increasing ventricular filling increases cardiac output. Increased preload increases sarcomere stretch inside cardiac myocytes which generate more force during contraction and thereby allows the heart to eject more blood. However, there is a limit to which this relationship can be maintained. In failing ventricles, overstretch can limit or decrease cardiac output. In these cases, reducing myocyte stretch to a more optimal length can improve overall cardiac function. Although the cellular basis has not been definitively determined, the most widely accepted mechanism is that as sarcomeres are stretched, there is a length-dependent reduction in the spacing between thick and thin filaments. As the filaments are stretched and get closer together, tropomyosin on the thin filament becomes more sensitive to calcium. When contraction occurs, the sarcoplasmic reticulum releases calcium. The more sensitive tropomyosin now allows more actin-myosin cross-bridges to form yielding greater force generation [1–3].

2. Multiple measurements have been developed to describe how well or efficiently a cardiac ventricle can pump. Essentially any measure that varies directly to cardiac output can be substituted on the y-axis. Some of the more popular metrics include venous return, stroke volume, cardiac index, and stroke work.

3. Measurements that are essentially synonyms for preload on a cardiac function curve include end-diastolic volume, end-diastolic pressure, right atrial pressure, and pulmonary capillary wedge pressure.

4. Cardiac output can change by moving between different points on a single curve or changing to different curves. Physiologic changes altering preload can cause movement along the same cardiac curve, while changes in inotropy can cause shifts to different curves. On the steep, positively sloped portion of a cardiac function curve (sometimes called the preload dependent segment), cardiac output increases as ventricular stretch increases. If preload continues to increase, the point of overstretch is reached and eventually passed. Cardiac output plateaus and then begins to fall. The plateaued segment is sometimes called the preload independent portion.
   (a) Moving from A to A2 shows an increase in cardiac output that is the result of increasing preload. Fluid resuscitation, passive leg raise, and decreasing PEEP are examples of interventions that can cause such a change.

   Point A2 also represents the end of the preload-dependent and the start of the preload-independent portion of the cardiac function curve. Cardiac output levels off beyond A2 and eventually drops as overdistension is reached.
   (b) Decreasing preload shifts the systems leftward. As ventricular filling approaches 0, so does the cardiac output. Physiologically, anything that decreases venous return will cause a move from A to A1. Examples include hemorrhage, dehydration, obstructive shock, and high levels of PEEP.
   (c) With preload being constant, moving from point A to B requires either an increase in cardiac inotropy or a decrease in afterload. Catecholamines (such

as epinephrine or dobutamine) that stimulate beta-1 adrenergic receptors in the heart can cause a more forceful contraction by a stretch-independent mechanism. Increasing intracellular calcium levels can also increase inotropy independent of preload. Administering calcium or a phosphodiesterase-3 inhibitor (PDE3), like milrinone, is a clinical way of achieving this.

Afterload is the pressure the ventricle must overcome in order to eject blood. Therefore, reducing afterload will also increase cardiac output independent of myocyte stretch. Clinically there are many pharmacologic agents that decrease afterload. Example drug classes include the following: nitric oxide inducers (such as nitroglycerin, nitroprusside, and isosorbide), alpha-1 adrenergic antagonists (such as prazosin), beta-2 adrenergic agonists, and PDE3 inhibitors.

Exercise, through multiple mechanisms including beta-1 and beta-2 receptor agonism, increases preload and decreases afterload simultaneously.

(d) Shifting to a lower cardiac function curve, such as from A to D, indicates that inotropy has dropped significantly independent of stretch. A clinical example of this is myocardial infarction causing myocyte damage or death. Fewer sarcomeres will be present, so less force will be generated. The result is a downward shift in the cardiac function curve as well as a decreased slope in the preload dependent portion.

5. Beta-1 adrenergic antagonists decrease cardiac chronotropy and inotropy. The overall effect will be a shift toward the right and toward a lower curve. Depending on the starting point, this can result in an increase or decrease in cardiac output:
   (a) Pure inotropy reduction will lead to less cardiac output at any fixed preload. Graphically, this will be a shift to a lower curve (such as from A to C).
   (b) However, there are situations when beta-1 antagonism can yield a net increase in cardiac output. If the ventricle is still in the preload-dependent segment of a given curve, a lower heart rate can allow for more time in diastole and therefore more filling. Also, beta-blockers can calm some cardiac arrhythmias. Better atrial-ventricular coordination preserves the function of atrial kick, which increases ventricular filling.
   (c) If starting at point A1, more preload will shift the ventricle toward point A. Inotropy reduction will drop the ventricle to a lower curve. Will it be as low as point C (or lower)? It depends on how sensitive the myocytes are and how much they are relying on beta stimulation in their current state. The final position will be lower than point A, but the net result could be a higher cardiac output than the original A1 starting point.

6. Following a PVC, there is a longer than usual time for diastole, more ventricular filling and myocyte stretch. More force will be generated during the next contraction, and the extra blood that entered the ventricle will be ejected.

7. Phenylephrine causes vasoconstriction via alpha-1 adrenergic agonism. This can cause an increase in afterload, which can decrease cardiac output. However, vasoconstriction can also shift pooled blood from peripheral and splanchnic

venous beds into central circulation; this can increase preload. The resulting net effect is controversial and may depend on the starting point on the cardiac function curve. Porcine models suggest that starting on the steep (preload dependent) part of a cardiac function curve causes a net increase in cardiac output [4]. While giving phenylephrine on the flatter (preload independent) part of the cardiac function curve causes a net decrease in cardiac output.

8. At point D2, the ventricle is overdistended and in failure. Additional fluid will not improve stroke volume. Decreasing myocyte stretch so that sarcomeres can get closer to their optimal length would be more helpful. Diuretics or hemoconcentration is more appropriate; the result will be moving from point D2 toward D. Adding inotropic support or significantly decreasing afterload with vasodilators can also improve cardiac output. These changes can shift the entire curve closer to curve C.

References

1. Hall J. Cardiac muscle: the heart as a pump and function of the valves. In: Hall J, editor. Guyton and Hall textbook of medical physiology. 13th ed. Philadelphia: Elsevier; 2016. p. 245–258
2. Noble MI. The Frank—Starling Curve. Clinical Science. 1978 Jan 1;54(1):1–7.
3. Kobirumaki-Shimozawa F, Inoue T, Shintani SA, et al. Cardiac thin filament regulation and the Frank–Starling mechanism. J Physiol Sci. 2014;64:221.
4. Maxime C, Zhongping J, et al. Effects of phenylephrine on cardiac output and venous return depend on the position of the heart on the Frank-Starling relationship. J Appl Physiol. 2012;113(2):281–9.

Chapter 76
West's Zones

Abhinava S. Madamangalam and Tilak D. Raj

Fig. 76.1

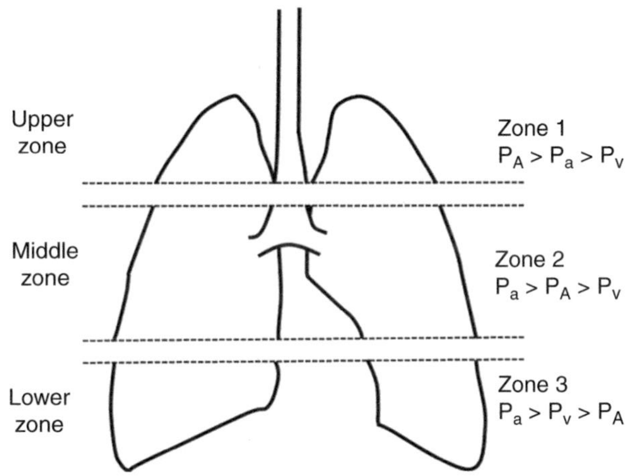

1. What does the above image depict, and what are the pressure profiles in the zones?
2. Describe the factors that affect pulmonary vascular resistance [1].
3. What are the clinical implications of the zones of west?

A.S. Madamangalam, MBBS, MD (✉)
Department of Anesthesiology and Perioperative Medicine, Augusta University Medical Center, 1120 15th Street, BI-2144, Augusta, GA 30912, USA
e-mail: amadamangalam@augusta.edu

T.D. Raj, MD, MRCP, FRCA
Department of Anesthesiology, Alliance Health Midwest, Midwest City, OK, USA
e-mail: tilakdraj@gmail.com

T.D. Raj (ed.), *Data Interpretation in Anesthesia*,
DOI 10.1007/978-3-319-55862-2_76

Answers

1. The image above depicts West's zones of the lung which describe the effects of gravity and the differing pressures within the alveoli, pulmonary arteries, and veins on ventilation and perfusion.

   When one views the vascular resistance in an upright individual, three lung perfusion zones are identified. The hydrostatic pressure in the pulmonary vascular system of an upright individual varies from the apex to the base of the lungs and therefore the perfusion characteristics vary as well. Pulmonary arterial pressure is 5 mmHg at the apex and 25 mmHg at the base, and pulmonary venous pressure is −5 mmHg at the apex and +15 mmHg at the bases.

   Zone 1 is not seen in normal lungs. It may be seen in positive pressure ventilation or after hemorrhage. Alveolar pressure exceeds pulmonary vascular pressures. Hence the pulmonary vessels are collapsed, and no flow occurs causing alveolar dead space.

   Zone 2 occurs about 3 cm above the level of the heart. P_v (venous pressure) is subatmospheric, and therefore the higher P_A (aveolar pressure) tends to compress the vessels on the venous side of the pulmonary circulation. Blood flow is driven by the gradient (P_a = arterial pressure) $P_a - P_A$. Flow occurs in pulses-starling resistor or waterfall effect.

   Zone 3 is in the bottom of the lungs below the level of the heart. When the pulmonary arterial and venous pressures are greater than the alveolar pressure, the alveolar pressure has no effect on circulation [2].

2. The pulmonary vascular circuit is a very low-resistance system. Many factors contribute to the control of this resistance. The largest contributor to the pulmonary vascular resistance (PVR) on the arterial side is from the capillaries. These vessels, at their most diminutive size are very thin walled and can therefore be affected by pressure exerted on them, either intra or extravascular pressure. The extravascular pressures are alveolar and interstitial pressures in the lung. PVR is lowest at functional residual capacity (FRC); at high lung volumes, the intra-alveolar vessels are compressed, and at low lung volumes, the extra-alveolar vessels are compressed.

   Large changes in cardiac output produce only small changes in PVR due to recruitment and distension of pulmonary vessels. Both acute and chronic lung diseases increase PVR. Other factors that influence PVR include autonomic factors (alpha-adrenergic, vasoconstriction; beta-adrenergic, vasodilatation) and local metabolic factors (vasodilators such as Nitric Oxide (NO) and prostacyclin; vasoconstrictors such as serotonin, histamine, noradrenaline and hypercapnia). Low PAO_2 produces vasoconstriction (HPV-hypoxic pulmonary vasoconstriction).

3. During measurement of the pulmonary wedge pressure, an assumption is made that there is a clear unobstructed communication between the pulmonary artery and veins, as the wedge pressure is measured from the right side of the heart. For the wedge pressure to be an accurate reflection of the left atrial pressure, the measurement needs to be performed in west's zone 3. If the wedge pressure is measured in west's zone 2, then the values reflect the pressure in the alveoli or extra-alveolar vessels and not the actual pulmonary venous pressure.

References

1. West, J.B. Ventilation/blood flow and gas exchange. 1st ed. Oxford: Blackwell Scientific Publications; Philadelphia: Lippincott; 1990. (5th ed., 1965).
2. West J, Dollery C, Naimark A. Distribution of blood flow in isolated lung; relation to vascular and alveolar pressures. J Appl Physiol. 1964;19:713–24.

Chapter 77
Spirometry

Daniel A. Biggs

The following are the results of spirometry testing performed on a patient:

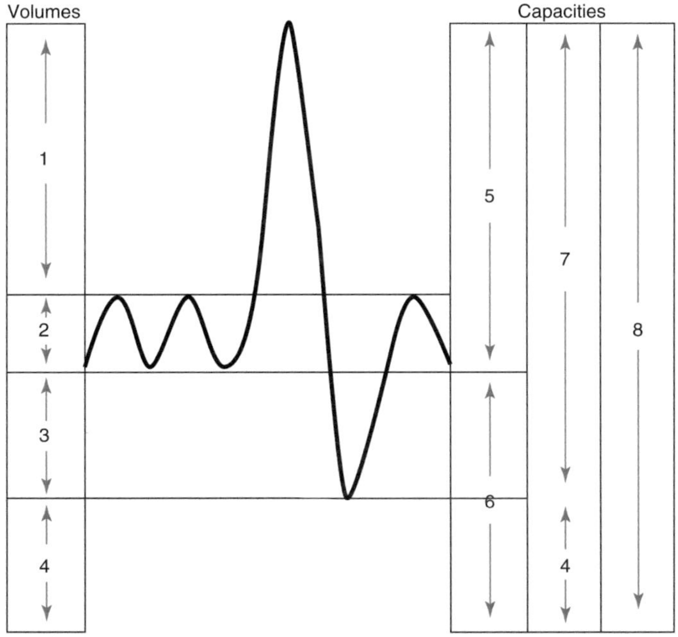

Fig. 77.1 Questions 1–8

D.A. Biggs, MD, MSc
Department of Anesthesiology, Oklahoma University Medical Center,
750 NE 13th Street, Suite 200, Oklahoma City, OK 73104, USA
e-mail: Daniel-biggs@ouhsc.edu

T.D. Raj (ed.), *Data Interpretation in Anesthesia*,
DOI 10.1007/978-3-319-55862-2_77

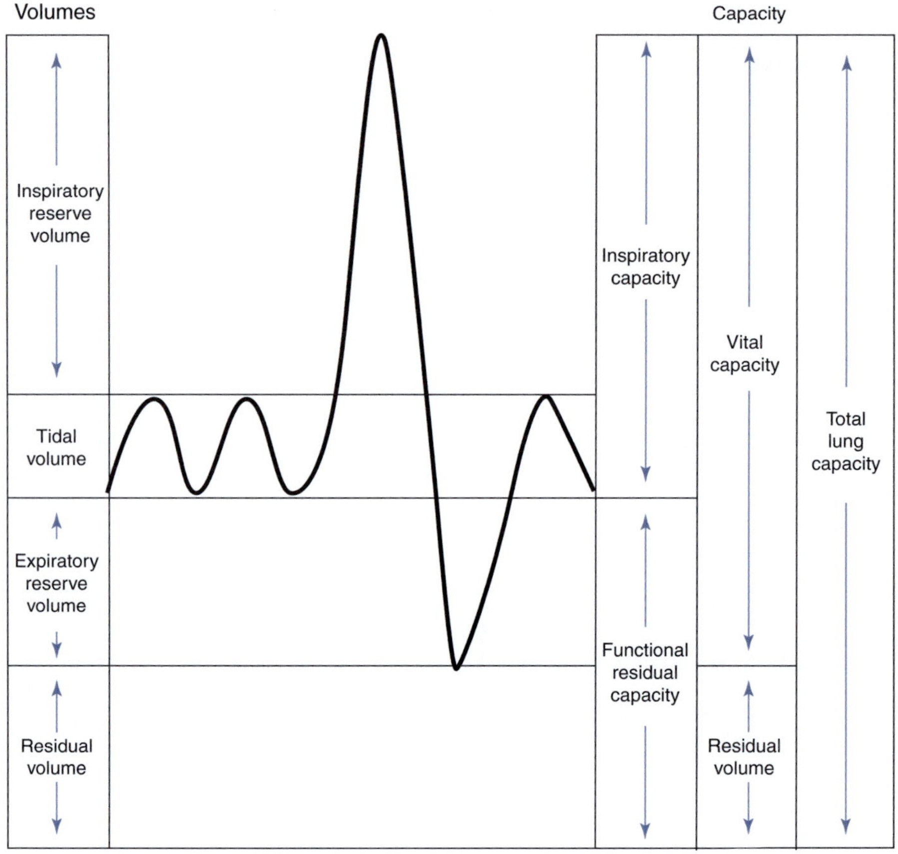

Fig. 77.2 Spirometry with labels

Questions

1–8. Label Fig. 77.1 and define each volume and capacity.
9. Which lung volume cannot be measured by spirometry and how can it be obtained?
10. What is the significance of the FRC and what factors influence it?
11. Define closing volume and closing capacity and what is their importance?

Answers

1. Inspiratory reserve volume (IRV)—maximum amount of air that can be inhaled after normal tidal inhalation [1].
2. Tidal volume (TV)—amount of air moved during breathing at rest [1].
3. Expiratory reserve volume (ERV)—maximum amount of air that can be exhaled after normal tidal exhalation [1].
4. Residual volume (RV)—amount of air in the lungs after complete expiration [1].
5. Inspiratory capacity (IC)—TV + IRV [1].
6. Functional residual capacity (FRC)—ERV + RV—the volume at the end of tidal expiration when the chest is at rest and inward lung and outward chest wall elastic recoil forces are equal [1].
7. Vital capacity (VC)—IRV + TV + ERV—total amount of air that can be moved into the lungs [1].
8. Total lung capacity [1].
9. The residual volume (RV) cannot be measured by spirometry. Radiographic planimetry, nitrogen washout, helium dilution, and body plethysmography may all be used to calculate residual volume [1].
10. FRC acts as the O_2 reserve when a patient becomes apneic. Factors that decrease the FRC include pregnancy, obesity, supine position, restrictive lung disease, general anesthesia, and muscle relaxants [2].
11. Closing volume (CV)—amount of gas remaining in the lungs, above the residual volume, when the bronchioles begin to collapse during expiration.
    Closing capacity (CC)—CV + RV [1].

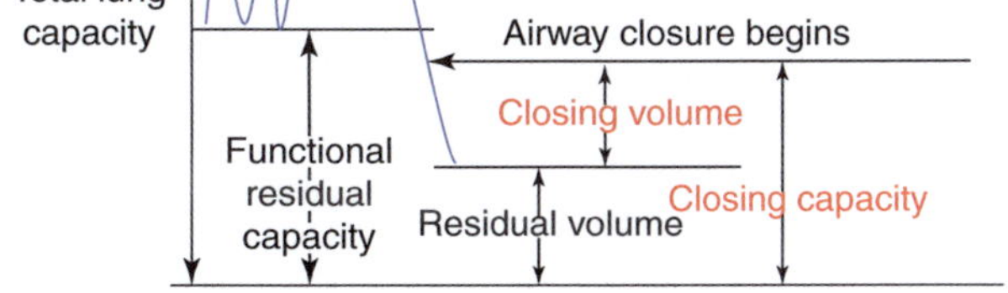

Fig. 77.3 Closing volume and capacity [3]

CV increases with increasing age, lung disease, and supine positioning. Airway closure usually occurs first in the dependent portions of the lungs. The closing capacity is usually less than FRC. In some patients, the closing volume can exceed the FRC. This produces a V/Q mismatch and may cause hypoxemia. Closing volume is measured by nitrogen washout.

References

1. Barash PG, Cullen BF, Stoelting RK, Cahalan MK, Stock MC, Ortega R. Clinical anesthesia. 7th ed. Philadelphia: Lippincott Williams & Wilkins; 2013.
2. Miller RD. Miller's anesthesia. 8th ed. Philadelphia: Elsevier Saunders; 2015.

Chapter 78
Autoregulation Curves

Abhinava S. Madamangalam

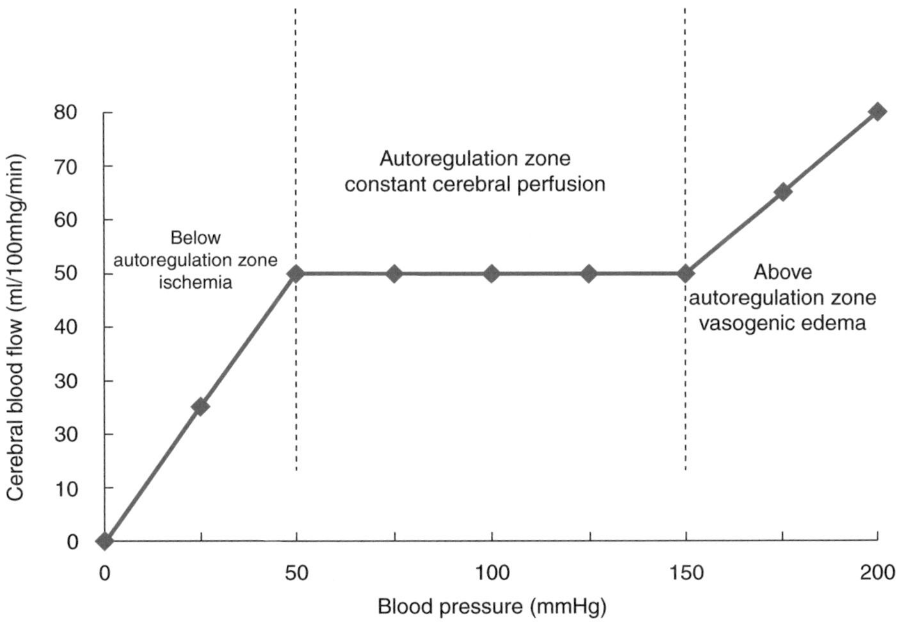

Fig. 78.1

A.S. Madamangalam, MBBS, MD
Department of Anesthesiology and Perioperative Medicine, Augusta University Medical Center, 1120 15th Street, BI-2144, Augusta, GA 30912, USA
e-mail: amadamangalam@augusta.edu

T.D. Raj (ed.), *Data Interpretation in Anesthesia*,
DOI 10.1007/978-3-319-55862-2_78

1. What does the above graph (Fig. 78.1) depict?
2. Define cerebral perfusion pressure, and how is it derived?
3. How is cerebral autoregulation achieved during normal states?
4. What are the conditions in which this balance of cerebral perfusion is upset?

Answers

1. The image depicts a normal cerebral autoregulation. The brain maintains a constant blood flow to itself despite changes in cerebral perfusion pressure. The ability of the organ to achieve this is called cerebral autoregulation.

2. Cerebral perfusion pressure (CPP) is defined as the difference between the mean arterial pressure (MAP) and intracranial pressure (ICP) {CPP = MAP − ICP}. If the central venous pressure (CVP) is greater than the ICP, then CPP = MAP − CVP. The cerebral flow is then modulated by the greater of the two pressures—CVP or ICP. The classic understanding is that autoregulation is maintained between MAPs of 50–150 mmHg [1]. As the ICP is generally in the range of 5–12 mmHg, MAP then becomes the main determinant of the cerebral blood flow. This can be affected by various factors such as sympathetic neural activity, the renin-angiotensin system, and changes in the arterial carbon dioxide partial pressure.

3. The primary mechanism of cerebral autoregulation is not clearly defined. Currently, it is believed to result from the interplay between the myogenic and metabolic responses of the vessels. The perivascular nerves and the vascular endothelium are also said to impact autoregulation.

4. Autoregulation is disrupted in both chronic and acute disease states. Severe head injury or acute ischemic stroke may disrupt autoregulation and expose the brain to further ill effects of altered blood pressure. Similarly, space-occupying lesions may impair autoregulation around the mass. Asphyxia and hypoxic injury as well as infections can disrupt the phenomenon [2].

   In chronic hypertension the autoregulatory curve is right shifted toward higher blood pressure. But in acute hypertension, there is failure of the autoregulation.

   Microvascular disease such as microangiopathy of long-standing diabetes can lead to a chronic loss in autoregulation.

   Several anesthetic drugs can affect autoregulation. Inhaled anesthetics tend to impair autoregulation, and the degree of the effect is dependent not only on the agent but also the partial pressure of the drug. Among the inhaled anesthetic agents, sevoflurane appears to preserve autoregulation at all doses [3]. In healthy individuals, propofol and remifentanil tend to maintain cerebral autoregulation [4].

References

1. Paulson OB, et al. Cerebral autoregulation. Cerebrovasc Brain Metab Rev. 1990;2(2):161–92.
2. Dagal A, et al. Cerebral autoregulation and anesthesia. Curr Opin Anaesthesiol. 2009;22(5):547–52. doi:10.1097/ACO.0b013e32833020be.
3. Pires PW, et al. The effects of hypertension on the cerebral circulation. Am J Physiol Heart Circ Physiol. 2013;304(12):h1598–614. doi:10.1152/ajpheart.00490.2012.
4. Morgan EG, Mikhail SM. Clinical anesthesiology. In: Neurophysiology and anesthesia. 4th ed. New York: McGraw-Hill; 2006.

Chapter 79
Anesthesia Circuits

Alberto J. de Armendi

Breathing System Questions

1. Identify the breathing systems labeled above as 1–5.
2. By what names are Mapleson systems also known as?
3. Name the components of the Mapleson breathing system?
4. What are the advantages of the Mapleson A system and how does it work?
5. Are there disadvantages of the Mapleson A system?
6. What are the advantages and disadvantages of the Mapleson D system?
7. What is the hardest system to scavenge anesthetic gases?
8. Are there advantages and disadvantages of the Mapleson F system?
9. What are the advantages and disadvantages of the circle system?

A.J. de Armendi, MD, PhD, MBA
Department of Anesthesiology, The Children's Hospital, University of Oklahoma Health Sciences Center, 750 NE 13th Street, Suite 200, PO Box 5318, Oklahoma City, OK 73104, USA
e-mail: Alberto-dearmendi@ouhsc.edu

T.D. Raj (ed.), *Data Interpretation in Anesthesia*,
DOI 10.1007/978-3-319-55862-2_79

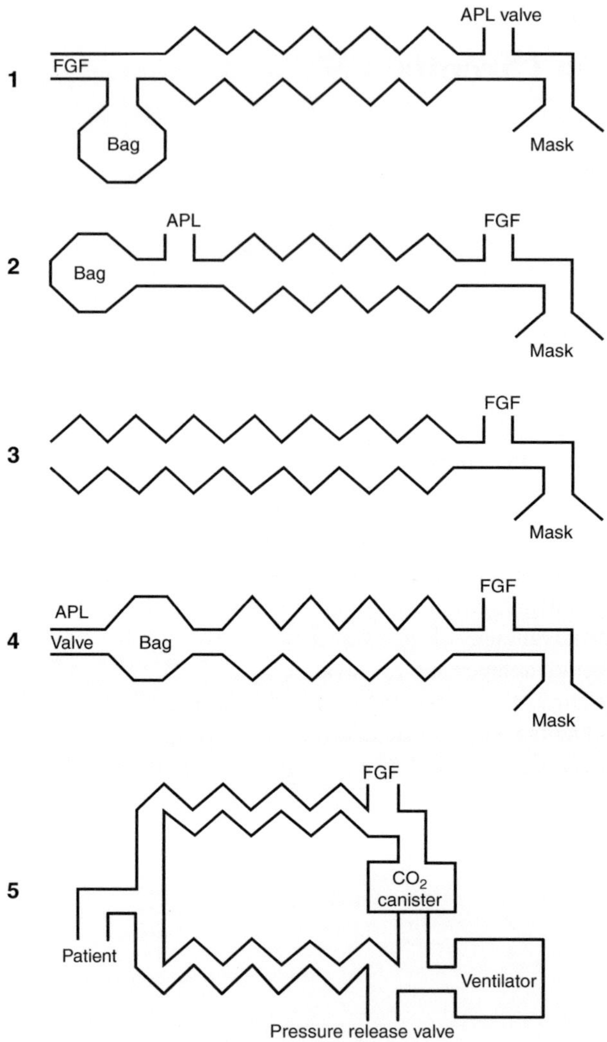

Fig. 79.1 Breathing systems

Answers/Discussion

1. They are Mapleson systems A, D, E, and F and the circle system (see Fig. 79.1) [1–5].

2. Mapleson systems are also known as carbon dioxide washout [depend on fresh gas flow (FGF) to wash out carbon dioxide] or flow-controlled breathing systems.

3. Components of the Mapleson breathing systems are (1) fresh gas flow, (2) breathing tube (corrugated for flexibility and kinking resistance), (3) mask, (4) reservoir bag (antistatic or low charged, monitors respiration, accommodates fresh gas flow during expiration, protects from excessive pressure generation), (5) connectors (increase dead space and resistance), (6) adaptors, and (7) adjustable pressure-limiting (APL) expiratory valve (spring-loaded adjustable one-way valve, and also known as pop-off valve, exhaust valve, overspill valve, pressure relief valve, scavenger valve, and expiratory valve).

4. The Mapleson A system is best for spontaneous respiration with the advantage of less waste of fresh gas flows. The APL valve is open during spontaneous respiration. Fresh gas flows equaling minute ventilation (75–100 ml/kg/min) are required for maximal efficiency. Higher fresh gas flows than minute ventilation will force alveolar gas to be vented, whereas lower fresh gas flows than minute ventilation will allow for rebreathing of alveolar gases to occur. Once the reservoir bag is full of fresh gas flow, the APL valve opens and the alveolar gas is vented [3].

5. The Mapleson A system should not be used for controlled ventilation. If the Mapleson A breathing systems are used during controlled ventilation, the APL valve is partially closed. Disadvantages of the Mapleson A system include (1) carbon dioxide must be monitored when used for controlled ventilation, (2) more waste of fresh gas flows, (3) scavenging is poor as the APL valve is near the patient, and (4) more operating room/atmospheric pollution [3].

6. In the Mapleson D breathing system, during spontaneously breathing with the APL valve open, the patient inhales mostly fresh gas flows delivered from the anesthesia machine. During exhalation, alveolar gases are vented at the APL valve. During controlled ventilation, the APL valve is partially closed, fresh gas flows are set at 1.5–2 times the minute ventilation, and alveolar gases are vented during inspiration as the reservoir bad is squeezed or the ventilator is activated (rates of 12–14 breaths/minute). The major disadvantage of the Mapleson D over the Mapleson A breathing system is that the fresh gas flows are set higher in order to avoid rebreathing of alveolar gases. Therefore, the Mapleson D system is less efficient (more costly) and causes more operating room/atmospheric pollution [3].

7. With an open end, the Mapleson E system is the most difficult for scavenging gases. The FGF depends not only on the patient's respiratory rate and minute volume but also on the capacity of the expiratory limb. If the latter is equal to the tidal volume, then an FGF rate of 2.5 times the patient's MV is sufficient. If the capacity is less, then the FGF should be increased.

8. The Mapleson F, also known as the Jackson Rees modification, helps monitor and assists ventilation. Major advantages of the Mapleson F breathing system are (1) can be used in neonates, (2) inexpensive, (3) lack of barotrauma potential, and (4) low resistance without any valves. During spontaneous respiration, the reservoir bag is left open and serves as a monitor by demonstrating breathing. During controlled ventilation, the open end of the reservoir bag is occluded and squeezed. Disadvantages of the Mapleson F system include (1) not efficient as high fresh gas flows are needed (1.5–3 times the minute ventilation), (2) increased rebreathing from the mixture of fresh gas flows and exhaled gas collection in the reservoir bag, (3) loss of heat, (4) lack of humidification, and (5) greater operating room/atmospheric pollution.

9. Advantages of the circle breathing system include (1) absorber and absorbent (carbon dioxide absorption, less fresh gas flows, diffuse rather than columnar gas spread, less turbulence, reduced resistance, bypass mechanism allows for carbon dioxide accumulation, and less canister dust), (2) improved economy, (3) less operating room and atmospheric pollution, (4) conservation of heat, (5) conservation of moisture, (6) controlled use of flammable gases/vapors, and (7) constant inhaled gas mixture deliveries (oxygen and gas analyzers). Disadvantages of the circle breathing system include (1) toxic product production (compound A due to CO_2 absorbent which can be reduced with calcium hydroxide free soda lime), (2) carbon monoxide production from desiccated soda lime, and (3) unidirectional valve problems (resistance, sticking, wetting, electrostatic, leaks).

References

1. Mapleson WW. The elimination of rebreathing in various semiclosed anaesthetic systems. Br J Anaesth. 1954;26:323–32.
2. Dorsch JA, Dorsch SE. Mapleson breathing system. In: Understanding anaesthesia equipment. 5th ed. New Delhi: William and Wilkins; 2008. p. 209–21.
3. Jonsson LO, Zetterstrom H. Fresh gas flow in coaxial Mapleson A and D systems during spontaneous breathing. Acta Anaesthesiol Scand. 1986;30:588–93.
4. http://www.anaesthesia.med.usyd.edu.au/resources/lectures/gas_supplies_clt/breathingsystems.html.
5. Kaul TK, Mittal G. Mapleson's breathing systems. Indian J Anaesth. 2013;57(5):507–15. doi:10.4103/0019-5049.120148.

Chapter 80
Flowmeters

John B. Carter

Fig. 80.1 Anesthesia flowmeter

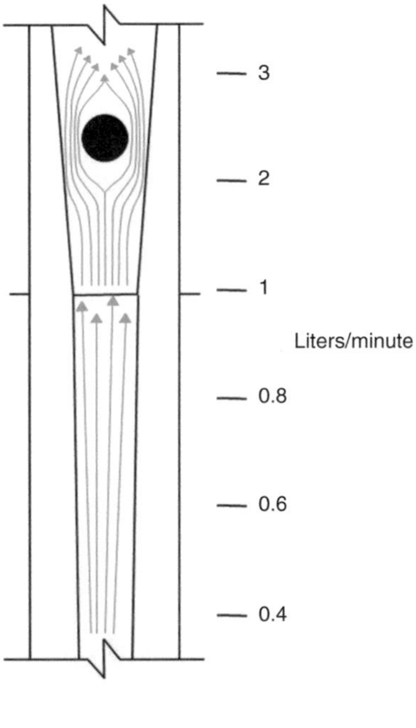

1. What are the physical principles of the anesthesia flowmeter?
2. Describe the components of the flowmeter assembly.
3. What are the concerns about flowmeter leaks?
4. List the causes of inaccuracy in flowmeters.

J.B. Carter, MD
Department of Anesthesiology, Oklahoma University Medical Center,
750 NE 13th Street, OAC 200, Oklahoma City, OK 73104, USA
e-mail: John-b-carter@ouhsc.edu

T.D. Raj (ed.), *Data Interpretation in Anesthesia*,
DOI 10.1007/978-3-319-55862-2_80

Answers

1. Operating principles of the conventional flowmeter
   (a) The anesthesia flowmeter is described as a constant pressure, variable orifice flow meter. Newer anesthesia machines may have electronic flowmeters; however, auxiliary O_2 flowmeters of the conventional type may be present.
   (b) The glass flowmeter or Thorpe tube is tapered, smaller at the bottom and wider at the top (Fig 80.1). Gas flows under the float raising it until the bobbin or ball stops as its weight is supported by the pressure difference above and below.
   (c) Flow tubes are specific to the physical characteristics of each gas.
   (d) Gas flow at low rates is laminar and viscosity of the gas is important. Laminar flow is predicted by the Hagen-Poiseuille formula:

$$Q = \frac{\pi \quad \mathrm{Pr}4}{8\eta l}$$

   where Q is flow, ΔP is the pressure gradient (unchanged), R is the radius (variable as tube widens), η is the viscosity (characteristic of each individual gas), and l is the length of the tube.

   At higher flow rates, flow becomes turbulent as the Reynolds' number exceeds 2000. With turbulent flow, the density becomes more important than viscosity:

$$\text{Reynolds number} = \frac{\upsilon \rho r}{\eta}$$

   υ, fluid linear velocity; r, radius; ρ, density; and η, viscosity [1]
   (e) Floats are meant to rotate, minimizing friction.

2. Components of flowmeter assembly
   (a) The flow control valve is manually controlled, turning counterclockwise. A needle valve disengages releasing the gas flow into the flowmeter. All gas flow from the flowmeter distally to the common gas outlet is in the low pressure circuit of the anesthesia machine.
   (b) The oxygen flow control is physically different; it is larger, has a fluted edge, and is color coded.
   (c) If a single gas has two flow tubes, they are placed in series and controlled by one valve.
   (d) The flow rate is read at the top of a bobbin and the middle of a ball. Float stops at the top and bottom of the tube to keep the float visible at high flows, giving an indication when flow is turned off, and prevent the float from becoming stuck at the top of the gas outlet.
   (e) Flowmeter scales are individually calibrated to the specific float and are gas specific. The tube, float, and scale are an inseparable unit [2].

3. Leaks
   (a) Flowmeter leaks are downstream from the oxygen failure cutoff valve or "fail safe" valve. Hypoxic gas mixtures from a leak in the flowmeter may be detected by the O_2 monitor, which is placed downstream.
   (b) Flowmeters are fragile and may leak from cracks or the O rings at either end. In the presence of a flowmeter leak, hypoxic mixtures are less likely when the oxygen flowmeter is placed downstream of the others. This is now the standard position. See Figs. 80.2 and 80.3. A crack in the O_2 flowmeter, even placed last, may still result in a hypoxic gas mixture.
   (c) Being in the low pressure circuit, specific tests may be necessary to detect leaks. In general, if the machine does not have a check valve at the common gas outlet, the low pressure circuit may be tested with a positive pressure leak test. Machines with a check valve must be tested with a negative pressure leak test [3].

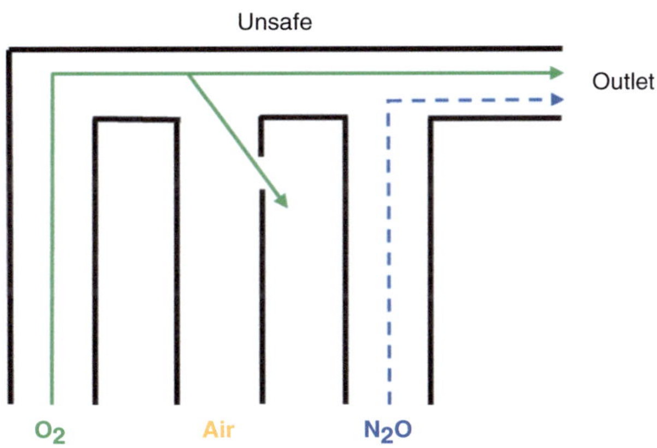

Fig. 80.2 Flowmeter leak with oxygen upstream of other gases

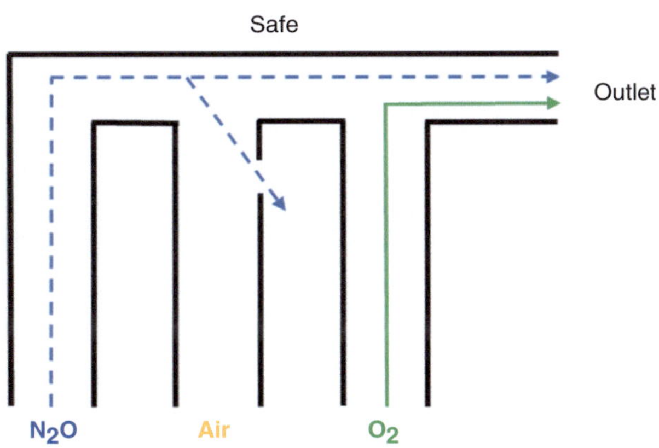

Fig. 80.3 Flowmeter leak with oxygen downstream of other gases

4. Causes of inaccuracy include:
   (a) The tube that is not vertical distorts the annular flow.
   (b) Back pressure from ventilator may cause the float to drop, measuring less than the actual flow.
   (c) A float may become sticky from either a dirty flow tube or static electricity.
   (d) Flowmeters are calibrated at 20 °C and 760 mm Hg. The effect of temperature is minor; however at decreased atmospheric pressure, the density will be less, and with higher, turbulent flow, the actual flow will be greater than the set flow.

References

1. Aitkenhead AR, Moppett IK, Thompson JP. Smith & Aitkenhead's textbook of anesthesia. 6th ed. Churchill Livingstone Elsevier; 2013.
2. Morgan EG, Mikhail MS. Clinical anesthesiology, Chapter 4, 4th ed.
3. Barash PG, Cullen BF. Clinical anesthesiology, Chapter 26, 6th ed. 2009.

Chapter 81
Cardiac Bypass Machines

Ranganathan Govindaraj

A 75-year-old white male is undergoing aortocoronary bypass grafting. On initiation of cardiopulmonary bypass (CPB), the alarm on the CPB machine goes off indicating high pressure in the arterial circuit.

1. Name some causes of high pressure on the arterial side.
2. List the components and functions of a CPB circuit.
3. What is extracorporeal circulation?
4. What are the types of oxygenators, their advantages, and disadvantages?
5. What types of filters are used on a bypass machine? Where are the filters located?
6. What is partial and total bypass?
7. What is left ventricular (LV) venting and why is it necessary?
8. What are the types of flow? What is the advantage of using pulsatile flow?
9. Name some complications during cardiopulmonary bypass.

R. Govindaraj, MD, FRCA
Associate Professor for Anesthesia and Pain, Department of Anesthesiology, UTMB, Galveston, TX, USA

Director for Ultrasound Guided Regional Anesthesia, Galveston, TX 77555, USA
e-mail: gorangan@utmb.edu

T.D. Raj (ed.), *Data Interpretation in Anesthesia*,
DOI 10.1007/978-3-319-55862-2_81

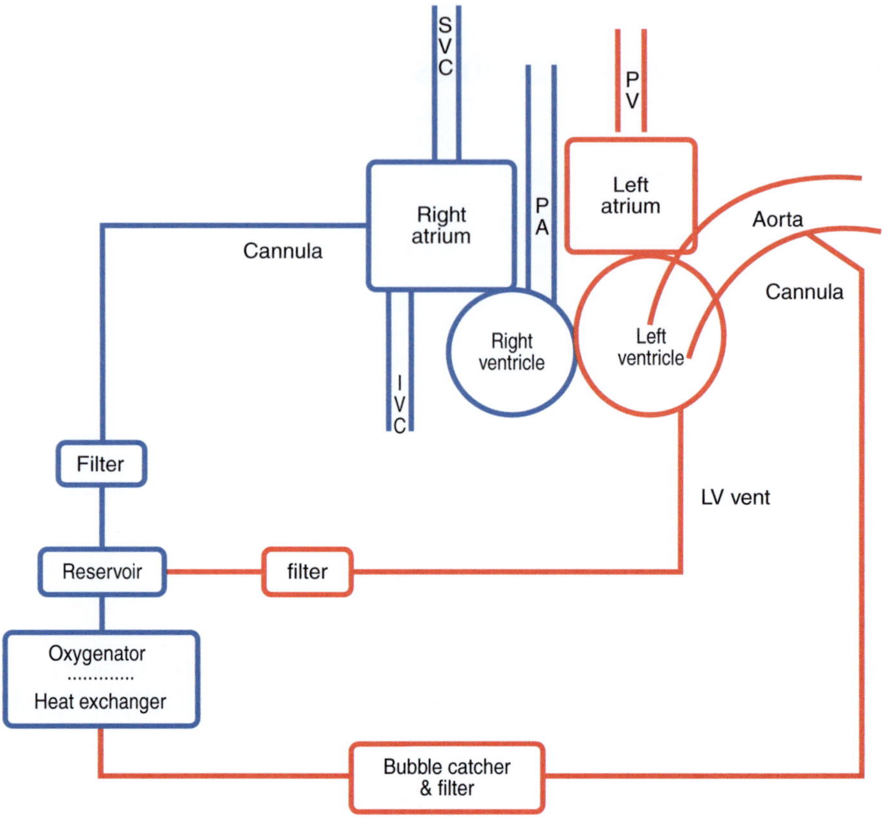

Fig. 81.1 Schematic diagram of Cardio pulmonary bypass machine

Answers

1. Systemic hypertension in the patient, occlusion and malposition of the aortic cannula and dissection of the aortic wall, an inadvertent clamp or kink in the line, and an obstructed arterial line filter can all cause high pressure on the arterial side.

2. Components [1]:
   (a) Venous reservoir
   (b) Membrane oxygenator bundle
   (c) Venous and arterial blood line/cannula
   (d) Arterial filter purge line
   (e) Arterial line filter
   (f) Venous blood pump (also called the arterial pump head; this pump forces venous blood through the membrane oxygenator and arterialized blood to the patient's aortic root)
   (g) Cardiotomy suction pump
   (h) Ventricular vent (left ventricular vent)

(i) Cardioplegia pump
(j) Crystalloid cardioplegia
(k) Water inlet line
(l) Water outlet line
(m) Gas inlet line

Functions:
(a) Oxygenation and carbon dioxide elimination
(b) Circulation of blood
(c) Systemic cooling and rewarming
(d) Diversion of blood from the heart to provide a bloodless surgical field

3. Extracorporeal circulation or extracorporeal life support is mechanical cardiopulmonary support. When it is used in the operating room to provide total support of heart and lung function to facilitate cardiac surgery, the technique is commonly called cardiopulmonary bypass (CPB). When used with extrathoracic cannulation for respiratory support, the technique is called extracorporeal membrane oxygenation (ECMO), and for renal support it is termed as hemodialysis [2].

4. There are two common types of oxygenators—bubble and membrane oxygenators.
   Bubble oxygenators are simple, low-cost oxygenators with greater efficiency that require lower priming volumes and are easy to assemble. The disadvantages are the production of microemboli and increased blood cell trauma as a result of turbulence and foaming which is created by bubbling oxygen through a column of blood.
   In a **membrane oxygenator**, gas exchange takes place through a thin membrane; hence there is minimal cellular trauma, but it requires a greater surface area and a larger priming volume. It is very expensive and difficult to clean.

5. There are two common types of filters used for blood filtration during CPB: depth and screen filters. **Depth filter** consists of packed fibers of Dacron with a significant amount of thickness but no defined pore size. Hence filtration depends on the thickness and tightness of the packing of the material. **Screen filter** is made of a woven mesh of polyester fibers with a defined pore size. The arterial line has a screen type filter, while the cardiotomy reservoir has a combination of both depth- and screen-type filters. Depth filters remove gaseous emboli and microemboli efficiently. The disadvantage with depth filter is it removes a lot of platelets. Screen filters, on the other hand, remove less platelets but also remove gaseous and microemboli less efficiently. Filters can also be placed in a number of other locations, including the ventilating gas line and the cardioplegia delivery circuit.

6. **Partial bypass** occurs when only a portion of systemic venous blood drains to the pump oxygenator while the remaining blood passes through the right heart and lungs to be ejected by the left ventricle. Partial bypass is employed in descending thoracic aortic surgery in order to provide perfusion to distal organs (spinal cord and visceral organs) while the aorta is cross-clamped. This is to decrease ischemia time especially to the spinal cord thereby minimizing the risk of neurologic complications (paraplegia).

Total bypass occurs when all the venous return from the right side of the heart is diverted into the pump oxygenator.

7. During CPB surgery, either no venting or LV venting via the cardioplegia cannula in the aortic root is practiced. The purpose of left ventricular venting is to prevent distension of the left ventricle and prevent cardiac ejection of air. Prevention of distension of the left ventricle is desirable to prevent mechanical damage to the muscle from excessive stretching, decreasing myocardial oxygen demand, facilitating subendocardial perfusion, and preventing pulmonary venous hypertension.
8. Pulsatile and nonpulsatile flows are the types used while on bypass. Pulsatile flow improves the quality of microcirculation and prevents systemic inflammatory response. But it has been calculated that very little of the pulsatile energy is actually delivered into the patient's arterial system.
9. The incidence of complications on CPB is about 1% with a death rate of about 0.04%.
   Aortic dissection. Best diagnosed by TEE or epi-aortic scanning.
   High arterial line pressure has already been discussed.
   Massive air embolism. On a smaller scale, air can entrain in some situations and can cause embolism in the arterial circuits. Microthrombi and air which cannot be filtered by the filters on the arterial side can embolize and cause postoperative confusion and delirium [3].
   Oxygenator failure. If the heart is still functioning, separation from CPB, or if the heart is arrested, the oxygenator needs replacing which requires interruption to circulation (consider cooling).
   Arterial pump failure either due to electrical or mechanical failure. Hand crank should be available.
   Clotting of the circuit from inadequate anticoagulation or inadvertent protamine administration while on bypass.
   Obstruction of venous return and air lock.
   Electrical failure. All CPB machines have a backup battery. If that fails, then hand cranking of the arterial pump is the option (not to forget the pump that operates the suction and vent).
   Hemolysis from trauma to the cells. This is increased when the pump run is long.
   Exsanguination due to disconnection of the tubing while on bypass.

References

1. Machin D, Allsager C. Principles of cardiopulmonary bypass. Contin Educ Anaesth Crit Care Pain. 2006;6(5):176–81. doi:10.1093/bjaceaccp/mkl043.
2. Hensley FA, Martin DE, Gravlee GP. A practical approach to cardiac anesthesia. 5th ed. Philadelphia: Lippincott Williams and Wilkins; 2013.
3. Stehouwer MC, Boers C, de Vroege R, C Kelder J, Yilmaz A, Bruins P. Clinical evaluation of the air removal characteristics of an oxygenator with integrated arterial filter in a minimized extracorporeal circuit. Int J Artif Organs. 2011;34(4):374–82. doi:10.5301/IJAO.2011.7749.

Chapter 82
Line Isolation Monitor

Abhinava S. Madamangalam and Tilak D. Raj

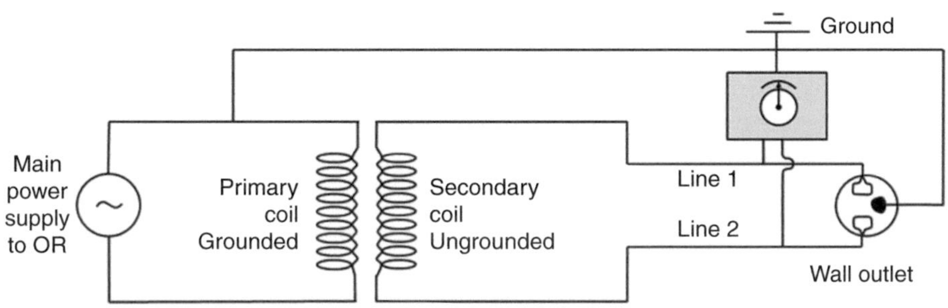

Fig. 82.1

1. What does the image show? Describe its function.
2. What are leakage currents?
3. What are line isolation monitors (LIM)?
4. List the locations where line-isolated electrical systems are required in a health-care facility.
5. What are the effects of differing current strengths?
6. Explain situations that enhance risks of electrical shock.

A.S. Madamangalam, MBBS, MD (✉)
Department of Anesthesiology and Perioperative Medicine, Augusta University Medical Center, 1120 15th Street, BI-2144, Augusta, GA 30912, USA
e-mail: amadamangalam@augusta.edu

T.D. Raj, MD, MRCP, FRCA
Department of Anesthesiology, Alliance Health Midwest, Midwest City, OK, USA
e-mail: Tilak-raj@ouhsc.edu

T.D. Raj (ed.), *Data Interpretation in Anesthesia*,
DOI 10.1007/978-3-319-55862-2_82

Answers

1. It shows an isolation transformer whose function is to allow electric power transmission between two circuits without a direct connection. On the left is the main power supply which is grounded and looped around the primary coil of the isolation transformer. The current flowing through this generates a magnetic field which creates an electrical potential difference in the secondary coil allowing current to flow from the primary to the secondary coil. By this arrangement an electrical fault on one side cannot spread to the other side. The isolation transformer transmits only the potential difference across the primary coil and not the absolute voltage. Hence a fault in a device plugged into the isolated power supply, which is not grounded, does not lead to an electric shock.

2. Perfectly working electrical equipment may yet produce leakage currents. This is defined as any current, not intended to be applied to a patient, but may pass from exposed metal parts of equipment to ground or to other parts of the instruments.

3. LIM detects electrical potential and leakage currents between the two lines of the isolated secondary system and ground. It is designed to alarm with audible and visual warnings when the secondary system degrades to the extent that there would be a 5 mA or greater electric shock with the next electric fault.

Things to remember:

- An alarm does **not** mean there is imminent danger to the patient or anyone else. The alarm therefore simply calls attention to the fact that the system has converted to a partially grounded system [1]. This is a situation that needs correction as soon as possible. No ongoing procedures need be halted.
- The LIM does **not** interrupt electrical service. All ungrounded systems will continue to work as usual [1, 2].
- An active alarm does not mean that there is a hazardous current flowing. It predicts that a current of at least 5 mA could flow from one conductor of the isolated system to ground if a path is provided. Therefore, a **second** fault or electric failure needs to occur before a true hazardous condition exists [2].

If the alarm on the LIM goes off, the last electrical equipment plugged into the system in an area is likely suspect and should be unplugged.

4. Electrically isolated systems are required in all wet locations [1]:
   (a) Intensive care units (ICUs)
   (b) Coronary care units (CCUs)
   (c) Emergency departments
   (d) Special procedure rooms
   (e) Electrophysiology laboratories
   (f) Dialysis locations

(g) Various other wet locations that involve patient care, such as GI labs

5. The human body is a large resistor to the flow of current. The flow which is dependent on the mass and the moisture content of the body.
   Macroshock
   1 mA—threshold of perception, a slight tingling at the fingertips.
   5 mA—maximum harmless current.
   10–20 mA—muscle contracture may prevent release of an electrode.
   50 mA—pain, fainting, and exhaustion.
   100 mA—ventricular fibrillation (VF) will likely result.
   Microshock
   As little as 100 μA can cause VF.

6. Patients undergoing thoracic surgery are at highest risk of electric shock as are those when cardiac catheters and dye injectors are being used. This is due to direct leakage of current in the circulatory system. A patient is most at risk when the heart is exposed directly to the conducting agent such as diagnostic catheters or pacing wires.

   Patients that are anesthetized or immobilized through illness or have restraints, or those on drug therapy are considered more susceptible to electrical hazards than normal individuals. These patients cannot disconnect themselves in the event of an electric shock. Thus they can be at a high risk for the ill effects of electrical leakage.

   Electrolyte imbalance, hypoxemia, elevated catecholamine levels, and some drugs such as digitalis also enhance the risk. Infants are at greater risk owing to their smaller body mass.

References

1. Barash PG, Cullen BF, Stoelting RK. Clinical anesthesia fundamentals. Wolters Kluwer Health; 2015. p. 803–5.
2. Butterworth JF, Mackey DC, Wasnick JD. Morgan & Mikhail's clinical anesthesiology. 5th ed. McGraw-Hill; 2013. p. 17–9.

Chapter 83
Machine: Schematic

Ranganathan Govindaraj

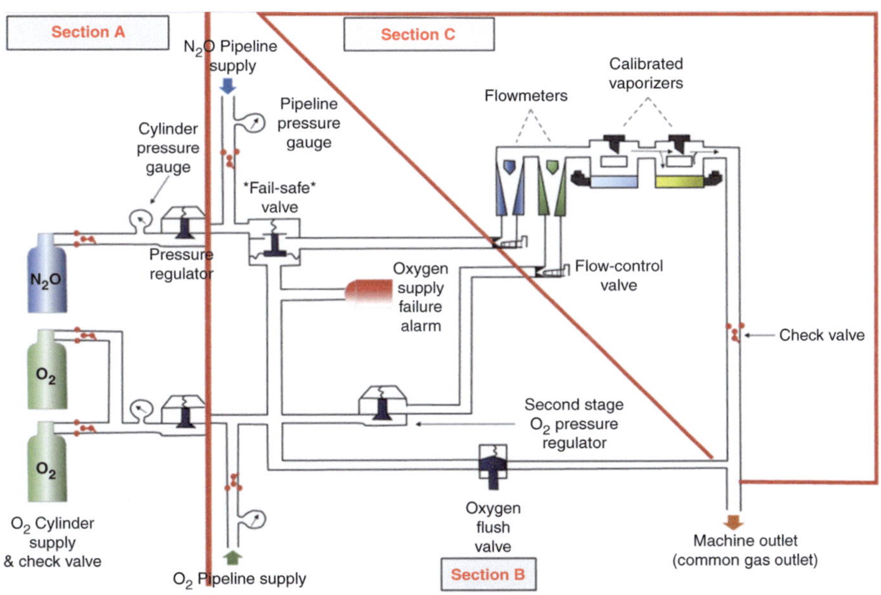

Fig. 83.1 Schematic diagram of an anesthesia machine

R. Govindaraj, MD, FRCA
Associate Professor for Anesthesia and Pain, Department of Anesthesiology, UTMB, Galveston, TX, USA

Director for Ultrasound Guided Regional Anesthesia, , Galveston, TX 77555, USA
e-mail: gorangan@utmb.edu

T.D. Raj (ed.), *Data Interpretation in Anesthesia*,
DOI 10.1007/978-3-319-55862-2_83

1. What is section A and what are its components?
2. What are the safety systems in the high-pressure system, and what is the pressure for the different gases in the high-pressure system?
3. What is section B and what are its components?
4. What is section C and what are its components?
5. What is a fail-safe valve and what is its function?
6. What are the mechanisms used to prevent delivering a hypoxic mixture at the fresh gas outlet?
7. What is the oxygen flush valve? What are the properties of the oxygen coming through the oxygen flush activation and what are the disadvantages?
8. How is the leak test performed?
9. How do we determine the presence of an oxygen pressure failure safety device or fail-safe valve?
10. What is an oxygen supply failure alarm?

Answers

1. This is the high-pressure system (cylinder to pressure regulators) in the anesthesia machine. Its components are:
   Hanger yoke, which includes the filter and unidirectional valve
   Yoke block
   Cylinders with safety features and pressure gauge
   Cylinder pressure regulators

2. Cylinder pressure can increase due to defective overfilling or when cylinders are exposed to high temperature. The increase in pressure can cause the cylinder to explode. Rupture disk device in the cylinder plays a safety role by rupturing the disk when the pressure in the cylinder increases beyond the safety range expelling the contents thereby avoiding an explosion. Thermally controlled fusible plug melts and releases the gas under high pressure due to expansion of gases when cylinders are exposed to higher temperature [1].
   Working pressure for the different gases in the high-pressure system are:
   Oxygen 1900 psig
   Nitrous Oxide 745 psig
   Air 1900 psig upstream of the pressure reducing valve

3. This is the intermediate pressure system (from pressure regulators to the flowmeter). Components include:
   Pipeline inlets for oxygen, nitrous oxide and air.
   Pipeline check valves and pressure gauges.
   Oxygen fail-safe (pressure-failure) valve.
   Oxygen flush valve.
   Second-stage pressure regulators in the Ohmeda machine but absent in the Narkomed machine.
   Flowmeter control valves.
   Pipeline pressure for oxygen is 50–55 psi, air 50–55 psi, and nitrous oxide 50 psi.
   The pipeline pressure of gases is usually slightly higher than cylinder pressure in order to preferentially enable use of pipeline gases. The intermediate zone working pressure for the gases ranges from 37 to 55 psig. When the pipeline pressure of oxygen falls below 30 psig, the low-pressure alarm gets activated. The second-stage pressure regulator in the Ohmeda machine reduces the pressure to 26 psig for nitrous oxide and 14 psig for oxygen.

4. It is the low-pressure system (flowmeters to the common gas outlet). The gases flow through flowmeters, vaporizers, and oxygen analyzer then through the fresh gas outlet to the patient.
   Components are:
   Flow meter tubes
   Vaporizer and its manifold
   Safety devices to prevent hypoxia (proportioning device)
   Check valve

Pressure relief devices like APL valve

Common gas outlet

Pressure in this section of the machine is slightly above atmospheric and not constant.

5. Fail-safe valve is located in the intermediate pressure zone of the machine. It prevents delivery of low FiO_2. When the oxygen pressure falls, the fail-safe valve which is kept open by the working pressure of oxygen gradually shuts off the other gas which is usually nitrous oxide. It then opens another valve due to the low pressure and directs the oxygen to an oxygen low pressure alarm. This safety facility is not available when oxygen and air mixture is being used.

6. Different machines use different mechanisms to prevent delivery of hypoxic mixtures such as:

   Mandatory minimum oxygen flow, minimum oxygen ratio settings, and

   proportionating systems are the different principles employed to prevent delivering hypoxic mixture.

   Ohmeda uses a Link-25 system, and the Narkomed uses an oxygen ratio monitor controller with a pneumatic oxygen/nitrous oxide interlock system to facilitate the process.

7. Oxygen flush valve is an emergency source of oxygen with high flows at high pressure. Flows of 30–70 l per minute are produced at a pressure of 60 psig (400 kPa):

   Oxygen flush can be activated regardless of whether the master switch is turned *on* or *off*. Oxygen flush activation may or may not result in other gas flows being shut *off* and may result in either a positive or negative pressure in the machine circuitry, depending on the design of the inlet and the flush line into the common gas outlet [2].

   Disadvantages associated with the oxygen flush include accidental activation and internal leakage, which can result in an oxygen-enriched mixture being delivered. The flush valve may stick in the *on* position. It may also stick and obstruct flow from the flowmeters. Barotrauma and awareness during anesthesia have resulted from its activation [3].

8. Low-pressure leak test checks the integrity of the back bar from the flow control valve to the common gas outlet. Methods used are:

   Common gas occlusion test to test high-pressure leaks

   Oxygen flush leak test for high-pressure leaks

   The abovementioned tests are good for North American Drager and Ohmeda 8000.

   Ohmeda-negative pressure leak test later came to be universal on every machine since 1993 and is known as the FDA universal negative pressure leak test. This test holds good on all anesthetic machines in current use. It does not require the presence or absence of check valves. The device used is a simple suction bulb to provide negative pressure [3].

   Machine master switch, flow control valves, and vaporizers are turned off. Suction bulb is attached to the common gas outlet and squeezed repeatedly until it is fully collapsed. This action creates low pressure in the circuit. Machine is leak free if the bulb remains collapsed for 10 s. A leak is present if the bulb reinflates within 10 s. Test is repeated with each vaporizer individually turned on.

9. The flow meter of oxygen and nitrous oxide is switched on, and as soon as the flows are registered, the oxygen source should be cut off. A proper functioning fail-safe valve will shut the flow of nitrous oxide immediately. Restoration of oxygen flow will restore the flow of nitrous oxide as well.

10. An oxygen supply pressure alarm will sound within 5 s of the oxygen pressure falling below 38 psig. In earlier machines, this was a pneumatic device called Ritchie whistle and is electronic in the present-day machines.

References

1. Gurudatt C. The basic anaesthesia machine. Indian J Anaesth. 2013;57(5):438–45. doi:10.4103/0019-5049.120138.
2. Dorsch JA, Dorsch SE. Hazards of anesthesia machines and breathing systems. In: Dorsch JA, Dorsch SE, editors. Understanding anesthesia equipment. 4th ed. Baltimore: Williams & Wilkins; 1999. p. 399.
3. Myers JA, Good ML, Andrews JJ. Comparison of tests for detecting leaks in the low-pressure system of anesthesia gas machines. Anesth Analg. 1997;84:179–84. PMID:8989021.

Index

T.D. Raj (ed.), *Data Interpretation in Anesthesia*,
DOI 10.1007/978-3-319-55862-2

N

O

P

MIX
Papier aus verantwortungsvollen Quellen
Paper from responsible sources
FSC® C105338

If you have any concerns about our products,
you can contact us on
ProductSafety@springernature.com

In case Publisher is established outside the EU,
the EU authorized representative is:
Springer Nature Customer Service Center GmbH
Europaplatz 3, 69115 Heidelberg, Germany

Printed by Libri Plureos GmbH
in Hamburg, Germany